Springer Nature More Media App

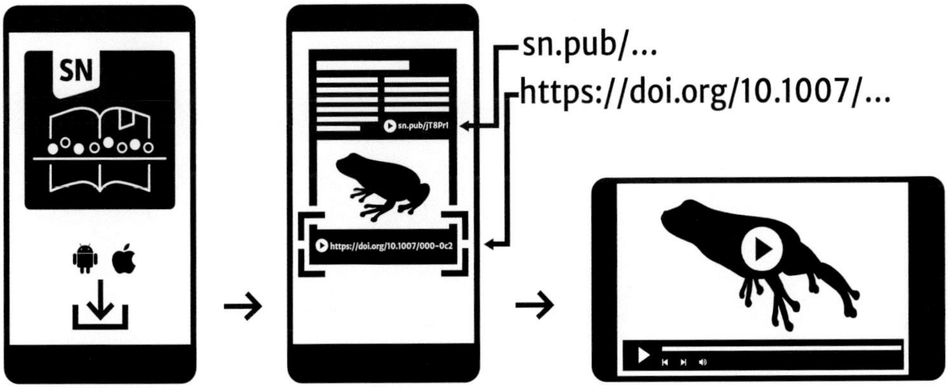

1.
Download

2.
Scan Link

3.
Enjoy Video

Support: customerservice@springernature.com

Neurosurgical Approaches Video Atlas

Helbert de Oliveira Manduca Palmiero
Eberval Gadelha Figueiredo

Neurosurgical Approaches Video Atlas

Springer

Helbert de Oliveira Manduca Palmiero, MD, PhD
Neurosurgery Department
Universidade de São Paulo
São Paulo, São Paulo, Brazil

Eberval Gadelha Figueiredo, MD, PhD
Neurosurgery Department
Universidade de São Paulo
São Paulo, São Paulo, Brazil

This work contains media enhancements, which are displayed with a "play" icon. Material in the print book can be viewed on a mobile device by downloading the Springer Nature "More Media" app available in the major app stores. The media enhancements in the online version of the work can be accessed directly by authorized users.

ISBN 978-3-032-04663-5 ISBN 978-3-032-04664-2 (eBook)
https://doi.org/10.1007/978-3-032-04664-2

This Springer imprint is published by the registered company Springer Nature Switzerland AG
The registered company address is: Gewerbestrasse 11, 6330 Cham, Switzerland

Preface: The Pursuit of Excellence

The primary objective of this book is to illustrate the most important surgical approaches to the skull, following the technical steps outlined in the literature and refined through continuous learning from our teachers, who, in turn, learned from their mentors and developed their techniques through books and experience. Neurosurgery originated from general surgery and, as such, retains core characteristics from other surgical specialties, including shared instruments and similar technical steps. However, neurosurgery has unique advantages, particularly the advancement of microsurgical techniques. Unlike any other specialty, this approach integrates general surgical and microsurgical steps. We begin with the craniotomy, progress through the microsurgical technical phases, and conclude by returning to the craniotomy to complete the operation.

This book is intended for neurosurgery residents, junior and senior fellows, and neurosurgeons who maintain a youthful mindset, are receptive to revision, and are capable of continuous improvement. While engaging with the chapters and watching the accompanying videos, readers may find several details that reflect their own practice, as well as others that might present enhanced techniques. Although neurosurgery has been informed by scientific advancements, its practitioners are continually refining our approach. Had this book been written 10 years ago, it would differ significantly from its current form—just as it will inevitably evolve over the next decade—as we continue to practice, read, observe, train in the lab, and pursue excellence.

Composed of 21 chapters, including the Introduction to Cranial Approaches and the Foundational Anatomy for Neurosurgical Approaches chapters, this volume covers procedures ranging from commonly performed surgeries, such as the pterional craniotomy, to more specialized approaches involving the posterior fossa and skull base. The procedural details are carefully described based on the literature on more than a century of neurosurgical practice. The references at the end of each chapter serve as a starting point for those seeking further mastery or as a concise summary for those wishing to review the technical steps. Craniotomies were recorded using an action video camera mounted on the surgeon's head, while microsurgical steps were captured using a smartphone attached to the neurosurgical microscope, and artificial intelligence provided voice for the videos. All procedures were conducted in our university laboratory using cadaveric specimens, adhering strictly to ethical standards and surgical technique protocols.

To make the most of this book, we recommend reading the chapters and some reference material before watching the videos. However, if you choose to view the videos first, you can still follow the technical steps, as each video starts with a summary of the chapter that outlines the surgical indications and operative setup prior to the craniotomy and microsurgery. It is important to acknowledge the limitations of this work due to the laboratory setting in which the procedures took place (without neuromonitoring, ultrasonic aspirators, or ultrasound devices) and the use of equipment that was reused multiple times. Additionally, while we illustrate the skin incisions, we do not display them in the videos to comply with the DVS protocol, which requires a standard bimastoid incision.

This book aims to enhance the quality of each chapter through scholarly rigor and practical insight. We encourage readers to engage in critical thinking, comparing our texts and videos with existing literature as well as their own experiences and practices. We hope this will be the first of many editions and actively welcome your feedback. The enduring principles of neurosurgery are just the starting point in our continuous pursuit of refinement.

São Paulo, Brazil — Helbert de Oliveira Manduca Palmiero, MD, PhD
São Paulo, Brazil — Eberval Gadelha Figueiredo, MD, PhD

Disclaimer The surgical videos in the supplementary material contain narration generated with the assistance of artificial intelligence. AI tools [Google], [Cloud TTS tool, version 2023–2024], [2025] were used to produce the narration (or parts of it). Every section has been carefully reviewed, revised, and approved by the author(s) to ensure accuracy, clarity, and alignment with the intended content, maintaining the integrity of the original material. The author takes full responsibility for the content of the final publication.

Acknowledgments

This book was conceived, produced, and reviewed for neurosurgery residents, young neurosurgeons, and all neurosurgeons seeking to enhance their technical mastery of cranial approaches. We are grateful for your interest in this work.

We are grateful to our professors and mentors who taught us neurosurgery, as well as to our colleagues from other specialties working alongside us, including otolaryngologists, ophthalmologists, head and neck surgeons, and general surgeons.

We would like to thank the ENT doctors and Fellows in Endonasal Endoscopic and Skull Base Surgery who assisted us with the transnasal transsphenoidal approach: Carolina Arcoverde de Oliveira, Guilherme Rodrigues Marinho, Igor Almeida Nascimento, and Marcio Ribeiro Studart da Fonseca Filho.

We extend our heartfelt thanks to the laboratory technicians of the Death Verification Service (DVS) at the University of São Paulo, Capital Campus, for their support and preparation of the cadaveric specimens.

This book was also made possible thanks to the generosity of patients' families who, after the end of life, permitted us to perform the dissections presented in this academic work for educational purposes. We extend our sincere gratitude.

Contents

Introduction to Cranial Approaches 1

1.1 Principles of Neurosurgery

Among the fundamental principles of neurosurgery, mastering neuroanatomy, and craniotomy techniques are cornerstone skills that we begin learning in medical school, refine during residency, and continue to hone until retirement. A deep understanding of neuroanatomy grants the neurosurgeon unparalleled precision, and to master this discipline, continuous practice is essential.

The execution of craniotomy using a defined technique began in 1889 with the introduction of temporary cranial resection, meticulously describing the step-by-step procedure. Most notably, Wagner practiced on cadavers before operating on a patient. The surgery was performed to evacuate an epidural hematoma, but despite the surgeon's efforts, the patient did not survive [1].

Neurosurgery has evolved as a specialty that originated from general surgery. When we compare our instrument tray with that of general surgery, we notice several similar instruments. However, performing craniotomy correctly requires specific surgical tools. Even in Wagner's time, manual trephines and gouges were used, and these were later followed by the Gigli saw [1]. Therefore, the advancement of craniotomy techniques has been associated with the development of specialized surgical instruments.

1.2 Pterional Craniotomy

One of the most essential neurosurgical procedures began to evolve in the nineteenth century. However, Yasargil formally described it in 1975 for the surgical treatment of vascular lesions in Willis's circle [2]. A simplified outline of the evolution of craniotomy techniques could be as follows:

H. de Oliveira Manduca Palmiero, E. G. Figueiredo, *Neurosurgical Approaches Video Atlas*, https://doi.org/10.1007/978-3-032-04664-2_1

(a) Development of craniotomy for hematoma evacuation (nineteenth century).
(b) Advances in craniotomy for intracranial tumor resection (early twentieth century).
(c) Transition to modern neurosurgery with the refinement of pterional craniotomy for cerebral aneurysm surgery (from the 1970s onward).

Currently, while we still use instruments similar to those from the nineteenth century, the addition of headholders, cranial drills, and operating microscopes has greatly advanced craniotomy techniques, allowing for procedures like awake brain surgery [3]. Moreover, with our expertise in craniotomy techniques, microsurgery, and careful brain retraction, we have refined methods to perform minimally invasive neurosurgical procedures [4].

1.3 Microsurgical View

The objective of craniotomy is to expose intracranial lesions, whether extradural, such as hematomas; intradural, such as meningiomas; or intra-axial, such as gliomas or vascular lesions (aneurysms, cavernomas, and vascular malformations). When operating on intradural lesions, we use a surgical microscope, which provides a cone-shaped view, with the cranial surface (craniotomy) as the base and deep structures as the vertex, where the surgical target is located. The wider the base, the greater the exposure, improving the illumination, expanding the conical view into a cylindrical perspective, and enhancing the working area and surgeon comfort [5].

A well-executed surgical approach, guided by anatomical landmarks and targeting the intracranial structures relevant to the procedure, along with proper patient positioning, enhances surgeon comfort and optimizes the operative workflow. This facilitates the main surgical objectives, whether brain decompression or hematoma evacuation in emergencies, or microsurgery such as tumor resection or aneurysm clipping. Once the patient is positioned, the next critical step in performing a craniotomy is identifying the key craniometric points, which serve as essential surgical landmarks.

1.4 Specimen Preparation

In this book, we used adult human cadavers with a post-mortem interval of less than 12 hours obtained from the Death Verification Service (DVS) in Sao Paulo. No additional preparation, such as vascular washing, immersion in alcohol solution, or chemical fixation, was performed to ensure that the physical properties of the skulls and brains remained as close as possible to those of in vivo surgical conditions. Anatomical dissections were conducted with family consent, following the DVS dissection protocol and Ofício 01 of the Discipline of Neurosurgery, as approved by the Research Ethics Committee of the School of Medicine, University of Sao Paulo.

1.5 Setting Up the Instruments Table

The arrangement of surgical instruments on the operating table must follow a systematic and reproducible methodology across procedures, aiming to optimize efficiency and facilitate intraoperative handling. To that end, the instruments table is typically organized according to the sequential order of use. Following the traditional paradigm in general surgery, the standard layout subdivides the table into specific sections: diaresis, grasping tissue and hemostasis, sponges and gauze (including drapes and instrument trays), special instruments, and finally, closure materials (Fig. 1.1) [6]. A practical demonstration of this setup is provided in the instructional video by the University of Sao Paulo (USP) e-Aulas platform [7].

Although neurosurgery initially emerged as a subspecialty of general surgery, it has evolved significantly since the 1970s, particularly with the advent of microsurgical techniques pioneered in part by Professor Yasargil. Consequently, the neurosurgical instrument table has been updated to include refined instruments for incision and dissection (the latter constituting a subset of the diaresis phase), marking the initial stage of the operation. Once the neurosurgical approach is established—the focus of this book—specialized instruments, including those for microsurgery, are incorporated (Fig. 1.2). In essence, the neurosurgical instrument layout maintains the procedural flow inherited from general surgery while integrating advanced tools designed for precise dissection and microsurgical manipulation (Fig. 1.3).

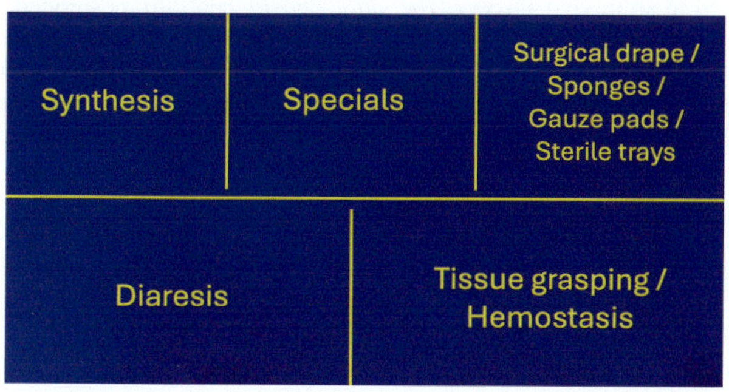

Fig. 1.1 Standardized layout of the surgical table based on traditional general surgery technique. The table is subdivided into five functional zones: (1) *Diaresis*—cutting and dissection instruments; (2) *Tissue grasping / Hemostasis*—forceps and clamps for manipulation and bleeding control; (3) *Surgical drape / Sponges / Gauze pads / Sterile trays*—materials for field preparation and fluid management; (4) *Specials—procedure-specific instruments*; and (5) *Synthesis*—suturing and closure instruments. This configuration supports systematic organization, anticipating instrument use and enhancing intraoperative efficiency (6, 7)

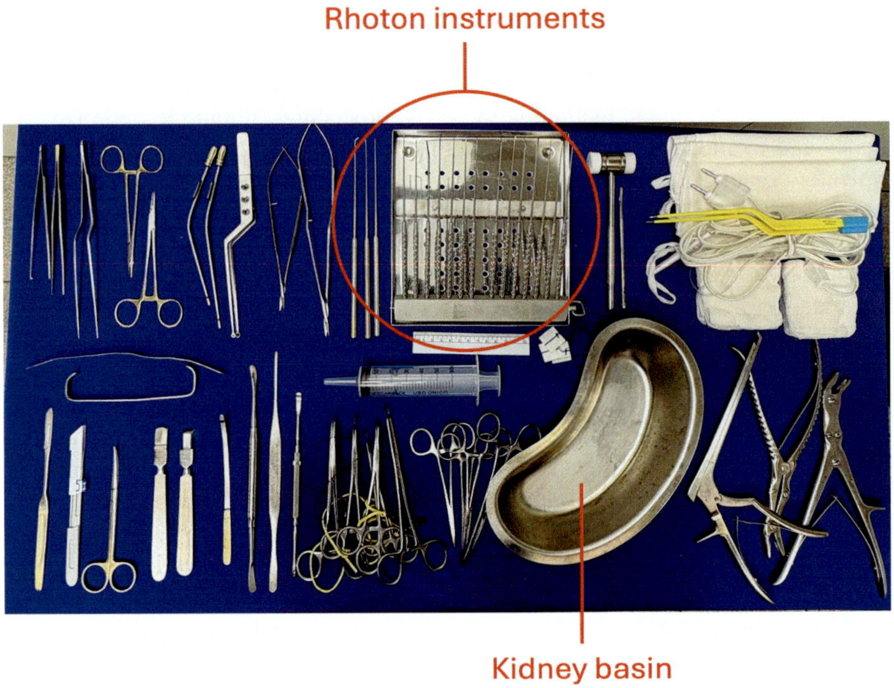

Fig. 1.2 An example of a neurosurgical instrument table prepared for a cranial procedure in this book and also used in an in vivo surgery. The *kidney basin*, centrally positioned, serves to safely contain the bone flap during surgery, preventing accidental falls and contamination. The *Rhoton instruments*, housed in a special zone, represent a set of highly specialized microsurgical tools used in the fine dissection phases of neurosurgical approaches. This configuration reflects the evolution of the traditional surgical table layout to accommodate the precision demands of modern neurosurgery

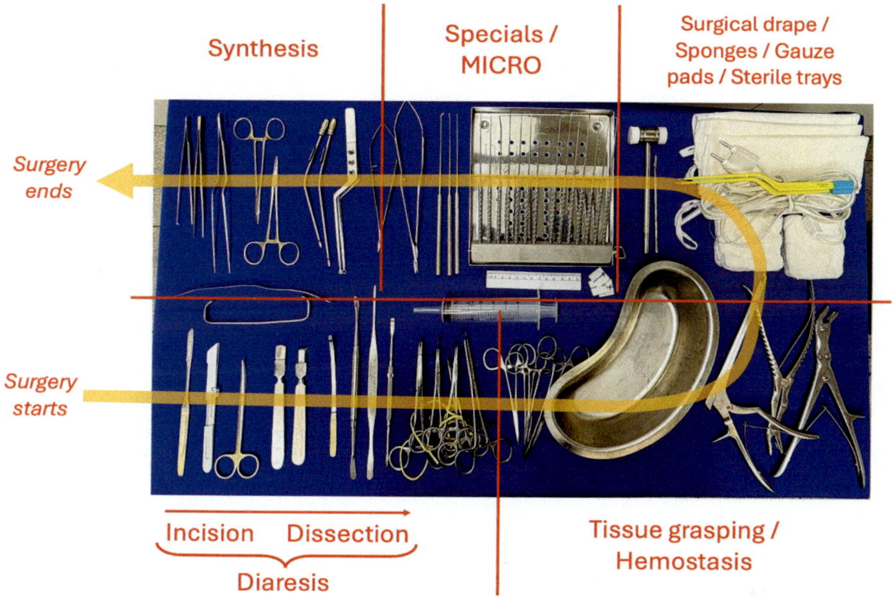

Fig. 1.3 Functional organization of the neurosurgical table reflecting the temporal sequence of surgical events. Instruments are organized to follow the logical progression of the procedure—from *diaresis* (*incision and dissection*) at the start, to *tissue grasping and hemostasis*, and culminating in *synthesis* (closure). The *special instruments/microsurgical set*, including Rhoton instruments, is integrated once the neurosurgical approach is established (craniotomy). Materials for field preparation (*drapes, sponges, gauze pads, and trays*) occupy the lateral zone. This systematic layout ensures ergonomic flow and minimizes cognitive and manual load during surgery

1.6 Laboratory Setup

The dissections were performed in the Neuroanatomy Laboratory of the Death Verification Service (DVS). Each cadaver underwent bi-coronal retromastoid (or bimastoid) incisions (Figs. 1.4 and 1.5) performed by DVS technicians following the institution's protocol. This incision technique preserves the specimen's original anatomical features at the end of the dissection, preventing alterations to the face or visible incisions outside the natural hairline. Additionally, throughout all craniotomies and dissections, anonymization and de-identification were strictly enforced in accordance with the institutional guidelines.

The cadavers were placed on a *Mercedes IMEC 1001* surgical table (Fig. 1.6). The heads were rigidly fixed using a *Sugita* head holder *(Sugita Fixator, Mizuho, Osaka, Japan)* (Fig. 1.7), a *Mayfield* head holder *(Integra LifeSciences, Princeton, New Jersey, USA)* (Fig. 1.8), or a horseshoe headrest, depending on the craniotomy technique applied and to simulate the surgical positioning.

Bone flap removal is performed using a cranial drill (craniotome) (Fig. 1.9) and appropriate neurosurgical instruments. Microsurgical procedures are conducted using a surgical microscope *(OP-Microscope—Carl Zeiss Contraves, Heidenheim, Germany)* (Fig. 1.10).

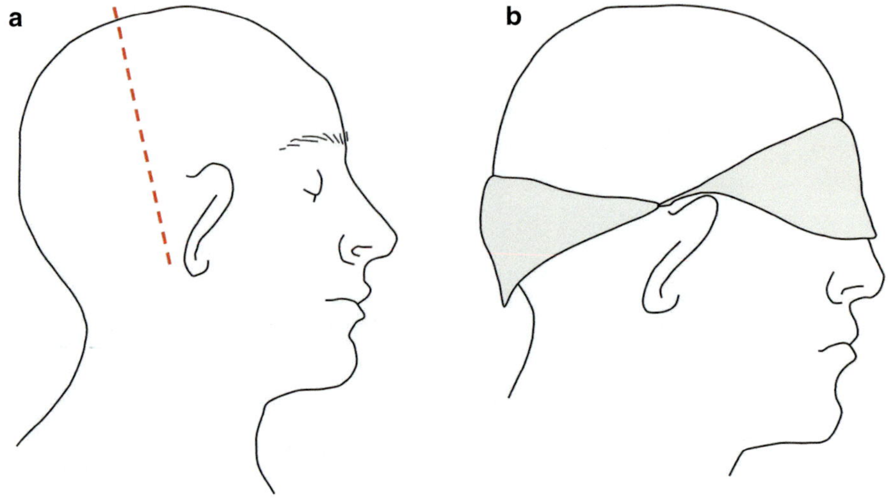

Fig. 1.4 Anatomical illustration depicting the bimastoid incision line (**a**) and the corresponding bitemporal scalp flap reflection (**b**), as standardized in the Death Verification Service protocol. It is important to note that the bimastoid incision is carried out by university technicians in accordance with institutional protocols and well-established descriptions in the scientific literature [8]

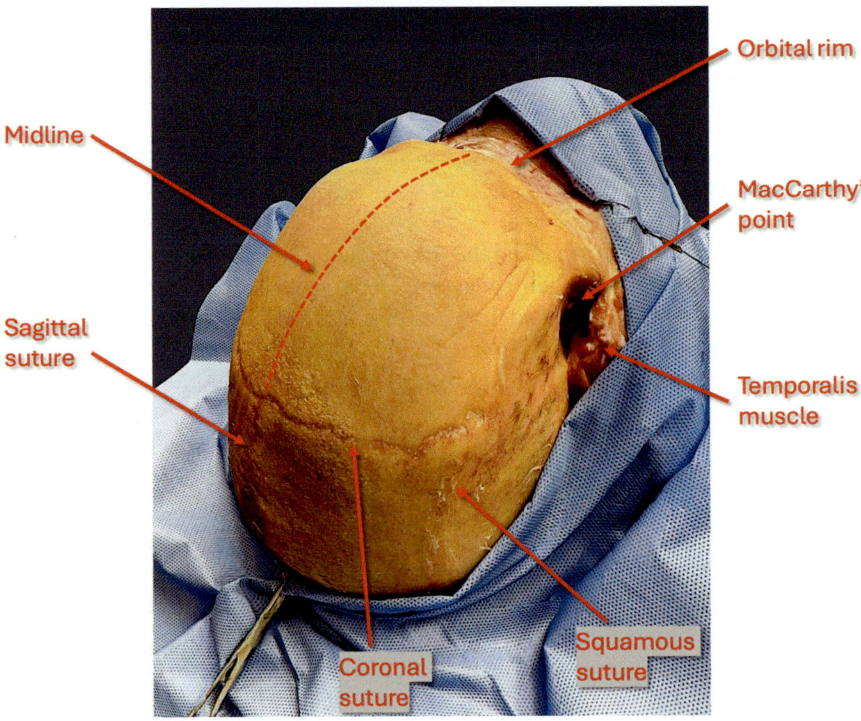

Fig. 1.5 Photogrammetry-based reconstruction of the cadaveric specimen prepared for surgical-anatomical dissection. Identify the anatomical landmarks such as the coronal, sagittal, and squamous sutures and the midline, orbital rim, temporalis muscle, and MacCarthy's point

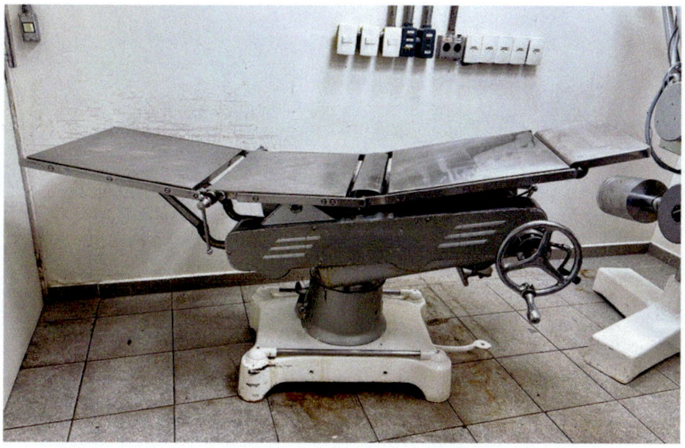

Fig. 1.6 The Mercedes IMEC 1001 surgical table is a manually operated model commonly used in neurosurgical settings. Its robust mechanical system allows for fine adjustments of the patient's position (or cadavers, as mentioned in this book) through lateral, Trendelenburg, and flexion-extension movements, utilizing a rotary crank mechanism. Despite its vintage design, this table remains reliable for precise intraoperative positioning, particularly in environments with limited access to automated systems

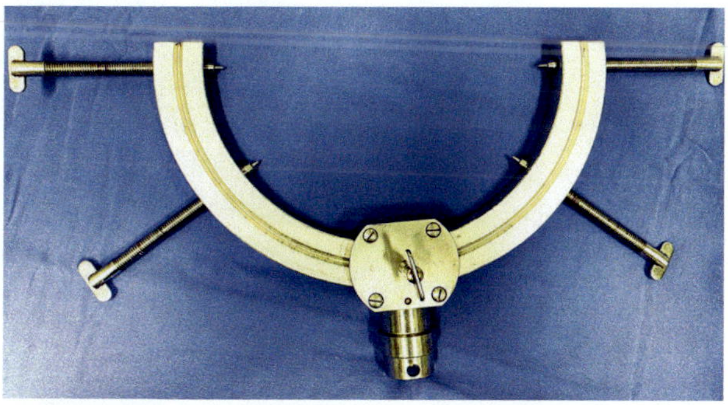

Fig. 1.7 *Sugita* head holder used for cadaveric dissections in this book. This rigid three-pin fixation system (the surgeon can use up to four pins in this system) provides stable cranial immobilization, enabling precise microsurgical training. While originally designed for live neurosurgical procedures, it is widely adopted in anatomical laboratories for high-fidelity simulations of operative approaches

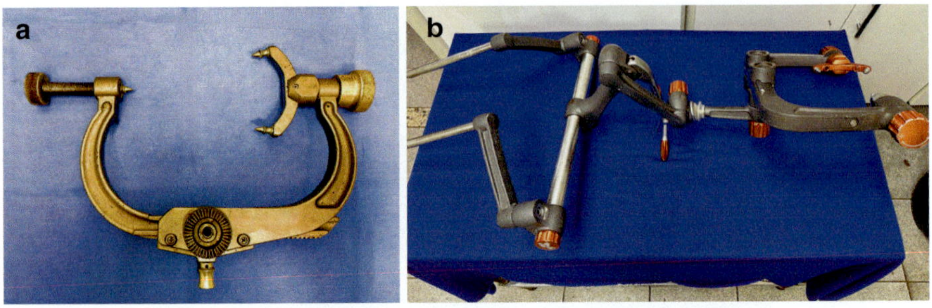

Fig. 1.8 Two models of the *Mayfield* head holder used in cadaveric laboratories. (**a**) The classic mechanical Mayfield clamp features a fixed three-pin configuration and a gear-based locking mechanism. (**b**) The articulated Mayfield frame has modular arms that allow for flexible positioning and enhanced ergonomics for microsurgical practice. Both systems provide rigid cranial fixation, which is essential for anatomical reproducibility and precision during skull base and intracranial dissections

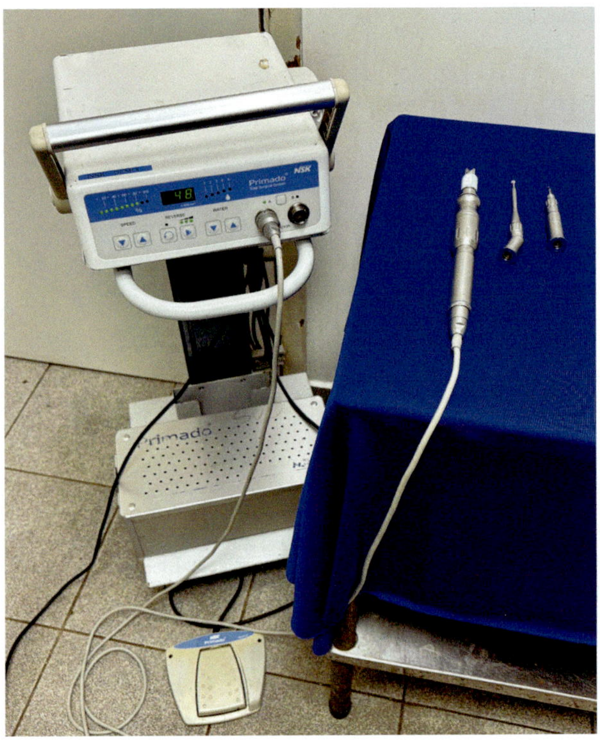

Fig. 1.9 *The NSK Primado* craniotome system used for performing craniotomies in the dissections presented in this book. This high-speed electric drill provides bone cutting with interchangeable handpieces and adjustable speed settings, controlled via foot pedal. Its ergonomic design and reliability make it ideal for anatomical studies and microsurgical training in cranial approaches

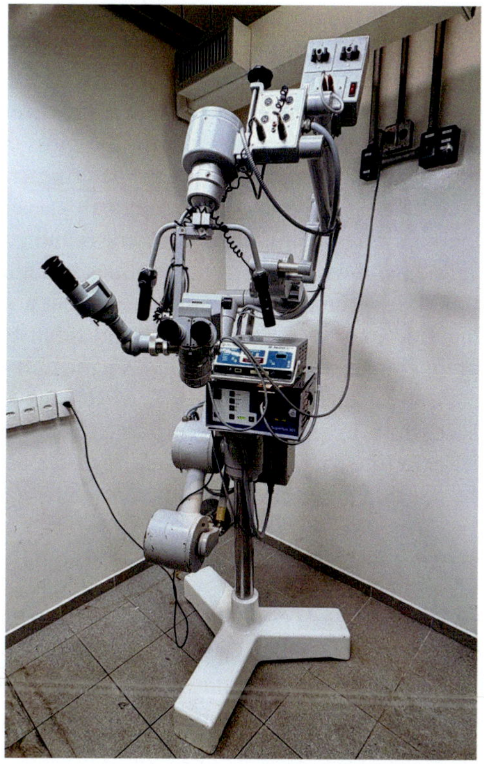

Fig. 1.10 *The operating microscope Carl Zeiss Contraves* used in our laboratory for all microsurgical dissections. Although this model is older, it offers stable optics and precise depth visualization for anatomical studies. We have adapted it with a custom recording system that utilizes an iPhone, enabling high-definition video capture of the dissections featured in this book

1.7 Patient Safety

Patient safety remains the foundation of neurosurgical practice, especially during craniotomy procedures. Before we begin studying craniotomy techniques, we highlight two critical errors and strategies to avoid or mitigate them: *wrong-side craniotomy* and *when the bone flap hits the floor*. We also review essential safety practices, including choosing the proper antiseptic (*Chlorhexidine* vs. *Povidone-Iodine*), using a *subgaleal drain* to prevent hematoma formation, and applying *dural tenting sutures* to reduce postoperative complications.

Wrong-Side Craniotomy Operating on the wrong side of a patient has devastating consequences for both the patient and the neurosurgeon. Among the surgical specialties susceptible to this error, neurosurgery and orthopedic surgery have a higher risk. Statistics from 2002 in the United States indicated an incidence of 2.2 wrong-side craniotomies per 10,000 craniotomies, within a total of 145,000 craniotomies, resulting in 32 wrong-side craniotomies that year [9]. Given the global volume of procedures, this number is likely to be significantly higher. Some procedures include hematoma evacuation, aneurysm clipping, and tumor resection. However, in ablative epilepsy surgeries, such as selective amygdalo-hippocampectomy, the consequences are irreversible, leading to permanent neurological deficits.

Several methods exist to prevent wrong-side craniotomies, including preoperative verification protocols, effective team communication, and checklists completed by multiple team members, such as nurses, anesthesiologists, and neurosurgeons. Additionally, thorough preoperative identification through multiple imaging reviews is essential [9]. However, one of the most significant factors is the neurosurgeon's vigilance and humility in acknowledging errors prompted by other team members. Quick recognition and correction can prevent catastrophic outcomes, underscoring the vital role of situational awareness and collaboration in surgical safety.

To avoid wrong-side craniotomies, we must adhere to protocols that include multiple cross-checks: (1) preoperative review of medical records, (2) confirmation of the side in front of the patient and relatives, (3) marking the surgical site in the preoperative area, (4) imaging verification emphasizing the need to confirm the patient ID in the images (CT, MRI), (5) keeping the patient's images open and accessible in the operative room, (6) surgical time-outs, and remaining humble enough to correct any potential mistakes before they occur [9, 10]. Is it human to err? YES. However, incorrect craniotomy can be prevented [9–11].

When a Bone Flap Hits the Floor From the beginning of neurosurgical residency, we are cautioned—just as medical interns are warned by both junior and senior residents—about the risks associated with bone flap drops. However, this concern is not limited to trainees; it affects all neurosurgeons, whether seasoned or in training, because it can arise in any surgical environment. Literature reports have indicated an incidence of approximately one bone flap drop per institution each year [12], which is consistent with typical observations in clinical practice. Furthermore, it is estimated that every neurosurgeon will encounter at least one such incident over the course of their career [12].

The first question is: how can it be prevented? A bone flap hits the floor when mishandled at three critical moments: (1) during elevation, when the flap is lifted from the skull; (2) during handling off the field, when it is transferred or repositioned; and (3) during closure, while securing the flap with plating [12]. To prevent this, both surgeons and surgical assistants should remain highly attentive. Awareness is the most effective tool for avoiding bone flap drops, thereby ensuring secure handling and proper communication throughout the procedure.

The second question is: what should be done if the bone flap drops? Managing an iatrogenically contaminated bone flap involves antibiotic irrigation and Betadine treatment, or alternatively, discarding and replacing the flap with cranioplasty material. Another option is to sterilize the bone to avoid and postpone cranioplasty by using autologous bone at a later stage [12, 13]. A bone flap falling to the floor is considered a "rare but ubiquitous complication" [12]. This finding highlights the importance of prevention and proper intraoperative management.

In summary, this study focuses on two critical errors and strategies to avoid or mitigate them:

1. Wrong-side craniotomy—Preoperative verification protocols, such as the "Time-Out" procedure, correct imaging review, and surgical site marking, can prevent this.
2. Bone flap dropping to the floor: This risk can be minimized by securing the bone flap with stay sutures, handling it with both hands and using a sterile tray to receive and store the flap safely.

For both wrong-side craniotomy and bone flap drops, documentation of the event in the medical record is essential and ensures that the entire surgical team is informed. Discussions in morbidity and mortality (MM) meetings are valuable from a didactic perspective, enabling surgeons to learn how to prevent such errors and how to manage them when they occur. Additionally, maintaining honesty with the patient and his/her family is crucial—clearly explaining what happened and addressing any concerns openly.

Chlorhexidine or Povidone-Iodine The comparative effectiveness of chlorhexidine (CHG) and povidone-iodine (PVI) for preoperative antisepsis in neurosurgery remains a subject of ongoing investigation [14–16]. Evidence suggests that CHG, particularly in alcoholic formulations, offers superior efficacy in reducing surgical site infections compared to PVI [14]. A systematic review and meta-analysis concluded that alcoholic CHG significantly lowers the risk of surgical site infections compared to PVI formulations, with CHG 4%–5% being the most effective [14]. Similarly, a large randomized controlled trial demonstrated that CHG-alcohol reduces overall surgical site infections rates compared to PVI, particularly for superficial and deep incisional infections [16]. However, in cranial neurosurgery, a study found no significant difference in surgical site infections rates between CHG and PVI alone but reported that combining both agents resulted in a significantly lower risk of infection [16]. While CHG demonstrates greater efficacy overall, the potential benefits of combination antisepsis strategies warrant further investigation in neurosurgical populations [14–16]. In our practice, we have been using both CHG and PVI in the surgical preparation of our patients.

Subgaleal Drain Periosteal, or subgaleal, drain insertion in supratentorial craniotomies remains a debated practice, often guided by surgeon preference rather than solid evidence. In a prospective observational study of 150 patients, Hamou et al. [17] analyzed the impact of subgaleal drains on postoperative outcomes, including fluid collections, wound healing, pain, and infection. They found that while subgaleal drains were more frequently used in cases involving larger craniotomies, longer incisions, or watertight dural closures, their use did not significantly affect rates of periorbital edema, subgaleal swelling, impaired wound healing, postoperative pain, or the need for surgical revision. Infections occurred in 7.3% of cases (total number) and were not linked to drain use. The study concluded that subgaleal fluid collections are common but generally self-limiting, and the presence of drains did not provide measurable clinical benefits in this cohort. Therefore, routine drain insertion may not be justified and should be based on intraoperative findings and individual case characteristics rather than a standardized protocol.

In our search on PubMed, we most often found articles referencing the use of subgaleal or subdural drains for treating chronic subdural hematoma, with very few mentions of subgaleal drains used in craniotomy procedures in general. We understand that the decision to use or not use a subgaleal drain usually depends on the neurosurgeon's personal experience or institutional preferences. In our dissections, we focused on the craniotomy technique in cadavers without emphasizing closure. However, it is in this context that one truly appreciates the saying: *I have never regretted placing a subperiosteal drain.*

Dural Tenting Sutures Dural tenting sutures were introduced by Walter Dandy in the early 1930s as a preventive measure against postoperative epidural hematomas (EDHs), a complication that was then a frequent cause of mortality due to unreliable hemostasis under hypotensive conditions [18, 19]. By anchoring the dura to the overlying bone or pericranium, the sutures were believed to reduce the potential epidural space and compress bleeding vessels. Over time, this technique became a nearly universal step in craniotomy closures.

However, in modern neurosurgery—with the availability of improved hemostatic techniques, normovolemic anesthesia, and careful monitoring—the prophylactic use of dural tenting sutures has been increasingly questioned. Large adult and pediatric series found that selective use of tenting sutures, only in the presence of active bleeding, resulted in low reoperation rates for EDH, challenging the dogmatic application of the technique [18–20]. Furthermore, complications such as cortex contusions, subdural hematomas, and cerebrospinal fluid (CSF) leaks have been reported in association with indiscriminate use of tenting sutures [20].

A recent randomized controlled trial showed that omitting prophylactic dural tenting in elective supratentorial craniotomies is not worse than routine tenting regarding reoperation for epidural hematoma, postoperative death, and neurological outcomes [21]. The study compared three approaches: dural tenting before durotomy, after durotomy under microscopic visualization, and no tenting at all. Most complications—such as cerebral contusions and hematomas—occurred in the group where the dura was anchored before opening. In contrast, the group where tenting was done after durotomy under direct microscopic visualization had no hematomas from venous injury or cortical contusions [20, 21].

In our dissections, dural anchoring was done before durotomy using the external leaflet of the dura mater. However, the overall evidence supports a more targeted, evidence-based approach—saving dural tenting for cases with a clear intraoperative bleeding risk rather than using it as a universal preventive measure. If dural tenting is considered necessary by the surgeon, the safer method seems to be performing it after durotomy, under direct visualization.

Our techniques typically originate from training during residency, peer exchange in surgical practice, and the neurosurgical literature. Still, nothing exceeds the value of personal experience—shaped through years of practice and lessons learned from managing our own complications.

1.8 Complications

There has been ongoing discussion among neurosurgeons regarding the inherent risks of operative intervention—not only concerning patient safety but also regarding medicolegal liability. From the earliest stages of residency, we are taught a core tenet of surgical maturity: only those who operate will face complications, yet rather than passively accepting this reality, neurosurgery has progressively developed strategies to enhance patient safety. These include the use of structured protocols like the time-out checklist—borrowed from aviation safety models—interdisciplinary teamwork with equal participation from anesthesiologists, nursing staff, and surgeons, and the integration of advanced intraoperative technologies such as neuronavigation, intraoperative ultrasound, intraoperative MRI, and neuromonitoring [22].

Despite these safeguards, risk can never be eliminated. Abandoning microsurgical techniques—still the definitive treatment for many cerebral aneurysms, the curative modality for selected tumors such as meningiomas, and the means of achieving maximal safe resection in gliomas—would ultimately harm patients rather than protect them [22]. Avoiding risk must never be mistaken for avoiding responsibility.

In this context, complications remain a powerful, albeit underutilized, pedagogical tool. As Heros elegantly noted, "I have learned more at M&M conferences than perhaps in any other setting" [23]. Unfortunately, the culture of open discourse about complications is increasingly hindered by legal concerns and academic incentives that prioritize flawless surgical narratives over authentic learning [24], yet it is precisely in the honest confrontation with adverse outcomes that surgical wisdom matures.

To contribute to this essential dialogue, each chapter of this book ends with a section on "*Pearls and Pitfalls*"—emphasizing intraoperative traps to avoid and practical lessons learned through direct surgical experience. This reflects the increasing call in the literature to adopt structured classifications for complications, such as the Landriel Ibañez system, to promote consistency and transparency in reporting [25]. As others have noted, complications should not be viewed as professional failures but rather as inevitable steps on the journey toward mastery, and sharing them openly remains our most ethical and educational commitment [23, 26].

1.9 Personal Protective Equipment

Personal protective equipment (PPE), including safety glasses, masks, gowns, and gloves, is crucial for craniotomy procedures. We consider surgical drapes to be part of personal protection for researchers; however, in actual surgical procedures, the sterile nature of drapes is primarily intended for patient safety.

1.10 Cranial Approaches to Philosophy

In Neurosurgery, the anatomical characteristics of various intracranial pathologies often dictate the surgical approaches used. For instance, tumors can create mass effects that facilitate surgical access, whereas aneurysms are typically located within subarachnoid cisterns, necessitating careful navigation through these spaces [27]. Hydrocephalus leads to dilation of the ventricular system, alters brain architecture, and influences surgical planning. Arteriovenous malformations (AVMs) often present as V-shaped structures, with the apex pointing toward the ventricles and the base extending toward the cortical surface [28]. Pioneers like Professor Yasargil have extensively studied these anatomical nuances, thereby enhancing the precision of microsurgical interventions. Professor Yasargil and other neurosurgeons who have followed his work in microneurosurgery have been instrumental in refining surgical techniques for aneurysms and AVMs, emphasizing the importance of understanding these anatomical relationships to optimize patient outcomes.

References

1. González-Darder JM. Historia de la craneotomía. Neurocirugia. 2016;229:1–13.
2. Vishteh AG, Spetzler RF, Lawton MT, et al. The pterional approach. Oper Tech Neurosurg. 1998;1(1):39–49.
3. Surbeck W, Hildebrandt G, Duffau H. The evolution of brain surgery on awake patients. Acta Neurochir. 2015;157:77–84.
4. Wong JHY, Poon WS, Yu SCH, Wai YK. Minimally invasive microsurgery for cerebral aneurysms. Stroke. 2015;46:2699–706.
5. Palmiero HOM. Avaliação anatômica, qualitativa e quantitativa das variantes do acesso supracerebelar infratentorial para o tálamo posterior [Doctoral thesis]. São Paulo: Faculdade de Medicina da Universidade de São Paulo; 2020.
6. Liehn M, Schlautmann H. 101 of surgical instruments: naming, recognizing, handling and presenting. Berlin: Springer; 2022.
7. Universidade de São Paulo. Montagem da mesa cirúrgica. e-Aulas USP. [video] 2020. Available from: https://eaulas.usp.br/portal/video.action?idItem=24976
8. Giannini C, Okazaki H. Nervous system. In: Ludwig J, editor. Handbook of autopsy practice. Totowa: Humana Press; 2002. https://doi.org/10.1007/978-1-59259-286-9_6.
9. Cohen FL, Britz GW, Adelson PD, et al. Wrong-site craniotomy: analysis of 35 cases and systems for prevention. J Neurosurg. 2010;113:461–73.
10. Kanat A. Wrong-site craniotomy: letters to the editor. J Neurosurg. 2013;119:1079–80.
11. Cima RR. Wrong-site craniotomy: editorial. J Neurosurg. 2010;113:458–60.
12. Jankowitz BT, Kondziolka DS. When the bone flap hits the floor. Neurosurgery. 2006;59:585–90.
13. Chernov M. When the bone flap hits the floor: correspondence. Neurosurgery. 2007;61(6):E1340.
14. Wade RG, Burr NE, McCauley G, Bourke G, Efthimiou O. The comparative efficacy of chlorhexidine gluconate and povidone-iodine antiseptics for the prevention of infection in clean surgery: a systematic review and network meta-analysis. Ann Surg. 2021;274(6):e481–8.
15. Darouiche RO, Wall MJ Jr, Itani KMF, Otterson MF, Webb AL, Carrick MM, et al. Chlorhexidine–alcohol versus povidone–iodine for surgical-site antisepsis. N Engl J Med. 2010;362(1):18–26.
16. Davies BM, Patel HC. Does chlorhexidine and povidone-iodine preoperative antisepsis reduce surgical site infection in cranial neurosurgery? Ann R Coll Surg Engl. 2016;98(6):405–8.

17. Hamou HA, Kotliar K, Tan SK, Weiß C, Christian B, Clusmann H, et al. Surgical nuances and placement of subgaleal drains for supratentorial procedures—a prospective analysis of efficacy and outcome in 150 craniotomies. Acta Neurochir. 2020;162(4):729–36.
18. Winston KR. Dural tenting sutures in pediatric neurosurgery. Pediatr Neurosurg. 1998;28(5):230–5.
19. Winston KR. Efficacy of dural tenting sutures. J Neurosurg. 1999;91(2):180–4.
20. Eroglu U, Zaimoğlu M, Sayacı EY, et al. Is placing prophylactic dural tenting sutures a dogma? World Neurosurg. 2021;153:e403–7.
21. Przepiórka Ł, Wójtowicz K, Kujawski S, et al. Dural tenting in elective craniotomies: a randomized clinical trial. Neurosurgery. 2025;00:1–10.
22. Jean WC, Charbel FT, Cohen-Gadol AA, Couldwell WT, Lawton MT, McDermott M, et al. Complications: skull base and cerebrovascular. Neurosurg Focus. 2024;57(4):E2.
23. Heros RC. Complications: our best way to learn. Neurosurg Focus. 2024;57(4):E1.
24. Spetzler RF, McDermott MW, Couldwell WT, Jean WC, van Loveren HR. Complications in neurosurgery—the need for a common language. J Neurosurg. 2017;126(4):1045–7.
25. Landriel Ibañez FA, Hem S, Ajler P, Vecchi E, Ciraolo C, Baccanelli M, et al. A new classification of complications in neurosurgery. World Neurosurg. 2011;75(5–6):709–15.
26. Spetzler RF, Sanai N, Zabramski JM. Complications in skull base and cerebrovascular surgery: lessons learned and future directions. Neurosurg Focus. 2024;57(4):E4.
27. Krayenbühl HA, Yasargil MG, Flamm ES, Tew JM Jr. Microsurgical treatment of intracranial saccular aneurysms. J Neurosurg. 1975;37(6):678–86.
28. Lawton MT. Exposure. In: Seven AVMs: tenets and techniques for resection. New York: Thieme; 2014. p. 3–20.

Foundational Anatomy for Neurosurgical Approaches

2

When considering cranial surgical approaches, it is tempting to reduce the concept to merely removing a portion of bone to access the brain and perform the procedure. However, what distinguishes neurosurgery from other disciplines is the intricate, multilayered nature of the tissues encountered during cranial access. The neurosurgeon must navigate not only the scalp and skull but also specialized anatomical layers such as the galea aponeurotica, temporalis fascia, dura mater, and neurovascular structures, all of which require precise handling to preserve function and minimize morbidity.

Each surgical corridor demands a tailored dissection strategy that respects the natural planes of these tissues, reflecting a deep understanding of their structural and functional relationships. Moreover, the complexity increases in regions such as the skull base, where the anatomy is densely compacted and the margin for error is minimal. Thus, cranial approaches in neurosurgery are not merely technical maneuvers—they are anatomical dialogues between the surgeon and the patient's unique topography. This highlights the vital importance of revisiting and mastering thorough anatomical knowledge when planning neurosurgical procedures. It is through this anatomical literacy that safe, effective, and elegant surgeries become possible.

2.1 Cranium and Skull Base

The cranium comprises eight principal bones—frontal, parietal, temporal, occipital, sphenoid, and ethmoid—that form a rigid protective vault and serve as the foundation for neurosurgical navigation. These bones are interconnected by fibrous sutures that function as growth sites during development and serve as landmarks during surgical planning [1–4] (Fig. 2.1).

The skull base is a structurally complex area divided into anterior, middle, and posterior cranial fossae, composed of the ethmoid, sphenoid, temporal, and occipital bones. This region includes multiple foramina for cranial nerves and vessels, and craniometric points [5] (Figs. 2.2 and 2.3).

H. de Oliveira Manduca Palmiero, E. G. Figueiredo, *Neurosurgical Approaches Video Atlas*, https://doi.org/10.1007/978-3-032-04664-2_2

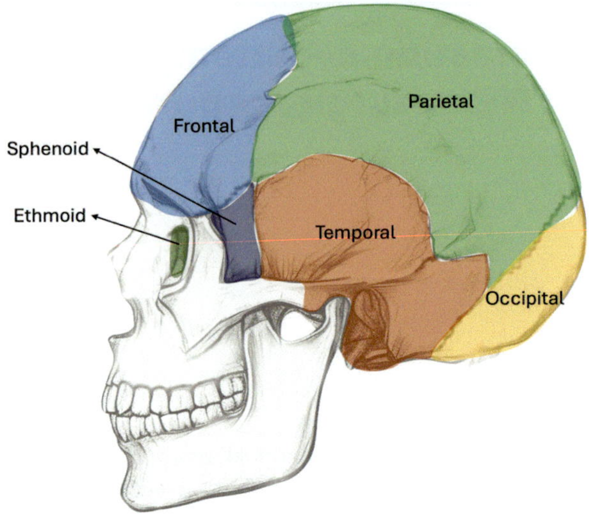

Fig. 2.1 Lateral view of the adult human skull illustrating the eight cranial bones relevant to neurosurgical approaches. The frontal, parietal, temporal, occipital, sphenoid, and ethmoid bones form the structural foundation for planning cranial access routes. There are spatial relationships and sutural boundaries that need to be mastered for the safe execution of neurosurgical procedures

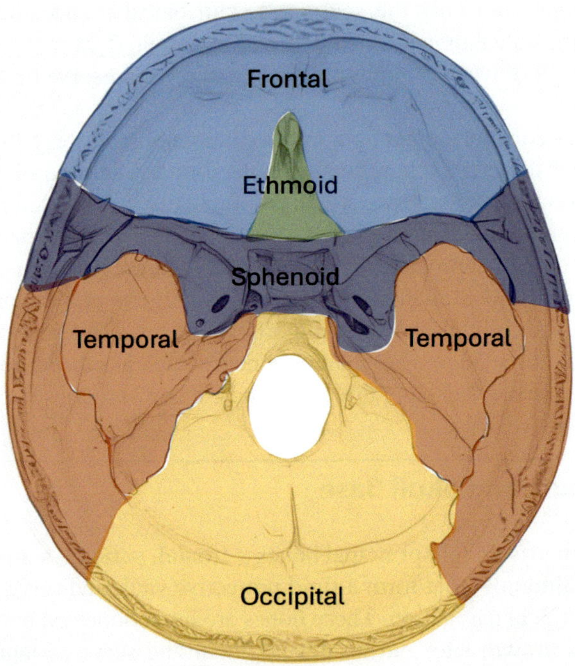

Fig. 2.2 Superior view of the skull base highlighting the frontal, ethmoid, sphenoid, temporal, and occipital bones—central structures in anterior, middle, and posterior cranial fossa surgery. The anterior cranial fossa is formed by the frontal, ethmoid, and sphenoid bones; the middle cranial fossa is composed of the sphenoid and temporal bones; and the posterior cranial fossa is primarily formed by the occipital bone, with contributions from the temporal and sphenoid bones This topographic layout is significant for planning transnasal, pterional, retrosigmoid, and far-lateral approaches, with each bone containing foramina and neurovascular corridors that facilitate surgical access to deep-seated intracranial structures. Additionally, these relationships between the bones are vital for safe navigation in skull base surgery, particularly in approaches targeting the sellar, parasellar, and clival regions

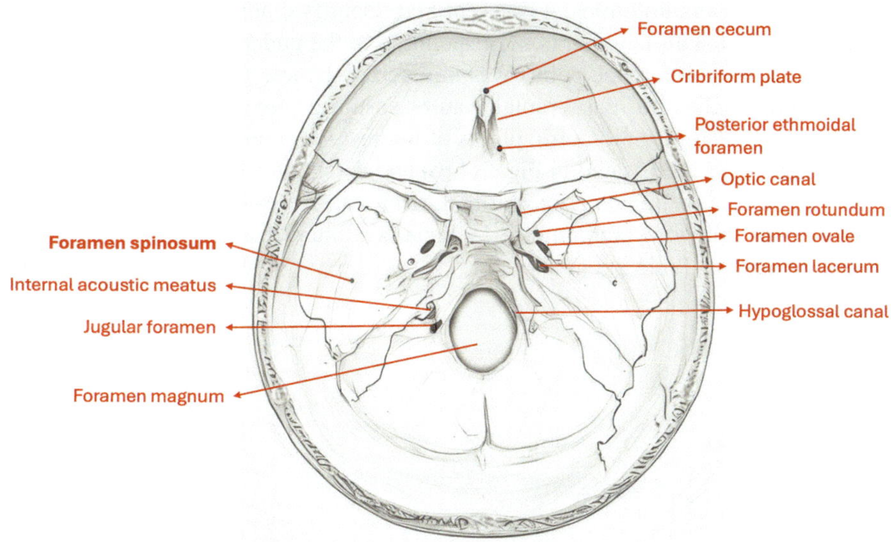

Fig. 2.3 Basal view of the skull illustrating the major foramina critical to neurosurgical approaches. These anatomical apertures serve as essential conduits for cranial nerves and vascular structures. For instance, the optic canal transmits the optic nerve and ophthalmic artery; the foramen rotundum allows the passage of the maxillary division (V2) of the trigeminal nerve; the foramen ovale transmits the mandibular division (V3) of the trigeminal nerve along with accessory vascular structures; and the foramen spinosum conveys the middle meningeal artery and vein. The jugular foramen and hypoglossal canal serve as exit points for the lower cranial nerves. This anatomical configuration of the foramina and their relationship within the anterior, middle, and posterior cranial fossae facilitates approaches to the cavernous sinus, clivus, petroclival region, and craniocervical junction

The paranasal sinuses—frontal, ethmoid, sphenoid, and maxillary—are pneumatized cavities that reduce cranial weight and influence transnasal approaches. Their proximity to critical neurovascular structures necessitates careful anatomical planning in skull base surgery [4, 5].

2.2 Craniometric Points

In all surgical procedures, surgeons rely on anatomical landmarks for precise orientation. Nowadays, we have tools like neuronavigation that assist us throughout surgery, from positioning and craniotomy to microsurgical dissection. Although neuronavigation enhances surgical safety, it is operator-dependent and prone to technical failures. A thorough understanding of neuroanatomy can ensure precise neurosurgical navigation. Therefore, a dedicated study of anatomical atlases and surgical technique books is crucial for mastering neurosurgical approaches.

For executing craniotomies, it is essential to identify craniometric points, which serve as external skull landmarks corresponding to the underlying brain structures. The study of these reference points was initiated by Broca. These landmarks guide surgical approaches to the cranial vault, ensuring precise and safe access. Accordingly, the key craniometric points of interest for cranial surgical approaches were delineated, as illustrated in Fig. 2.4 [6] and detailed in Table 2.1 [7–9].

Furthermore, for the posterior, parietal, occipital, and suboccipital approaches, we outline the following craniometric landmarks of interest, as illustrated in Fig. 2.5 [6] and detailed in Table 2.2 [7–9].

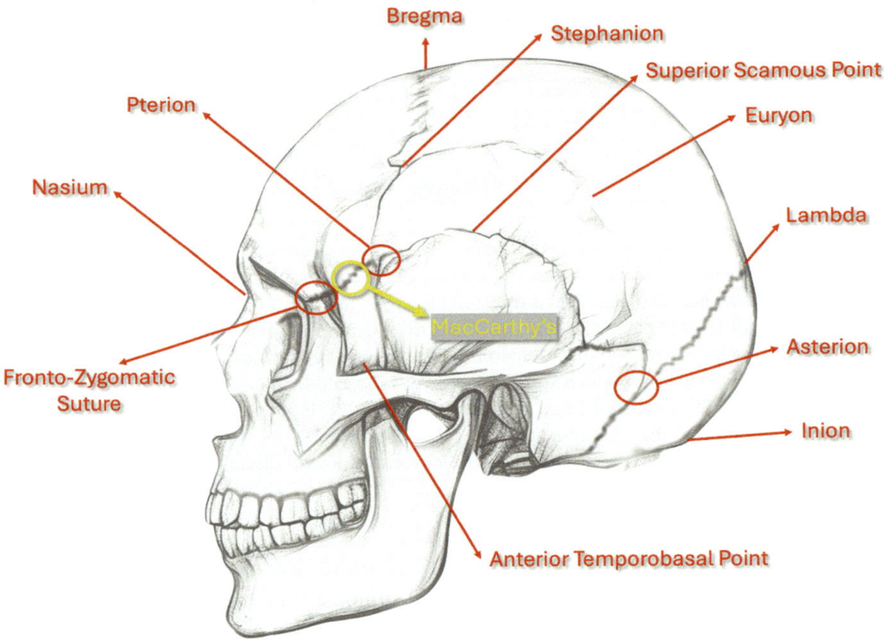

Fig. 2.4 Lateral view of the skull showing the identification of key craniometric landmarks relevant for performing craniotomies [6]

Table 2.1 Identification of craniometric points and anatomical landmarks on the lateral aspect of the skull, followed by their anatomical description

Craniometric points	Anatomical description
Na: Nasium	Midpoints at the frontal and nasal bones
P: Pterion	Four bones meet: the frontal, parietal, temporal, and sphenoid levels
SSP: Superior scamous point	Related to the inferior rolandic point (where the central sulci and Sylvian fissure meet)
St: Stephanion	The coronal suture intersects the superior temporal line.
Eu: Euryon	Corresponds to the supramarginal gyri
λ: Lambda	Junction between the lambdoid and sagittal sutures
In: Inion	The most prominent point of the external occipital protuberance; the confluence of sinuses (superior sagittal sinus, straight sinus, occipital sinus, and transverse sinus meet at the torcular Herophili)
Ast: Asterion	Junction of three sutures: the lambdoid, parietomastoid, and occipitomastoid
Br: Bregma	The coronal and sagittal sutures meet at the top of the skull.
FZS: Frontozygomatic suture	Fronto-Zygomatic Sutures point of junction, referential for the OZ and Supra-Orbital-Zygomatic craniotomies
ATB: Anterior temprobasal point	Landmark of the anterior temporal fossa

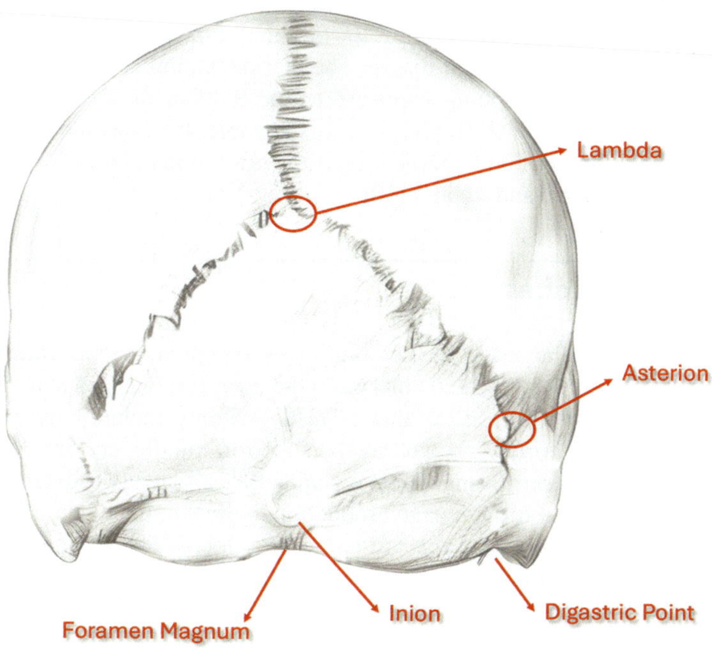

Fig. 2.5 Posterior view of the skull showing the identification of key craniometric landmarks relevant for performing parietal, occipital, suboccipital, retrosigmoid, and far-lateral craniotomies [6]

Table 2.2 Identification of craniometric points and anatomical landmarks on the posterior aspect of the skull, followed by their anatomical description

Craniometric points	Anatomical description
λ: Lambda	Junction between the lambdoid and sagittal sutures; the confluence of sinuses
Ast: Asterion	Junction of three sutures: the lambdoid, parietomastoid, and occipitomastoid
In: Inion	Confluence of the sinuses as a reference for torcular Herophili
D: Digastric point	At the mastoid notch, where the posterior belly of the digastric muscle originates on the medial side of the mastoid process of the temporal bone
M: Foramen magnum	The inferior limit of the occipital bone

2.3 The MacCarthy's Keyhole

The MacCarty keyhole, which is positioned over the frontosphenoidal suture near the frontozygomatic junction (in Fig. 2.4, see the yellow circle showing the MacCarthy's Keyhole), is essential for both the pterional and frontotemporo-orbitozygomatic (FtOZ) approaches. The suture is strategically placed over the frontosphenoidal suture, just behind the frontozygomatic junction, allowing optimal exposure of the periorbita and frontal dura. This positioning facilitates a wider surgical corridor, thereby reducing brain retraction and improving access to the anterior, middle, and posterior cranial fossae. The pterional approach benefits from the MacCarty keyhole by enhancing exposure to the Sylvian fissure and skull base structures. Similarly, in FtOZ craniotomy, this keyhole serves as the primary burr hole for removing the roof and lateral wall of the orbit, maximizing access to skull base lesions, aneurysms, and tumors [10].

2.4 Cerebral Lobes

The *frontal lobe* is the largest of the cerebral lobes, comprising approximately 35% of the cerebral cortex. It is situated anterior to the central sulcus and superior to the lateral (Sylvian) fissure (Figs. 2.6 and 2.7). Its anatomy includes the precentral gyrus (primary motor cortex), as well as the superior, middle, and inferior frontal gyri (Fig. 2.8). The inferior frontal gyrus contains Broca's area (Brodmann areas 44 and 45), which is critical for language production in the dominant hemisphere [11]. Medially, the superior frontal gyrus and paracentral lobule extend onto the medial surface, adjacent to the cingulate gyrus—part of the limbic system (Fig. 2.9). The orbital surface features gyri involved in decision-making and emotional regulation [12].

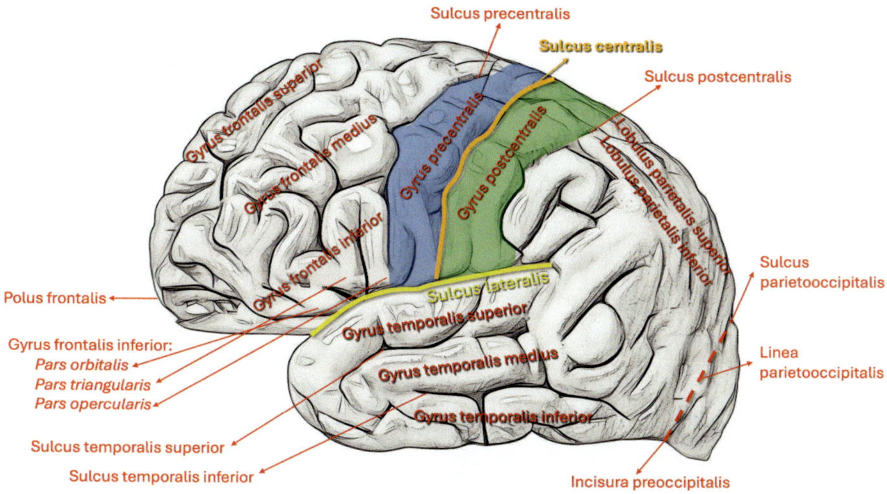

Fig. 2.6 Lateral view of the cerebral hemisphere, illustrating the major sulci and gyri of the frontal, parietal, and temporal lobes. Anatomical landmarks include the central sulcus (sulcus centralis, separating the frontal and parietal lobes), precentral and postcentral gyri, as well as the superior, middle, and inferior frontal gyri, and the superior, middle, and inferior temporal gyri. The lateral sulcus (Sylvian fissure) separates the frontal and parietal lobes from the temporal lobe. The inferior frontal gyrus is further divided into pars opercularis, pars triangularis, and pars orbitalis—regions that are critical for language processing. See the motor gyrus (Gyrus precentralis) highlighted in light blue and the sensory gyrus (Gyrus postcentralis) in light green

The *temporal lobe* is located below the lateral sulcus and has three main gyri on its lateral surface—superior, middle, and inferior. The superior temporal gyrus contains Heschl's gyrus (primary auditory cortex) and nearby language-processing areas. Medially, the mesial temporal structures include the hippocampus, parahippocampal gyrus, amygdala, and uncus—essential for memory and emotion [13] (Figs. 2.6 and 2.10). The fusiform gyrus on the inferior surface aids high-level visual recognition [14].

The *parietal lobe*, located behind the central sulcus, is divided by the intraparietal sulcus into superior and inferior parietal lobules. The postcentral gyrus (Brodmann areas 3, 1, 2) contains the primary somatosensory cortex, organized somatotopically into the sensory homunculus [15]. The supramarginal (area 40) and angular (area 39) gyri play roles in language and visuospatial integration. Medially, the precuneus is involved in self-referential processing and default mode network functions (Figs. 2.9, 2.10, and 2.11) [16].

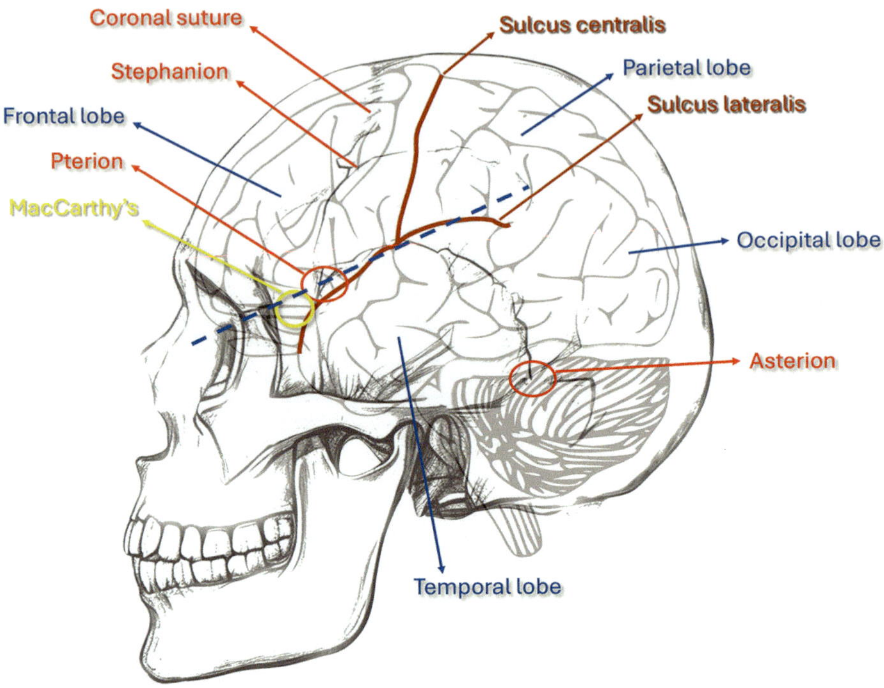

Fig. 2.7 This illustration superimposes the cranium onto an anatomical drawing of the brain to correlate key craniometric landmarks with the underlying encephalic structures. The red labels highlight surface landmarks of the cranium, such as the coronal suture, stephanion, pterion, and asterion, while the orange labels indicate the major cortical sulci. The blue dashed line approximates the course of the Sylvian fissure, extending from the lateral orbital rim through MacCarthy's point and the pterion, following the depression formed at the junction of the frontal and temporal bones over the sphenoid wing

The *occipital lobe* serves as the visual processing center. On its medial surface, the calcarine sulcus delineates the primary visual cortex (area 17), bordered by the cuneus and lingual gyrus. The lateral surface showcases the lateral occipital gyri, which are involved in object and motion perception. Inferiorly, it transitions into the fusiform gyrus, which is critical for face and object recognition (Figs. 2.6, 2.10, and 2.12) [17].

The *insula*, often referred to as the fifth lobe, is situated within the lateral sulcus and covered by the opercula. It is divided into anterior (affective-cognitive) and posterior (sensorimotor) regions. The insular cortex lies above the extreme capsule, claustrum, and basal ganglia. It serves as a central hub for multisensory integration and autonomic regulation. In neurosurgical procedures, it is accessed via the trans-sylvian route and is bordered by branches of the middle cerebral artery [18] (Fig. 2.13).

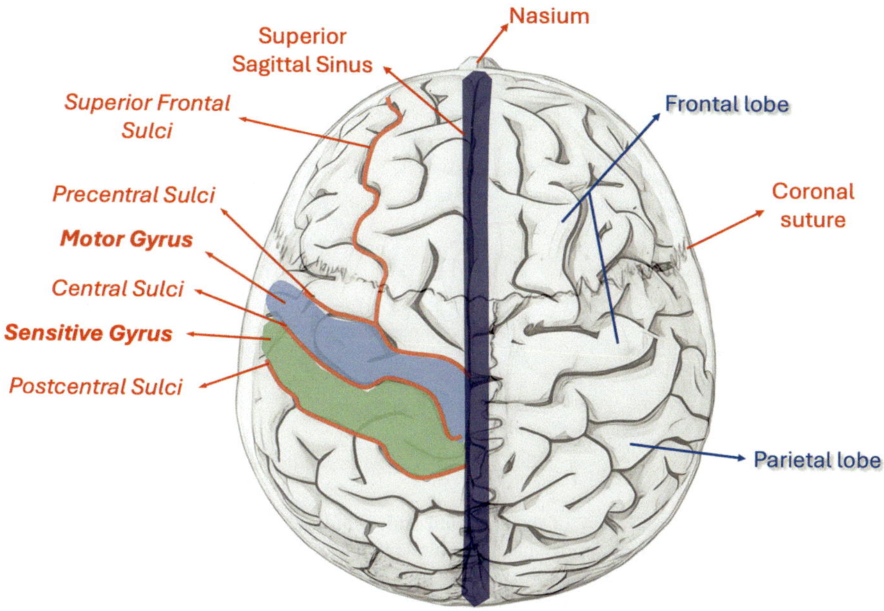

Fig. 2.8 Superior view of the cerebral hemispheres highlighting the motor gyrus (precentral gyrus) in light blue and the sensitive gyrus (postcentral gyrus) in light green. Anatomical landmarks include the central sulcus, precentral sulcus, postcentral sulcus, superior frontal sulci, superior sagittal sinus, coronal suture, and nasium

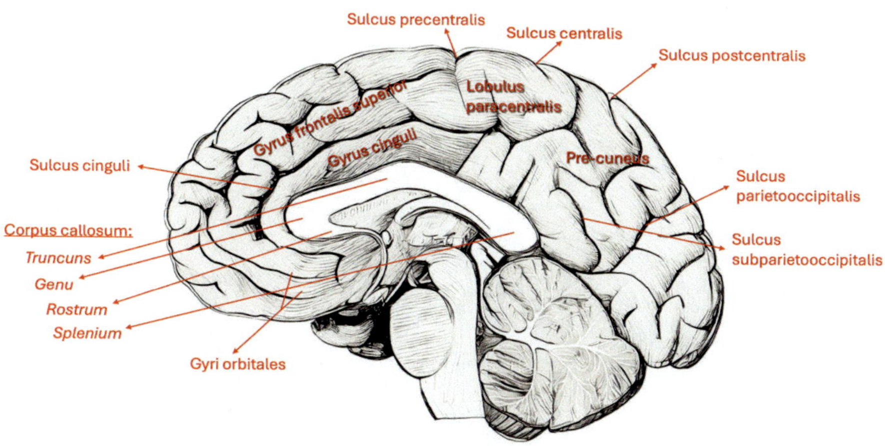

Fig. 2.9 Medial view of the cerebral hemisphere highlights the anatomical landmarks of the frontal and parietal lobes, as well as limbic and callosal structures. Notable features include the superior frontal gyrus, cingulate gyrus and sulcus, paracentral lobule, precuneus, and parieto-occipital sulcus. The corpus callosum is shown with its subdivisions: rostrum, genu, truncus (body), and splenium. This perspective is essential for interhemispheric approaches, corpus callosotomy, and understanding medial cortical topography in procedures involving the cingulate cortex

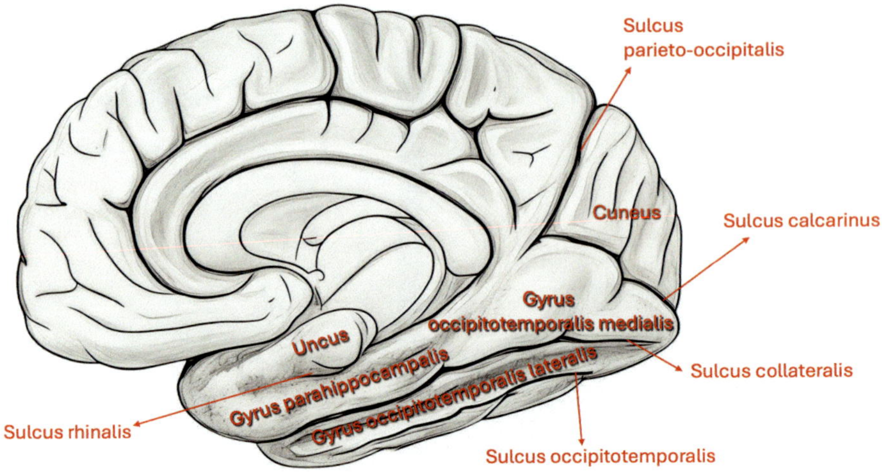

Fig. 2.10 Medial and basal view of the temporal and occipital lobes highlighting mesial structures relevant to neurosurgical approaches. Notable landmarks include the uncus, parahippocampal gyrus, and medial and lateral occipitotemporal gyri (fusiform gyrus), bordered by the collateral and occipitotemporal gyri. The calcarine and parieto-occipital sulci delimit the cuneus, which houses the primary visual cortex. These regions are central to limbic, visual, and memory processing and are involved in approaches to mesial temporal epilepsy, occipital tumors, and parahippocampal resections

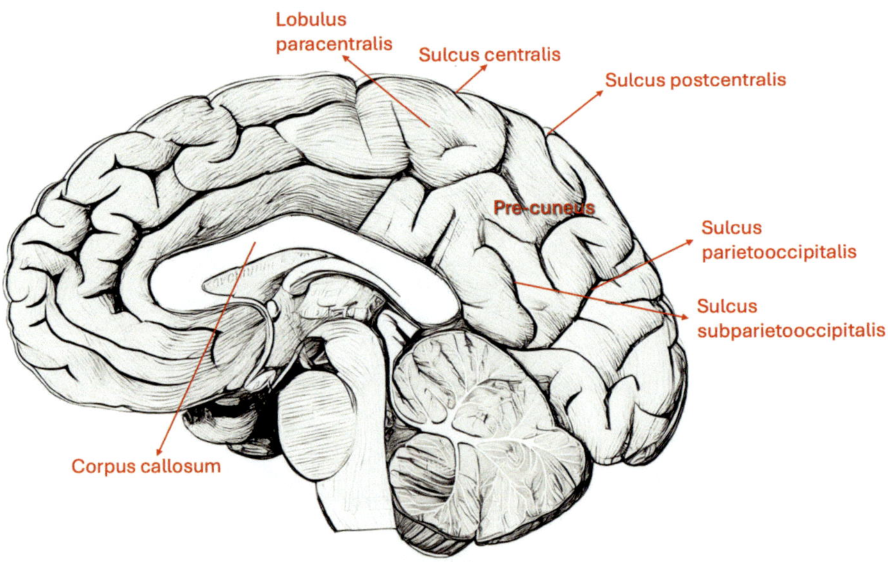

Fig. 2.11 Medial view of the parietal lobe illustrating the paracentral lobule, precuneus, and associated sulci. The paracentral lobule bridges the frontal and parietal lobes around the central sulcus and contains motor and sensory areas for the lower limbs. Posteriorly, the precuneus is bordered by the parieto-occipital and subparieto-occipital sulci and is involved in visuospatial integration. This regions is especially relevant in interhemispheric approaches and callosal surgeries due to its proximity to the corpus callosum and medial vascular structures

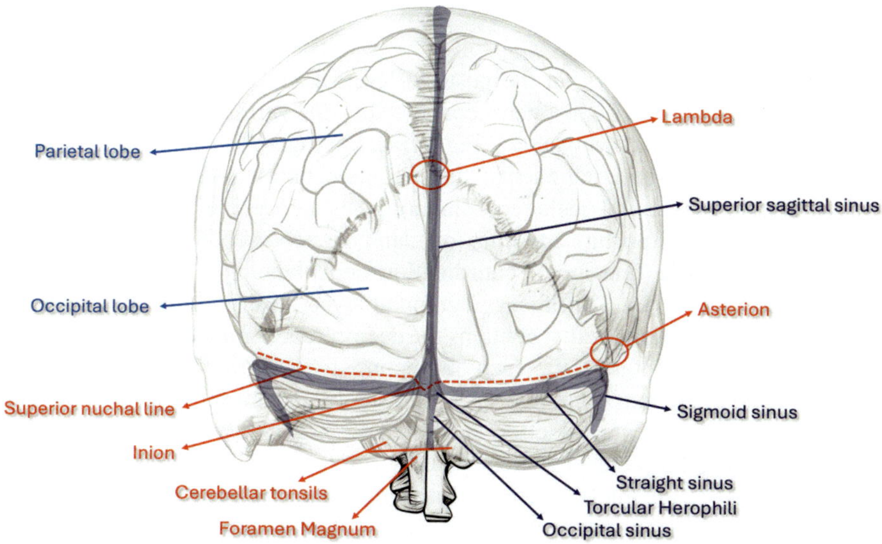

Fig. 2.12 This illustration superimposes the external surface of the cranium with a posterior view of the brain, highlighting the parietal and occipital lobes, cerebellum, and brainstem. Neuroanatomical and craniometric landmarks—such as the lambda, asterion, inion, superior nuchal line, and foramen magnum—are identified to correlate surface anatomy with the underlying neural structures

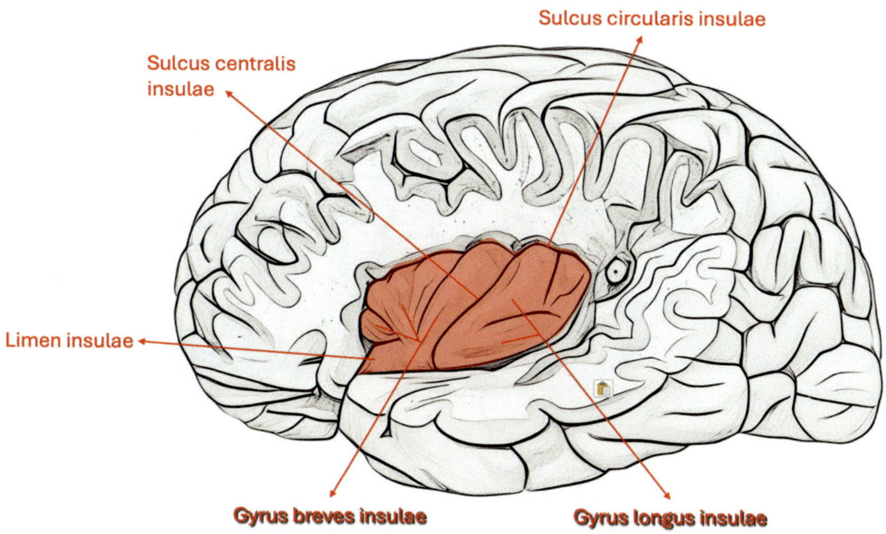

Fig. 2.13 Lateral view of the insular lobe with overlying opercular removed to reveal its detailed anatomy. The insula is bounded by the circular sulcus (sulcus circularis insulae) and divided by the central insular sulcus into anterior gyri breves insulae and posterior gyrus longus insulae. The limen insulae mark the transition between the temporal lobe and the insular cortex. This hidden cortical region plays a key role in sensory integration, emotion, and autonomic regulation, and is critically accessed in transsylvian approaches for insular glioma resection and vascular procedures involving the middle cerebral artery branches

2.5 Cerebellum

The cerebellum, located within the posterior cranial fossa beneath the tentorium cerebelli, consists of two hemispheres connected by the vermis and is layered into a cortex, white matter, and deep nuclei (Fig. 2.14). Phylogenetically and functionally, it is divided into three components: the archicerebellum (vestibulocerebellum), which governs balance and ocular coordination; the paleocerebellum (spinocerebellum), which regulates posture and limb tone; and the neocerebellum (pontocerebellum), responsible for fine motor coordination and planning [19–23]. Its cortex, organized into molecular, Purkinje, and granular layers, overlays the arbor vitae—a branching white matter core that contains the deep cerebellar nuclei (dentate, emboliform, globose, and fastigial), each projecting to specific functional systems [24–26]. The cerebellum communicates with the brainstem through three peduncles, integrating afferent and efferent pathways critical for motor modulation. Lesions affecting the cerebellar hemispheres result in ipsilateral incoordination, whereas damage to the midline vermis causes truncal ataxia and gait disturbance. In neurosurgery, careful navigation around the cerebellar nuclei and peduncles is essential during posterior fossa tumor resections, Chiari decompressions, and vascular procedures [27, 28]. Beyond motor control, the cerebellum plays a pivotal role in cognition and emotion, contributing to the so-called cerebellar cognitive affective syndrome [21, 29, 30].

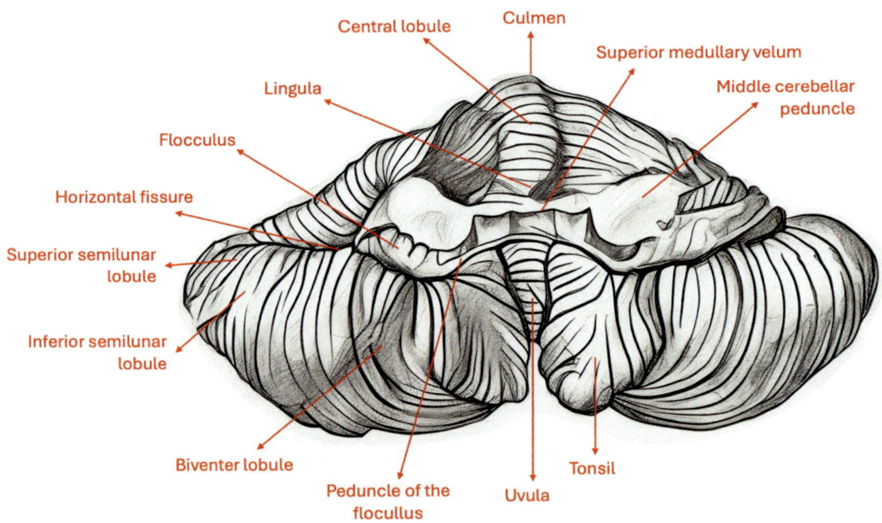

Fig. 2.14 Anterior view of the cerebellum illustrating its anatomical subdivisions. Midline vermian structures—such as the lingula, central lobule, culmen, uvula, and nodule—are flanked by paired hemispheric lobules, including the superior and inferior semilunar, biventral, and tonsillar regions. The horizontal fissure demarcates the dorsal cerebellar lobes, while the middle cerebellar peduncle serves as a major conduit for pontocerebellar fibers. The flocculus and its peduncle are components of the vestibulocerebellum, which is important for balance and eye movement coordination

2.6 Brainstem

The brainstem, continuous with the diencephalon rostrally and the spinal cord caudally, serves as a compact conduit for ascending and descending tracts and houses the nuclei of cranial nerves III–XII [31, 32] (Figs. 2.15 and 2.16). Structurally, it comprises the midbrain, pons, and medulla oblongata. The midbrain contains the tectum (superior and inferior colliculi for reflexes), tegmentum (with the red nucleus and periaqueductal gray), and cerebral peduncles (including the substantia nigra) [19, 33, 34]. The pons bridges the midbrain and medulla, transmitting signals via transverse pontocerebellar fibers to the cerebellum, and houses the cranial nerve nuclei V–VIII (See the *CPA Angle* in Fig. 2.17). The medulla, where pyramidal decussation occurs, contains the nuclei for cranial nerves IX–XII and is crucial for vital autonomic functions [35–37]. Clinically, localized lesions can manifest as distinct syndromes: Weber (midbrain infarct), Millard-Gubler (ventral pons), Wallenberg (lateral medulla), and locked-in syndrome (pontine infarction with preserved cognition and eye movements) [38, 39]. Given its dense anatomy, millimetric precision is essential during approaches to intrinsic lesions or vascular malformations, particularly around the floor of the fourth ventricle and cranial nerve root entry zones.

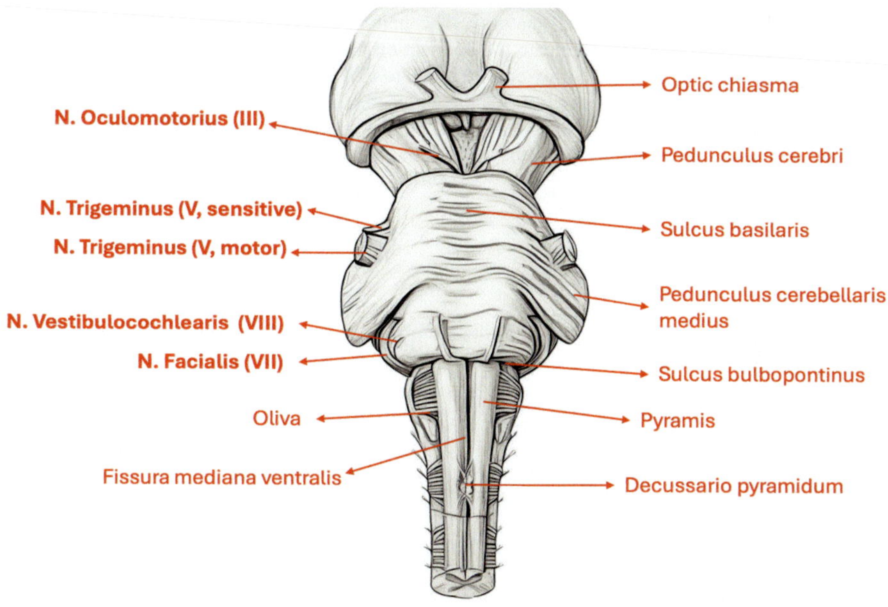

Fig. 2.15 Anterior (ventral) view of the brainstem demonstrating the emergence of cranial nerves and anatomical landmarks relevant to neurosurgical approaches. The optic chiasm marks the rostral limit near the diencephalon. The oculomotor nerve (CN III) emerges from the interpeduncular fossa, while the trigeminal nerve (CN V) has distinct motor and sensory roots originating from the pons. At the pontomedullary junction, the facial (CN VII) and vestibulocochlear (CN VIII) nerves are observed. The pyramids and olives define the medulla, with the pyramidal decussation marking the crossing or corticospinal fibers. Structures such as the pedunculi cerebri and middle cerebellar peduncles delineate major white matter tracts

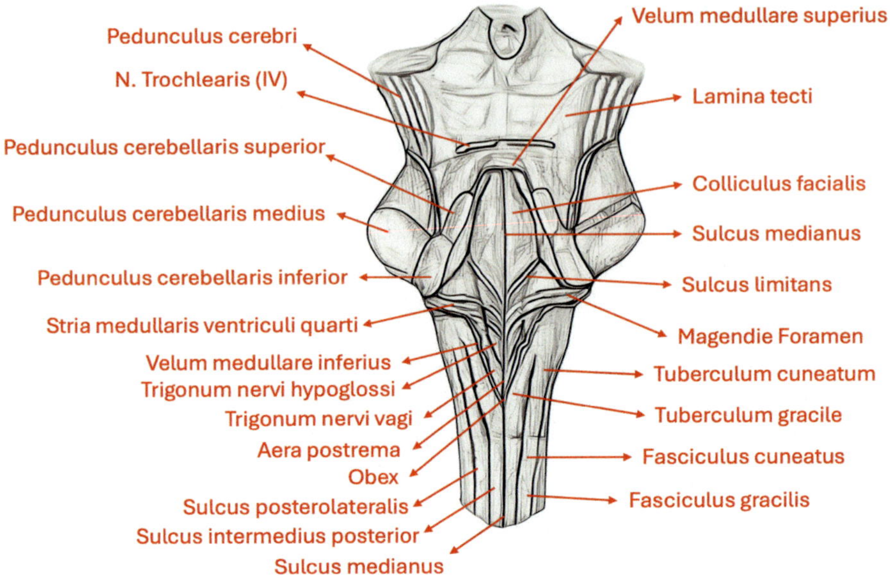

Fig. 2.16 Posterior (dorsal) view of the brainstem and floor of the fourth ventricle, illustrating landmarks relevant to neurosurgical anatomy. The pedunculi cerebri and cerebellar peduncles (superior, middle, and inferior) delineate the connection between the brainstem and cerebellum. The trochlear nerve (CN IV) is the only cranial nerve to exit dorsally. The lamina tecti houses the colliculi, while the colliculus facialis overlies the abducens nucleus and internal genu of the facial nerve. The sulcus limitans, median sulcus, and area postrema are important for safe dissection during fourth ventricle surgeries. Inferiorly, the tubercles and fasciculi (gracile and cuneate) reflect the ascending somatosensory pathways

a

b

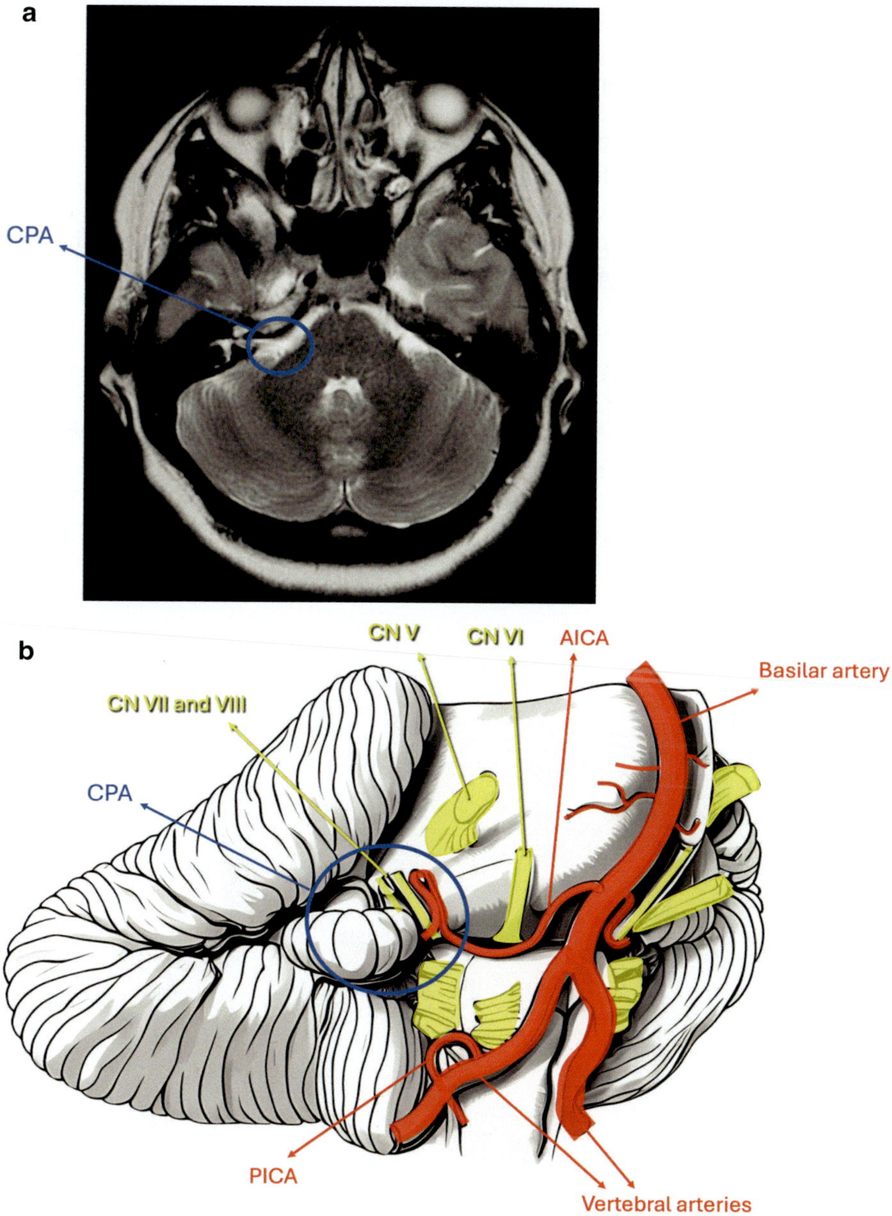

Fig. 2.17 (**a**) Anatomical illustration of the right CPA, highlighting its neurovascular relationships, including cranial nerves V–VIII, the anterior inferior cerebellar artery (AICA), posterior inferior cerebellar artery (PICA), and the basilar and vertebral arteries. Surgical access to this region is generally obtained through retrosigmoid or presigmoid approaches. (**b**) Axial T2-weighted MRI depicting the right cerebellopontine angle (CPA) cistern (blue circle), where cranial nerves VII and VIII enter the internal auditory canal

2.7 Arteries

The central nervous system's arterial supply is bifurcated into two major systems: the internal carotid arteries (ICA) and the vertebrobasilar system. The ICA system provides approximately 80% of cerebral blood flow, supplying the anterior and lateral regions of the brain through the anterior cerebral artery (ACA) and middle cerebral artery (MCA). The vertebral arteries converge to form the basilar artery, which bifurcates into the posterior cerebral arteries (PCA), delivering blood to the occipital lobes, thalamus, and medial temporal lobes [19, 40–42]. These systems form the Circle of Willis, a critical anastomotic network that enables collateral flow in cases of vascular compromise [43].

The ICA is anatomically subdivided into seven segments (C1–C7), with a simplified four-segment model (C1–C4) often adopted in surgical contexts. The terminal ICA bifurcates into the ACA and MCA. The ACA is segmented into A1–A5 and irrigates the medial frontal and parietal lobes and corpus callosum [44] (Fig. 2.18). The MCA, the most frequently affected vessel in ischemic stroke, spans M1–M4 and supplies the lateral cerebral cortex and deep structures like the basal ganglia via lenticulostriate arteries [45] (Fig. 2.19). The PCA, segmented as P1–P4, supplies visual and medial temporal regions and arises from the basilar artery [46, 47] (Fig. 2.20).

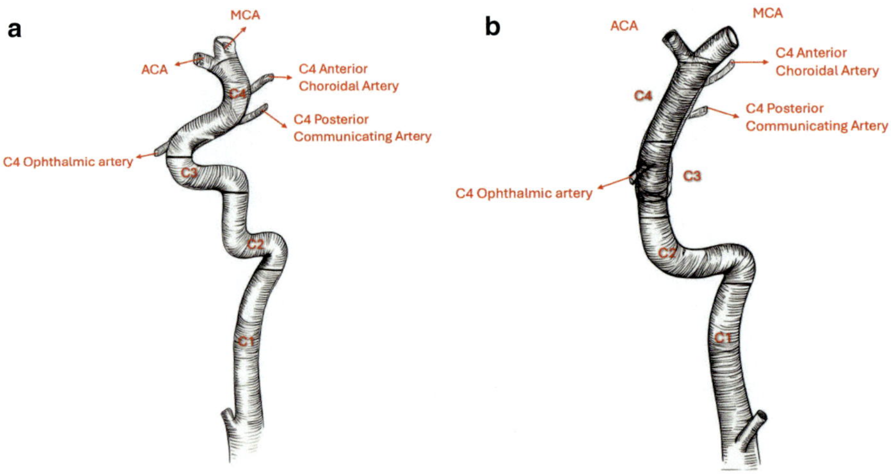

Fig. 2.18 Lateral (**a**) and oblique (**b**) views of the internal carotid artery (ICA) illustrating its segmentation and major intracranial branches relevant to neurosurgical approaches. The ICA is shown divided into four segments: C1 (cervical), C2 (petrous), C3 (lacerum), and C4 (cavernous and supraclinoid). At the C4 segment, the ICA gives rise to critical branches including the ophthalmic artery, posterior communicating artery, anterior choroidal artery, anterior cerebral artery (ACA), and middle cerebral artery (MCA). These branches supply major territories of the brain and are commonly involved in aneurysms and vascular malformations. Familiarity with this segmental anatomy is essential for skull base and vascular neurosurgery, especially in procedures involving the cavernous sinus, clinoid segment, and circle of Willis

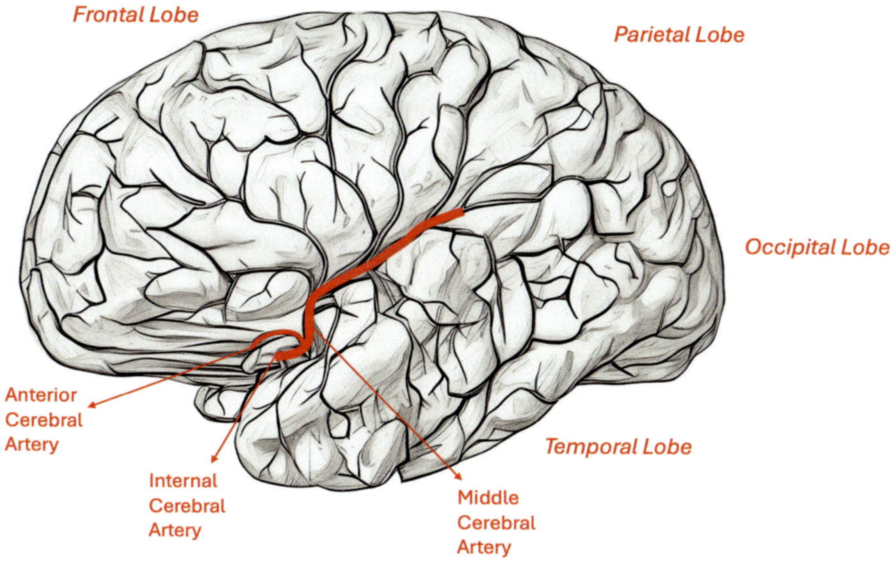

Fig. 2.19 Lateral view of the cerebral hemispheres highlighting the major cortical branches of the internal carotid artery system. The internal cerebral artery (ACA) bifurcates into the anterior cerebral artery (ACA) and middle cerebral artery (MCA). The ACA courses medially to supply the medial aspects of the frontal and parietal lobes, while the MCA extends laterally through the Sylvian fissure to perfuse the lateral surfaces of the frontal, parietal, and temporal lobes

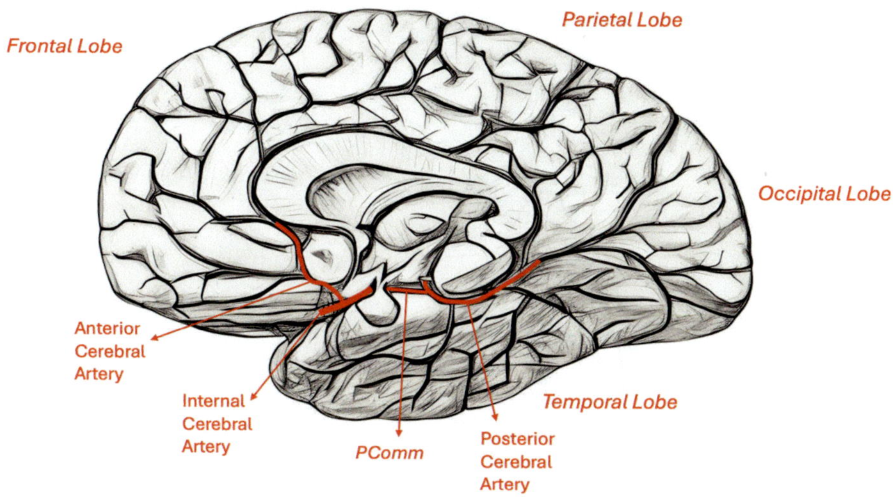

Fig. 2.20 Medial-inferior view of the cerebral hemisphere highlighting the main components of the anterior and posterior circulation. The internal cerebral artery (ICA) ascends and bifurcates into the anterior cerebral artery (ACA) and middle cerebral artery. The posterior communicating artery (PComm) bridges the ICA to the posterior cerebral artery (PCA), forming part of the Circle of Willis. The ACA curves anteriorly and superiorly along the medial surface of the frontal and parietal lobes, while the PCA courses posteriorly, supplying the medial temporal and occipital lobes

The vertebrobasilar circulation provides essential perfusion to the brainstem, cerebellum, and occipital lobes (Fig. 2.21). Vertebral arteries give rise to the posterior inferior cerebellar artery (PICA) and merge into the basilar artery, which branches into the anterior inferior cerebellar artery (AICA) and superior cerebellar artery (SCA) before terminating in the PCA [47]. This posterior circulation is vital for autonomic control and sensorimotor function, and its anatomy is a cornerstone in skull base surgery.

The Circle of Willis includes anterior and posterior communicating arteries and is often anatomically variant, such as in the fetal-type PCA, in which the PCA arises from the ICA via a dominant posterior communicating artery [48, 49] (Fig. 2.21). Surgeons must also recognize persistent embryonic arteries—notably the persistent trigeminal and hypoglossal arteries—which can complicate endovascular or skull base procedures [47, 48].

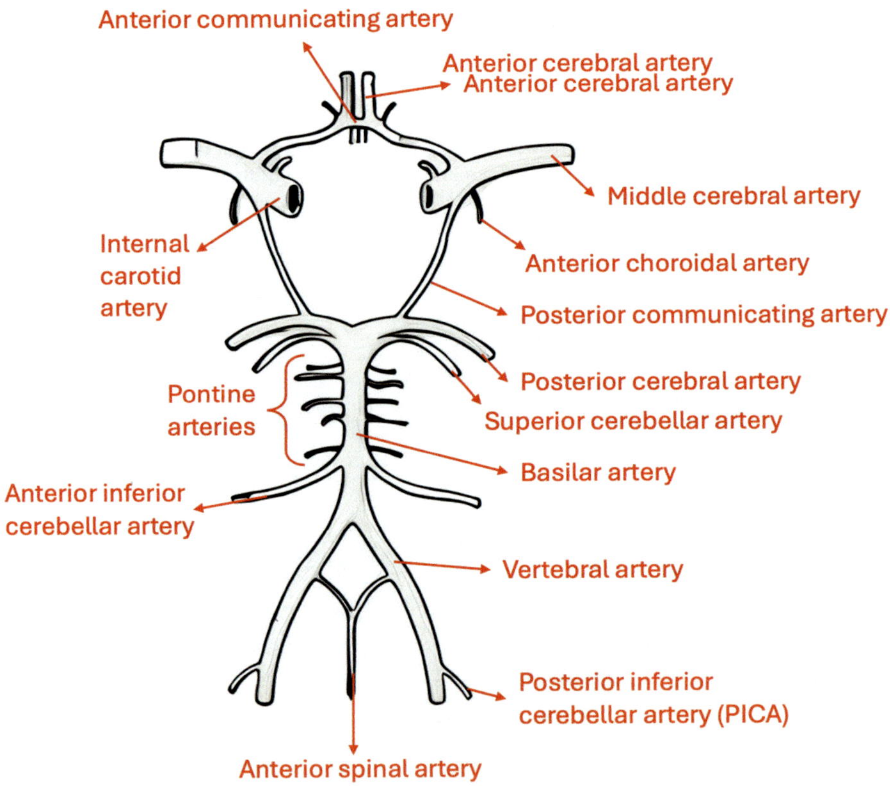

Fig. 2.21 Schematic illustration of the Circle of Willis and brainstem arterial network, showing both anterior and posterior circulations. The internal carotid arteries give rise to the anterior cerebral arteries (ACA), joined by the anterior communicating artery, and to the middle cerebral arteries (MCA). The posterior communicating arteries (PComm) connect the ICA system to the posterior cerebral arteries (PCA), which arise from the basilar artery—formed by the confluence of the vertebral arteries. Branches of the vertebrobasilar system include the posterior inferior cerebellar artery (PICA), anterior inferior cerebellar artery (AICA), superior cerebellar artery (SCA), and numerous pontine arteries. The anterior spinal artery arises from vertebral contributions

2.8 The Venous Sinuses and Veins

Understanding the venous structures is crucial for safe craniotomy. The bridging veins between the cortex and dural sinuses are especially vulnerable during interhemispheric, parasagittal, and subtemporal approaches. Their disruption can result in venous hypertension, brain swelling, and hemorrhage. Additionally, variations in venous anatomy, such as an enlarged *Labbé vein* or a dominant *Trolard vein*, may require adjustments in surgical planning (Fig. 2.22). The *Trolard vein* is directly associated with the frontal and parietal lobes because it runs along the central sulcus, connecting the superior sagittal sinus to the superficial middle cerebral vein. The *Labbé vein* is directly related to the temporal lobe, as it drains into the transverse sinus, providing a critical venous pathway for the lateral aspect of the brain [50].

Another important anatomical consideration is the lateralization of the Superior Sagittal Sinus. The Superior Sagittal Sinus is an unpaired dural venous sinus that typically runs along the midline within the superior margin of the falx cerebri

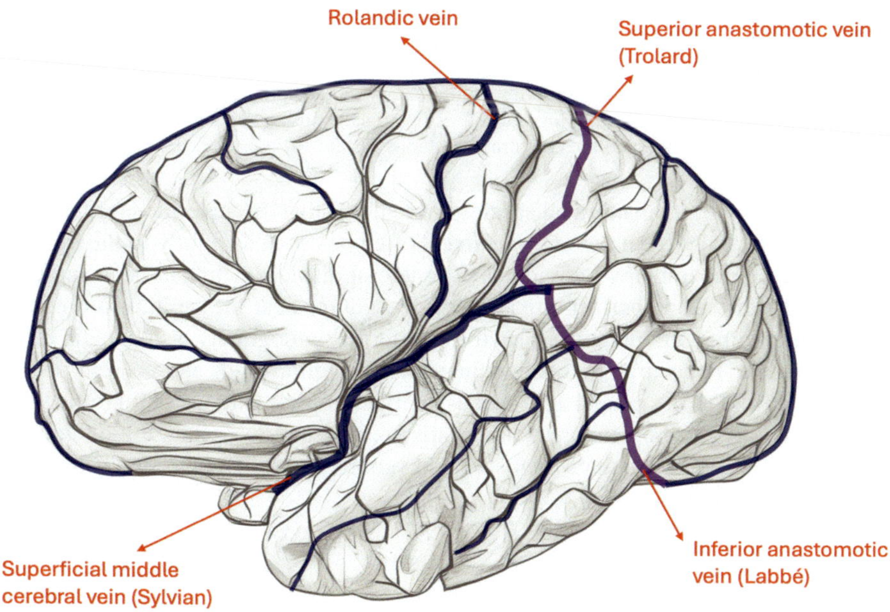

Fig. 2.22 The superficial middle cerebral vein (the *Sylvian* vein) runs along the lateral fissure, mainly over the insula and opercular surfaces of the frontal, parietal, and temporal lobes; it drains into either the cavernous sinus, sphenoparietal sinus, or anastomoses with the veins of Trolard and Labbé. The *Trolard* vein—also known as the superior—typically lies over the parietal lobe, where it connects the superficial middle cerebral vein to the superior sagittal sinus. The vein of *Labbé*—also called the inferior anastomotic vein of Labbé—runs over the temporal lobe, connecting the superficial middle cerebral vein to the transverse sinus. The *Rolandic* vein, or the central sulcal vein, lies over the central sulcus, draining parts of both the precentral (frontal lobe) and postcentral (parietal lobe) gyri, and typically drains into the superior sagittal sinus

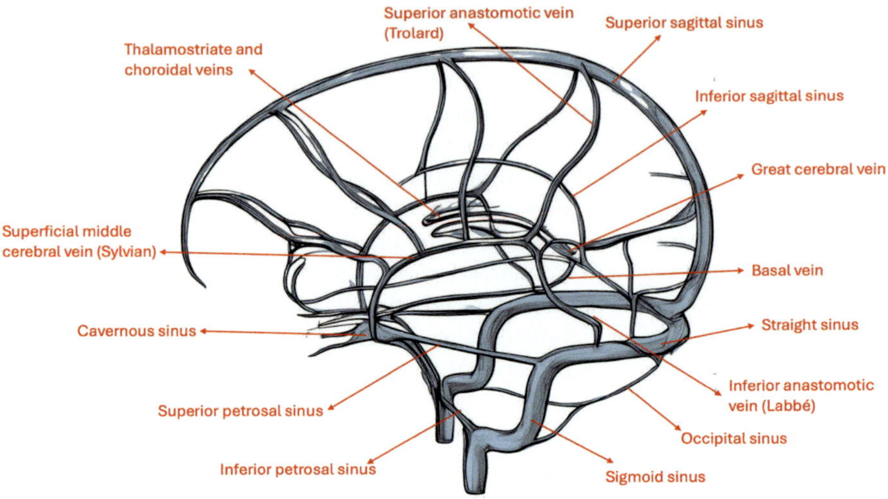

Fig. 2.23 Cerebral venous system highlighting the superficial and deep venous drainage pathways. Superficial veins include the superficial middle cerebral vein (Sylvian), superior anastomotic vein (of Trolard), and inferior anastomotic vein (of Labbé). Deep venous structures such as the great cerebral vein (of Galen), basal vein, and thalamostriate and choroidal veins converge into the straight sinus, which joins the superior sagittal sinus and occipital sinus at the confluence of sinuses. The cavernous sinus, superior and inferior petrosal sinuses, and sigmoid sinus drain the base of the brain and connect to the extracranial venous system

(Fig. 2.23). However, anatomical studies have shown that the superior sagittal sinus can deviate laterally from the midline and is often positioned slightly to the right of the sagittal suture in many individuals. The lateral displacement can be as large as 1 cm. Therefore, when performing surgical procedures near the sagittal suture, it is crucial to use imaging modalities, such as computed tomography or magnetic resonance imaging, to accurately localize the superior sagittal sinus and prevent potential injury [51]. During cranial approaches, meticulous dissection, careful retraction, and preservation of the venous anatomy are fundamental to optimizing outcomes. The balance between adequate exposure and venous protection determines the success of cranial approaches.

2.9 Ventricles

During specific neurosurgical procedures, it is necessary to access the lateral ventricles or the third ventricle for CSF drainage, promoting brain relaxation, or serving as a landmark for accessing lesions (Fig. 2.24) [37, 52–54]. *Kocher's point* is a commonly utilized entry site for accessing the lateral ventricle through the frontal lobe, positioned 2–3 cm lateral to the midline at the level of the coronal suture through the cranium. *Kocher's point* is also anatomically referenced using the sulci and gyri on the surface of the frontal lobe. At the junction of the superior frontal gyrus and precentral gyrus, typically aligned with the superior frontal sulcus. This positioning ensures a direct and safe trajectory into the frontal horn of the lateral ventricle, minimizing damage to the eloquent cortex and subcortical structures.

Accessing the third ventricle through the *lamina terminalis* provides a direct and safe route, which is often used in endoscopic third ventriculostomy (ETV) and tumor resection. We can also access the *lamina terminalis* through the Sylvian fissure following the optic nerve toward the chiasma and the *lamina terminals*.

The *temporal horn* of the lateral ventricle is accessed following the incisura line, which is an imaginary trajectory along the tentorial incisura that helps avoid critical neurovascular structures. This access is useful during amygdalo-hippocampectomy through an anterior approach to the Sylvian fissure via supraorbital, supraorbital-zygomatic, and pterional craniotomies.

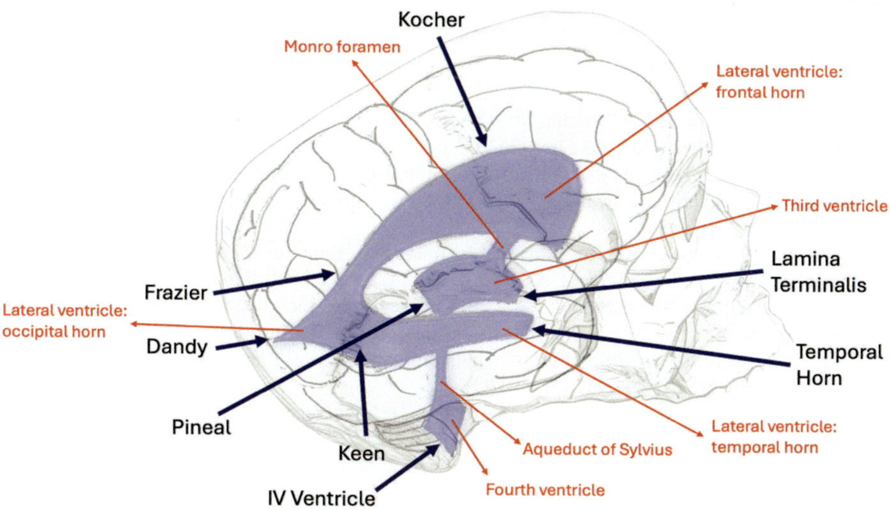

Fig. 2.24 Illustration showing access to the frontal horn of the lateral ventricles through Kocher's point (11–13 cm along the nasion-to-inion line and 3 cm lateral to the midline for EVD; or 1 cm anterior to the coronal suture and 3 cm lateral to the midline for endoscopic access), access to the lateral ventricles via the parietal and occipital approaches through Frazier's point (3–4 cm from the midline and 6–7 cm above the inion), Dandy's point (3 cm above the inion and 2 cm lateral to the midline), and Keen's point (2.5–3 cm posterior and 2.5–3 cm superior to the top of the pinna); lamina terminalis and pineal region are identified, as well as the access to the fourth ventricle via the telovelar or endoscopic approach

To access the lateral ventricles from the parietal and occipital lobes, whether for ventriculoperitoneal shunt (VPS) placement or during neurosurgical approaches to these lobes, two ventricular access points are commonly used: *Keen's point* and *Frazier's point*.

The Keen's point is located 3 cm lateral to the midline and 3 cm above the inion. This entry point is used for posterior ventricular access, particularly for ventriculoperitoneal (VP) shunt placement into the atrium of the lateral ventricle. The Frazier's point is positioned 2–3 cm lateral to the midline and 4 cm above the external auditory meatus. This approach is also used for ventricular access, often in cases requiring posterior or occipital approaches. Both points provide posterior entry to the lateral ventricle, commonly for shunt procedures or external ventricular drains (EVDs), when the anterior approach is contraindicated.

Access to the fourth ventricle relies on the underlying pathology and the required exposure. The most common approaches in cranial procedures include the median suboccipital (telovelar) approach, which is the standard route. This method involves midline pathology and exposure to the bulbar medullary fissure by dissecting the uvulotonsillar cleft and mobilizing the tonsils without splitting the vermis, thereby providing broad access to the ventricular floor while preserving cerebellar function. The far-lateral approach is used for lateral recess lesions, extending access through the foramen of Luschka by opening the cerebellomedullary cistern and mobilizing the tonsils.

References

1. Moore KL, Persaud TVN, Torchia MG. The developing human: clinically oriented embryology. 11th ed. Philadelphia: Elsevier; 2020.
2. Sperber GH. Craniofacial development. Hamilton: BC Decker Inc.; 2001.
3. Williams PL, Bannister LH, Berry MM, et al. Gray's anatomy. 38th ed. Edinburgh: Churchill Livingstone; 1995.
4. Kennedy DW, Zinreich SJ, Rosenbaum AE, Johns ME. Functional endoscopic sinus surgery: theory and diagnostic evaluation. Arch Otolaryngol. 1985;111(9):576–82.
5. Lund VJ, Stammberger H, Nicolai P, et al. European position paper on endoscopic management of tumors of the nose, paranasal sinuses and skull base. Rhinol Suppl. 2010;22:1–143.
6. Paulsen F, Waschke J. Sobotta atlas of anatomy: head, neck, and neuroanatomy. 16th ed. Munich: Elsevier; 2019. p. 11, 13.
7. Gusmão S, Silveira RL, Arantes A. Pontos referenciais nos acessos cranianos. Arq Neuropsiquiatr. 2003;61(2-A):305–8.
8. Reis CV, Arantes AA, Nicolato A, Gusmão S. Delimitação dos acessos cranianos. Arq Bras Neurocir. 2012;31(3):135–45.
9. Ribas GC, Rhoton AL Jr, Cruz OR, Peace D. Surgical anatomy of microneurosurgical sulcal key points. Neurosurgery. 2006;59:177–211.
10. Jumah F, Adeeb N, Dossani RH. Collin S. MacCarty (1915–2003): inventor of the "MacCarty Keyhole" as the starting burr hole for orbitozygomatic craniotomy. World Neurosurg. 2018;111:269–74.
11. Petrides M. The anatomy of the frontal lobe. In: Mai JK, Paxinos G, editors. The human nervous system. 3rd ed. San Diego: Academic Press; 2012. p. 988–1011.
12. Ongur D, Price JL. The organization of networks within the orbital and medial prefrontal cortex of rats, monkeys and humans. Cereb Cortex. 2000;10(3):206–19.

13. Amaral DG, Insausti R. The hippocampal formation. In: Paxinos G, Mai JK, editors. The human nervous system. 3rd ed. London: Elsevier; 2012. p. 896–942.
14. Kanwisher N, Yovel G. The fusiform face area: a cortical region specialized for the perception of faces. Philos Trans R Soc Lond Ser B Biol Sci. 2006;361(1476):2109–28.
15. Penfield W, Boldrey E. Somatic motor and sensory representation in the cerebral cortex of man as studied by electrical stimulation. Brain. 1937;60(4):389–443.
16. Cavanna AE, Trimble MR. The precuneus: a review of its functional anatomy and behavioural correlates. Brain. 2006;129(3):564–83.
17. Zeki S. The visual image in mind and brain. Sci Am. 1992;267(3):68–76.
18. Türe U, Yaşargil MG, Al-Mefty O. The transsylvian surgical approach to the insula in the human brain: an anatomical study. Neurosurgery. 1999;45(4):1066–75.
19. Standring S, editor. Gray's anatomy: the anatomical basis of clinical practice. 42nd ed. New York/Philadelphia: Elsevier; 2020.
20. Manto M, et al. Consensus paper: roles of the cerebellum in motor control. Cerebellum. 2012;11(2):457–87.
21. Schmahmann JD, Sherman JC. The cerebellar cognitive affective syndrome. Brain. 1998;121(4):561–79.
22. Haines DE. Neuroanatomy: an atlas of structures, sections, and systems. 9th ed. Philadelphia: Wolters Kluwer; 2019.
23. Voogd J, Glickstein M. The anatomy of the cerebellum. Trends Neurosci. 1998;21(9):370–5.
24. Bastian AJ. Learning to predict the future: the cerebellum adapts feedforward movement control. Curr Opin Neurobiol. 2006;16(6):645–9.
25. Nolte J. The human brain: an introduction to its functional anatomy. 7th ed. Philadelphia: Elsevier; 2015.
26. Ito M. Control of mental activities by internal models in the cerebellum. Nat Rev Neurosci. 2008;9(4):304–13.
27. Stoodley CJ, Schmahmann JD. Functional topography in the human cerebellum. NeuroImage. 2009;44(2):489–501.
28. Timmann D, Daum I. Cerebellar contributions to cognitive functions. Cerebellum. 2007;6(3):159–62.
29. Bastian AJ. Cerebellar ataxia: assessment and treatment. Phys Ther. 1997;77(6):672–82.
30. Schmahmann JD. Disorders of the cerebellum. J Neuropsychiatry Clin Neurosci. 2004;16(3):367–78.
31. Klockgether T. Sporadic ataxia with adult onset: classification and diagnostic criteria. Lancet Neurol. 2010;9(1):94–104.
32. Yasargil MG. Microneurosurgery, Volume IVB: CNS tumors. Stuttgart: Thieme; 1996.
33. Samii M, Gerganov V, Samii A. Functional outcome after resection of cerebellar tumors. Neurosurgery. 2010;66(6):1074–81.
34. Nolte J. The human brain: an introduction to its functional anatomy. 7th ed. Philadelphia: Elsevier; 2020.
35. Parent A, Carpenter MB. Carpenter's human neuroanatomy. 9th ed. Baltimore: Williams & Wilkins; 1995.
36. Duvernoy HM. The human brainstem and cerebellum. Vienna: Springer; 2009.
37. Greenberg MS. Handbook of neurosurgery. 9th ed. New York: Thieme; 2020.
38. Kim JS. Pure lateral medullary infarction. Brain. 2003;126(8):1864–72.
39. Plum F, Posner JB. The diagnosis of stupor and coma. 3rd ed. Oxford: Oxford University Press; 1982.
40. Osborn AG. Osborn's brain: imaging, pathology, and anatomy. 2nd ed. Elsevier; 2017.
41. Tatu L, Vuillier F, Moulin T, Bogousslavsky J. Arterial territories of the human brain. Neurology. 1998;50(6):1699–708.
42. Duvernoy HM. The human brain: surface, sectional anatomy with MRI, and blood supply. 2nd ed. Springer; 1999.
43. Liebeskind DS. Collateral circulation. Stroke. 2003;34(9):2279–84.
44. Rhoton AL Jr. The cerebral arteries. Neurosurgery. 2002;51(4 Suppl):S53–S120.

45. Gibo H, Lenkey C, Rhoton AL Jr. Microsurgical anatomy of the middle cerebral artery. J Neurosurg. 1981;54(2):151–69.
46. Zeal AA, Rhoton AL Jr. Microsurgical anatomy of the posterior cerebral artery. J Neurosurg. 1978;48(4):534–59.
47. Rhoton AL Jr. The posterior circulation: microsurgical anatomy and surgical approaches. Neurosurgery. 2002;51(4 Suppl):S121–58.
48. Lasjaunias P, Berenstein A, Ter Brugge K. Surgical neuroangiography, vol. 1. 2nd ed. Springer; 2001.
49. Kapoor K, Singh B, Dewan LI. Variations in the configuration of the circle of Willis. Anat Cell Biol. 2008;41(3):155–60.
50. Rhoton AL Jr. The cerebral veins. In: Rhoton's cranial anatomy and surgical approaches. 2nd ed. New York: Oxford University Press; 2019. p. 47–66.
51. Ghosh A, Chi J, Holsgrove D. Neuroanatomy, superior sagittal sinus. In: StatPearls [Internet]. Treasure Island: StatPearls Publishing; 2023.
52. Rhoton AL Jr. The lateral and third ventricles. Neurosurgery. 2002;51(4 Suppl):S207–71.
53. Winn HR, Youmans JR. Youmans and Winn neurological surgery. 8th ed. Philadelphia: Elsevier; 2023.
54. Lozier AP, Cohen-Gadol AA. Operative techniques in neurosurgery: neurosurgical operative atlas, vol. 2. New York: Thieme; 2019.

3 Frontal and Transbasal Approaches

3.1 Introduction

The frontal lobe is routinely accessed in neurosurgical practice. It can be used for the treatment of vascular, neoplastic, infectious, functional disorders, and epilepsy. With the patient in the supine position, the skull is secured in a head holder, and adjustments made in flexion and rotation allow the frontal lobe and adjacent structures to be accessed unilaterally or bilaterally, reaching the subfrontal skull base (Fig. 3.1).

The frontal, bifrontal, and frontobasal approaches are essential for accessing lesions in the anterior cranial fossa and surrounding areas. The frontal approach involves a unilateral craniotomy, allowing access to the ipsilateral frontal lobe and subfrontal region, and is commonly used for tumors like olfactory groove meningiomas. The bifrontal approach consists of a bilateral frontal craniotomy, providing wider exposure of the anterior cranial fossa, and is suitable for midline lesions, such as large meningiomas or esthesioneuroblastomas. The frontobasal approach, also known as the transbasal approach, entails a bifrontal craniotomy along with additional osteotomies of the orbital rims and nasal bones, enabling access to the anterior and paranasal sinuses, and is used for extensive tumors affecting the sinonasal region and anterior skull base [1, 2]. Some authors characterize the frontobasal approach as an intradural route to the skull base via the frontal lobe only, whereas the transbasal approach is viewed as extradural, involving the frontal bone, orbital roofs, and part of the nasal bone [1].

The transbasal approach is an extensive modification of the frontobasal approach by integrating bifrontal craniotomy with frontonasoorbital osteotomies, which include the orbital rims and nasal bones, to create an extradural midline skull base

Supplementary Information The online version contains supplementary material available at https://doi.org/10.1007/978-3-032-04664-2_3. The videos can be accessed individually by clicking the DOI link in the accompanying figure caption or by scanning this link with the SN More Media App.

H. de Oliveira Manduca Palmiero, E. G. Figueiredo, *Neurosurgical Approaches Video Atlas*, https://doi.org/10.1007/978-3-032-04664-2_3

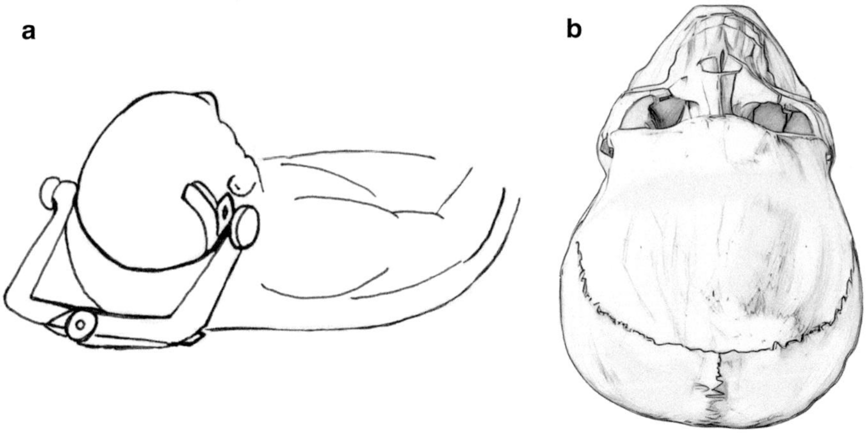

Fig. 3.1 Anatomical illustration showing on the left (**a**) the patient positioned in supine with the head elevated and flexed, and on the right (**b**) the skull from a vertex perspective to the orbito-nasal region, passing through the frontal lobes. This is the neurosurgeon's view when approaching the frontal lobes and the skull base through these structures

working corridor. This technique enhances exposure to the anterior cranial fossa and the central skull base and can be extended to the nasal cavity and paranasal sinuses, making it suitable for resecting complex sinonasal and midline skull base tumors. The key steps include a bicoronal scalp incision, harvest of the pericranial flap, bifrontal craniotomy, orbital rim osteotomy, and microsurgical dissection of the sellar region. Adding craniofacial osteotomies further increases access to the sinonasal cavities, clivus, and craniocervical junction [1, 2]. This chapter focuses on the frontal, frontobasal, and transbasal approaches from a neurosurgeon's perspective.

3.2 Indications for the Approach

Based on the descriptions provided so far, the approach to the frontal lobe and, consequently, to the basal skull region enables the surgical treatment of vascular lesions such as cavernomas and AVMs; tumors including metastases, gliomas, and meningiomas; intraventricular conditions such as hydrocephalus and tumors; trauma-related injuries like depressed fractures, hematomas, and contusions; infections including empyemas and abscesses; parasitic lesions such as neurocysticercosis and hydatid cysts; epilepsy; and neurofunctional treatments, which encompass movement disorders [3, 4].

3.3 Operative Set-Up

Patient Positioning The patient is placed in the supine position on the operating table, and a *Mayfield* or *Sugita* head holder is used to stabilize the head.

Head Positioning The head positioning in the frontal and frontobasal approaches follows the same principles as the frontotemporal approaches. Nevertheless, it includes specific adjustments depending on the craniotomy type—whether unilateral frontal, bifrontal, frontobasal, or transbasal) as follows:

(a) *Elevation.* The head is elevated 15° above the level of the heart to facilitate venous drainage and reduce intracranial pressure [5].
(b) *Rotation.* Typically kept in a neutral or slightly contralateral position (5–15°) depending on the side and extent of exposure required [5].
(c) *Extension:* Mild extension (10–15°) to optimize the surgical angle and minimize frontal lobe retraction. Flexion may be increased slightly for deeper subfrontal access but should be adjusted carefully to avoid excessive frontal lobe pressure [5].

Skin Preparation The entire scalp, forehead, and upper eyelid region were treated with an antiseptic solution (shampoo and chlorhexidine, or povidone-iodine). Draping includes isolating the surgical field, ensuring the planned incision site, and protecting the eyes.

3.4 Surgical Technique (Video 3.1)

3.4.1 The Frontal Approach

For unilateral frontal craniotomy, the head is rotated 5°–15° contralateral to the craniotomy side to center the surgical field for the neurosurgeon [6]. In this approach, preoperative imaging is essential to assess the lesion's relationship with contiguous bony structures, such as the coronal and sagittal sutures and the superior temporal line, which serve as landmarks for frontal bone localization. Additionally, an important anatomical consideration is the lateralization of the superior sagittal sinus.

The superior sagittal sinus is an unpaired dural venous sinus that typically runs along the midline within the falx cerebri's superior margin. However, anatomical studies have shown that the superior sagittal sinus can deviate laterally from the midline, with a tendency to be slightly positioned to the right of the sagittal suture in many individuals. The lateral displacement can be up to 1 cm. Therefore, when performing surgical procedures near the sagittal suture, it is crucial to study preoperative imaging modalities, such as computed tomography, magnetic resonance imaging, or neuronavigation, to accurately localize the superior sagittal sinus and avoid potential injury [7].

Another important point is that we often perceive the target lesion as more posterior than it actually is, forgetting that the frontal lobe extends up to the supraorbital margin. At the same time, craniotomies should not focus on the forehead to avoid esthetic complications. Therefore, the craniotomy area should be expanded by increasing the exposure area to enhance surgical access, microscope illumination, and reconstruction feasibility.

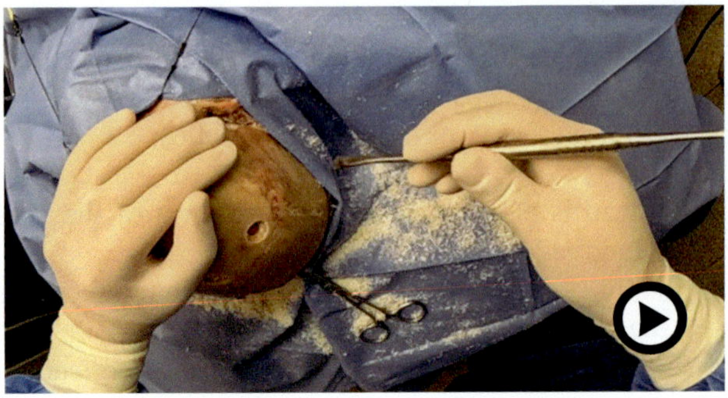

Video 3.1 This video demonstrates the step-by-step process of performing unilateral frontal and bifrontal craniotomies, highlighting important anatomical landmarks, technical details, and surgical strategies essential for reaching lesions in the anterior cranial fossa and midline skull base, including tumors, vascular malformations, and traumatic pathologies (▶ https://doi.org/10.1007/000-hst)

Therefore, the unilateral frontal approach is a surgical technique that involves the following steps:

Skin Incision The center of the incision should be aligned with the surgical target. Straight or C-shaped incisions with the base oriented toward the midline are recommended for smaller craniotomies (Fig. 3.2). In selected cases, extension to the contralateral midpupillary line may be recommended.

Muscle Flap In general, unilateral frontal craniotomy is performed within the frontal bone above the superior temporal line. However, if craniotomy expansion to the temporal bone is necessary, the temporalis muscle should be dissected while preserving a muscle cuff at the superior temporal line to facilitate proper reconstruction at the end of the procedure.

Craniotomy We recommend two burr holes, ensuring that the burr holes are positioned parallel to midline. The rationale for placing one burr hole at the midline is to facilitate dural dissection over the superior sagittal sinus. If a burr hole is made directly over the sinus, it allows for easier dural separation. In cases of sinus injury, an adjacent burr hole should be created to facilitate dural repair. Ultimately, craniotomy should be centered on the target lesion (Figs. 3.2 and 3.3).

Dural Opening The dura mater is incised in a curvilinear fashion with the base oriented toward the midline and reflected toward the midline to expose the underlying brain tissue. It is recommended to keep the base of the dural incision along the midline due to the location of the superior sagittal sinus, as this positioning facilitates repair in the event of an accidental sinus opening, making the procedure less complex and more controlled (Fig. 3.4).

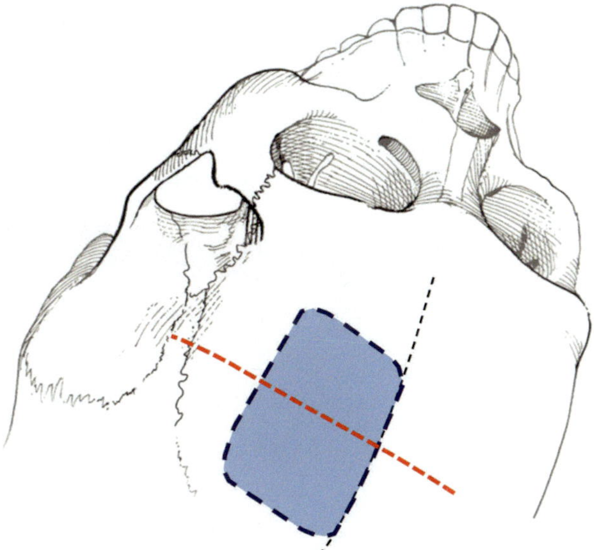

Fig. 3.2 Illustration showing an example of a left unilateral frontal craniotomy, noting the medial border of the craniotomy along the midline. The surgeon may choose to create two burr holes at the midline for safe dural detachment over the venous sinus or laterally. In this example, the craniotomy has a quadrilateral shape due to the four trephination points. Additionally, the straight red dashed line represents the linear incision. A C-shaped incision is also used for this type of craniotomy, but in this example, the craniotomy is located near the parasagittal frontal region

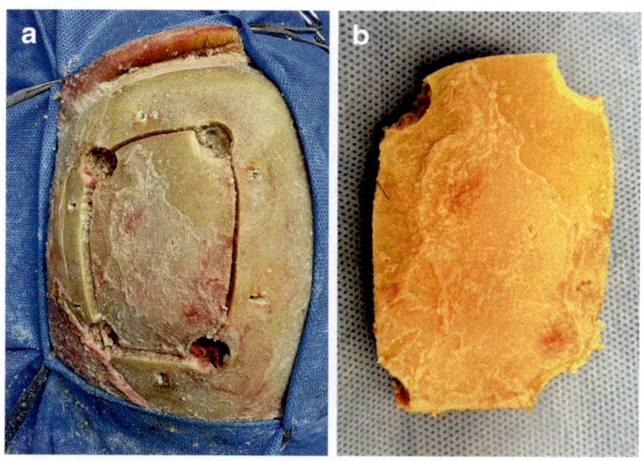

Fig. 3.3 Photographs show the frontal unilateral craniotomy in **a** and the bone flap in **b**

Closure The dura was sutured closed after addressing the lesion. The bone flap is secured with a miniplate and screws. The muscle is sutured, and the skin layers are then sutured in anatomical positions using staples or Nylon stitches.

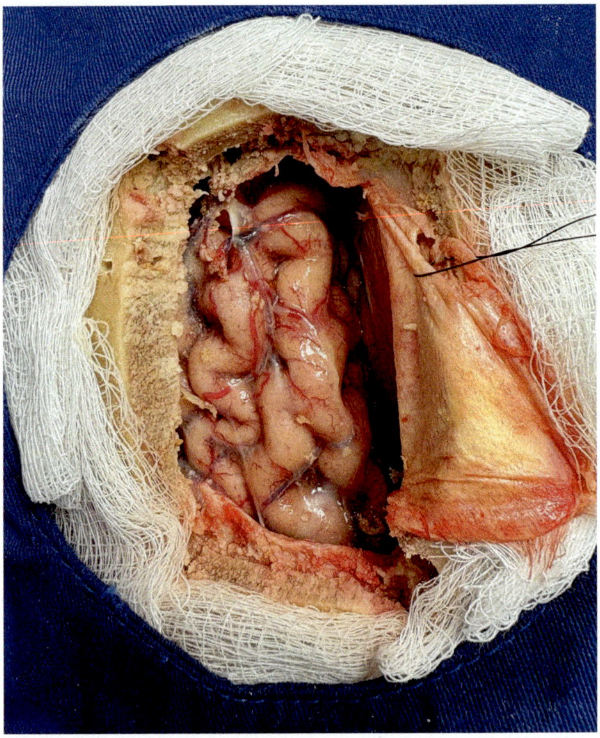

Fig. 3.4 Photograph showing the unilateral frontal craniotomy and the dural opening

3.4.2 The Bifrontal and Frontalbasal Approaches

The bifrontal and frontobasal approaches provide broad exposure to the anterior cranial fossa, facilitating access to anterior skull base lesions with minimal brain retraction [8–10]. These techniques are particularly useful for treating tumors, vascular lesions, reconstructive procedures, and trauma. Below is the step-by-step surgical technique (Figs. 3.5 and 3.6):

Skin Incision A bicoronal incision is made, extending from one zygomatic arch to the other, approximately 2–3 cm posterior to the hairline, to preserve the pericranial flap. The pericranium was carefully preserved for later use in the reconstruction. The dissection is carried down to the supraorbital rim, ensuring the protection of the supraorbital and supratrochlear nerves by mobilizing them if necessary. The scalp flap is retracted anteriorly to expose the frontal bone (the coronal and sagittal sutures are important landmarks) and the superior orbital rims.

Muscle Flap The temporalis muscle is detached from its anterior insertion along the superior temporal line and retracted posteriorly to improve access to key burr hole sites. Care should be taken to preserve the vascular supply to the pericranial flap for reconstruction.

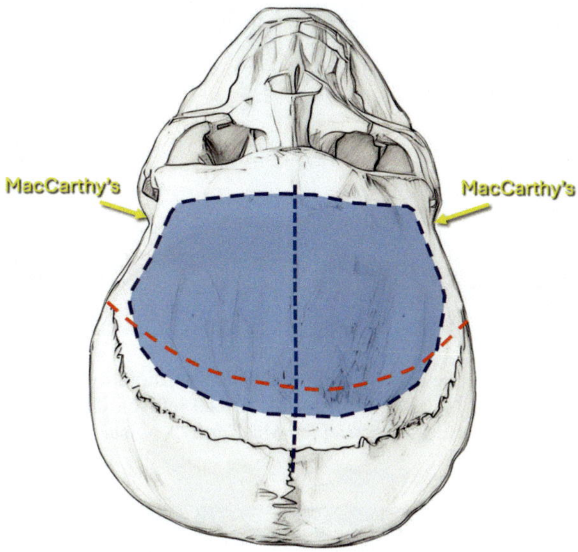

Fig. 3.5 Illustration showing an example of a bifrontal craniotomy where the surgeon can create two trephination points laterally at MacCarthy's point and one or two at the midline. The red dashed line corresponds to the bicoronal incision

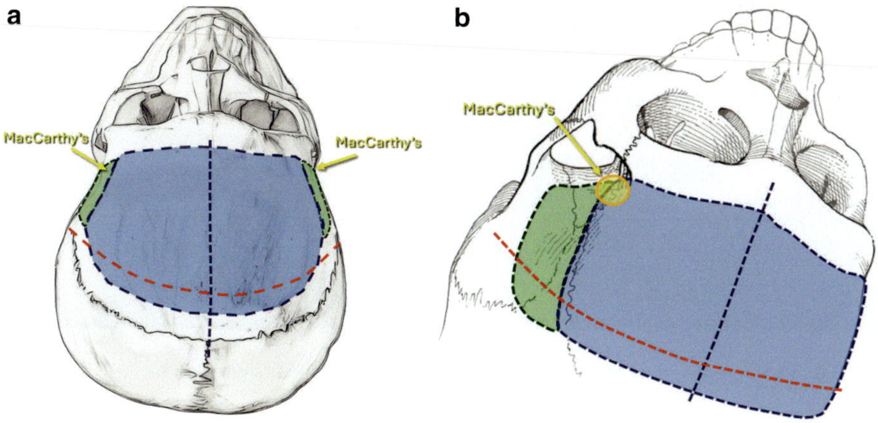

Fig. 3.6 These illustrations show how much we can extend the bifrontal craniotomy toward the temporal bone (green area in **a**). In **b**, we see MacCarthy's point as a reference for the bifrontal craniotomy (blue area) and also for the extension to the temporal region (green area)

3.4.2.1 Craniotomy

Burr Hole Placement Two bilateral key burr holes are placed in the pterional region, at the MacCarthy's key hole. Parasagittal burr holes (one or two) are placed 1–2 cm lateral to the midline, over the slope where the frontal bone curves downward to the forehead.

Bone cuts: a low-profile bifrontal craniotomy is performed, connecting the parasagittal and pterional burr holes with the craniotome. The bone cut extends

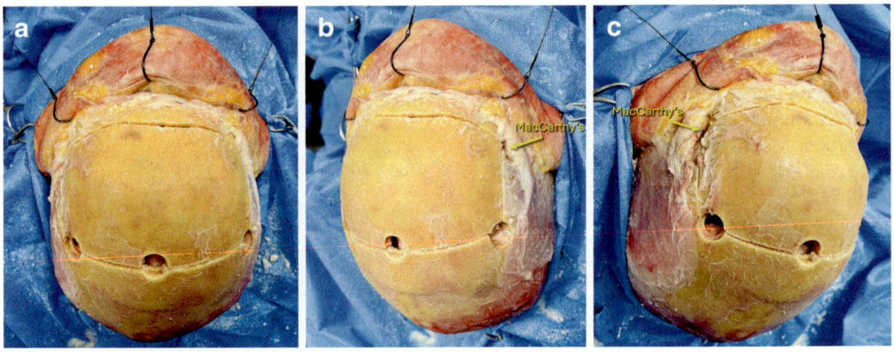

Fig. 3.7 See the bone flap of the bifrontal craniotomy over the craniotomy area, viewed from the front (**a**) and laterally on the right (**b**) and left (**c**). Observe the temporalis muscle partially dissected on the sides, exposing the MacCarthy's points

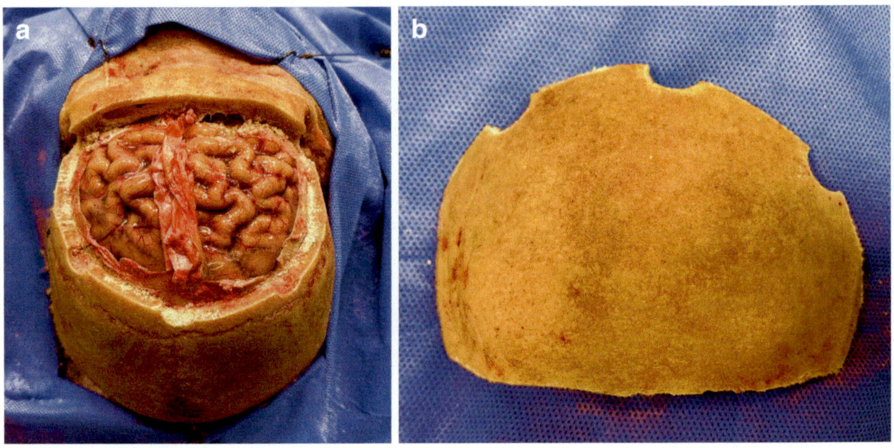

Fig. 3.8 Photographs show the bifrontal craniotomy in **a** and the bone flap in **b**

inferiorly through the superior orbital bar and anterior wall of the frontal sinus, allowing for *en bloc* removal of the frontal bone, frontal sinus, and supraorbital bar. The frontal sinus is cranialize (posterior wall removed), and the nasofrontal ducts are plugged using a small muscle graft wrapped in surgicel to prevent cerebrospinal fluid leakage (Figs. 3.7, 3.8, and 3.9).

Brian Relaxation Administration of mannitol and cerebrospinal fluid drainage (via lumbar drain or cisternal opening) may be used to minimize frontal lobe retraction.

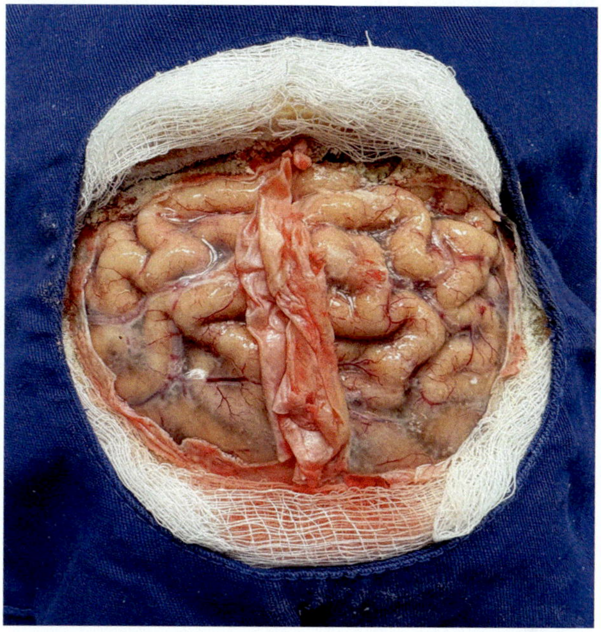

Fig. 3.9 Photograph showing the bifrontal craniotomy and the Two-Piece dural opening

Dural Opening The dura was opened in a U-shaped or curvilinear fashion, with the base of the flap along the superior sagittal sinus (Fig. 3.9). The superior sagittal sinus is either preserved or ligated, depending on the extent of exposure required. The frontal lobes are gently retracted using microsurgical techniques, allowing a subfrontal approach to the anterior skull base.

3.4.2.2 Closure

Dural Closure A watertight dural closure is achieved using primary suturing or duraplasty with the fascia lata, pericranial flap, or synthetic dural substitutes. A pericranial flap may be needed to reconstruct the skull base, depending on the case.

Bone Reconstruction The bone flap is repositioned and secured using a miniplate. Any remaining defects in the anterior skull base will be reconstructed using autologous bone grafts, hydroxyapatite cement, or titanium mesh.

Soft Tissue and Skin Closure The pericranial flap is placed over the anterior skull base to reinforce the closure and prevent cerebrospinal fluid leaks. The scalp is reapproximated using resorbable sutures or staples.

Postoperative Drains Two subgaleal drains may be placed to prevent subcutaneous fluid collection and left for 24–48 hours, avoiding excessive negative pressure (*see* Figs. 3.5, 3.6, 3.7, 3.8, and 3.9).

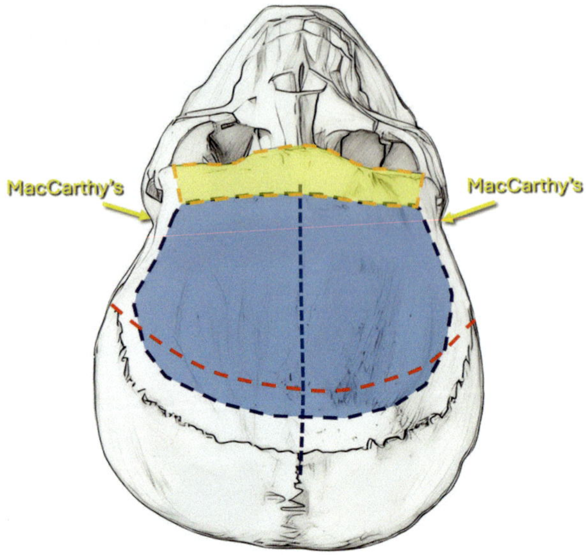

Fig. 3.10 Illustration of the transbasal approach from a two-piece craniotomy, with the frontal craniotomy (blue area) and the supraorbital bar with orbital roof osteotomies (yellow area); the red dashed line corresponds to the bicoronal incision

3.4.3 The Transbasal Approach

The transbasal approach is an advanced skull base technique that provides extensive exposure to the anterior skull base, paranasal sinuses, and upper clivus [10–14]. It is used for treating complex tumors, trauma, infections, and vascular lesions involving the anterior cranial fossa, ethmoidal region, sphenoid sinus, and clivus. The following steps outline the surgical technique, incorporating important details to improve the approach (Fig. 3.10):

Skin Incision A bicoronal incision is performed 2–3 cm posterior to the hairline, extending from one zygomatic arch to the other. The pericranial flap is preserved for reconstruction and cerebrospinal fluid leak prevention. The scalp is elevated anteriorly to the supraorbital rims to ensure that the supraorbital and supratrochlear nerves are carefully preserved or mobilized, if necessary.

Muscle Flap The temporalis muscle was elevated laterally, following the superior temporal line, to expose the key craniotomy landmarks. The muscle is reflected posteriorly to maintain vascularization and minimize devascularization of the pericranial flap, which is essential for reconstruction.

3.4.3.1 Craniotomy

In the first piece, bilateral frontal craniotomy is performed using two parasagittal burr holes (1–2 cm lateral to the midline); two lateral burr holes above the orbital rims, near the pterional region, at MacCarthy's points. A high-speed craniotome is used to create a single bone flap that extends from the supraorbital ridge to the coronal suture. The posterior wall of the frontal sinus was removed with a high-speed drill to cranialize the sinus and avoid postoperative mucocele formation.

In the second section, orbital rim osteotomy and nasal bone resection are performed to further expose the anterior skull base.

Dural Opening According to some authors, a key advantage of the transbasal approach is extradural access to the subfrontal basal region; however, a hybrid extra- and intradural approach can be performed to reach the regions of interest [1]. The dura was opened in a U-shaped manner, with the base of the flap along the anterior cranial base. The subfrontal and interhemispheric cisterns were opened for cerebrospinal fluid drainage and frontal lobe relaxation to minimize retraction. Mannitol, similarly as hypertonic saline, plays an important role in brain relaxation. The olfactory tracts are carefully dissected or sacrificed, depending on the tumor location and extent.

3.4.3.2 Closure

Dural Closure Watertight dural closure is performed using autologous fascial lata, pericranial flap, or synthetic dural substitutes. The pericranial flap is rotated and sutured to cover the cranial defect, thereby reducing the risk of cerebrospinal fluid leakage.

Bone Reconstruction The bone flap is repositioned and secured using titanium plates or sutures. If extensive resection of the anterior skull base is performed, bone grafts, hydroxyapatite cement, or a titanium mesh may be required.

Soft Tissue and Skin Closure The pericranial flap reinforces the skull base and prevents cerebrospinal fluid leakage. The scalp is reapproximated using sutures or staples to ensure tension-free closure.

3.4.3.3 Preserving Olfaction in the Transbasal Approach

The preservation of olfaction after anterior skull base surgery is challenging because olfactory tracts and bulbs often remain in the surgical corridor [15, 16]. To minimize olfactory loss: a. The cribriform plate is preserved whenever possible, avoiding extensive drilling near the fovea ethmoidalis; b. *En bloc* mobilization of the olfactory bulbs and tracts can be performed, ensuring gentle dissection from the frontal lobes; c. Neuronavigation is used to guide osteotomies anterior to the crista galli, thereby reducing the risk of iatrogenic olfactory injury; d. A limited transbasal approach that spares the cribriform plate and superior ethmoidal region can help preserve olfaction.

3.5 Pearls and Pitfalls

- *Optimize Patient Positioning.* Elevating the head 15° above the heart improves venous drainage and reduces intracranial pressure. A mild extension of 10°–15° optimizes the surgical angle and minimizes frontal lobe retraction. Failure to properly elevate the head may lead to venous congestion and increased intracranial pressure, making the procedure more challenging.

- *Perform Detailed Preoperative Planning.* Imaging studies, including CT and MRI, should be performed to assess the lesion's relationship to bony landmarks, such as the coronal and sagittal sutures, as well as the superior temporal line. Understanding the lateralization of the superior sagittal sinus is important for preventing unintentional injury during craniotomy.
- *Align the Skin Incision with the Surgical Target.* The incision should provide direct access to the lesion while minimizing unnecessary tissue dissection. A straight incision is preferred for smaller craniotomies, and a C-shaped incision with the base toward the midline is preferred.
- *Preserving the Pericranial Flap for Reconstruction.* The pericranium should be carefully elevated and preserved during a bicoronal incision, as it plays a critical role in preventing CSF leakage and reconstructing the skull base.
- *Strategically Place Burr Holes.* At least three to four burr holes should be used, with two placed near the midline to facilitate safe dural separation. If the superior sagittal sinus is encountered, an adjacent burr hole can be created to allow for controlled dural repair.
- *Expand the Craniotomy for Better Exposure.* The craniotomy should be centered on the target lesion and should be expanded as needed to improve illumination, visualization, and microsurgical maneuverability.
- *Achieving Brain Relaxation Before Dural Opening.* Mannitol and hypertonic saline administration, along with CSF drainage (via lumbar drain or cisternal opening), minimizes frontal lobe retraction and enhances surgical access.
- *Plan a Safe Dural Opening.* The dura should be incised in a U-shaped or curvilinear manner with the base toward the midline. This arrangement facilitates easier repair in cases of accidental sinus opening.
- *Dural Closure.* To prevent CSF leakage, secure, and watertight closure. If necessary, pericranial flaps, fascial lata, or synthetic dural substitutes should be used for additional reinforcement.
- *Frontal Sinus.* A persistent CSF leak may develop if the frontal sinus is not cranialized and sealed properly, increasing the risk of infection and tension pneumocephalus. The nasofrontal ducts should be obliterated using a muscle graft or other sealing technique.
- *Bone Reconstruction.* Improper bone flap repositioning or inadequate soft tissue handling may lead to forehead deformities, asymmetry, or frontal bossing, which can be cosmetically and functionally problematic.

References

1. Siqueira MG. Tratado de Neurocirurgia: Volume I. Barueri, Brazil: Manole; 2016. Chapter 5: p. 35–47; Chapter 6: p. 49–57.
2. Vilany L. Anatomical step-by-step dissection of complex skull base approaches for trainees: surgical anatomy of the bifrontal transbasal approach, surgical principles, and illustrative cases. J Neurol Surg B Skull Base. 2024;85:596–606.

3. Rao D, Tanriverdi T, Ulm AJ, et al. An illustrative review of common modern craniotomies. J Clin Imaging Sci. 2020;10(81):81.
4. Fernández-de Thomas RJ, Munakomi S, De Jesus O. Craniotomy. In: StatPearls [Internet]. Treasure Island: StatPearls Publishing; 2025.
5. Crowley RW, Tarapore PE, Rutledge C, et al. Positioning for cranial surgery. In: Winn HR, editor. Youmans and Winn neurological surgery. 8th ed. Philadelphia: Elsevier; 2023. p. 442–56.
6. Meyer FB. Atlas de Neurocirurgia: Acessos Básicos ao Crânio e Procedimentos Vascular. Rio de Janeiro: DiLivros; 2005. p. 83–123.
7. Ghosh A, Chi J, Holsgrove D. Neuroanatomy, superior sagittal sinus. In: StatPearls [Internet]. Treasure Island: StatPearls Publishing; 2023.
8. Fossett DT, Caputy AJ. Operative neurosurgical anatomy. New York and Stuttgart: Thieme; 2001. Chapter 6: p. 27–31
9. Ozlen F, Oguzoglu SA, Orhan M, et al. Low-profile 1-piece bifrontal craniotomy for anterior skull base approach and reconstruction. J Craniofac Surg. 2010;21(1):233–8.
10. Donald PJ. Frontobasal approach for trauma and tumor. Minim Invas Neurosurg. 1994;37(1):37–41.
11. Sekhar LN. The extended frontal approach to tumors of the anterior, middle, and posterior skull base. J Neurosurg. 1992;76:198–206.
12. Safaee MM, McDermott MW, Benet A, Theodosopoulos PV. Tailored extended bifrontal craniotomy for anterior skull base tumors: anatomic description of a modified surgical technique and case series. Oper Neurosurg (Hagerstown). 2017;14(4):386–94.
13. Raso JL, Gusmão S. Transbasal approach to skull base tumors: evaluation and proposal of classification. Surg Neurol. 2006;65(Suppl 1):S1:33–8.
14. Kurtsoy A, Menku A, Tucer B, Oktem IS, Akdemir H, Koc RK. Transbasal approaches: surgical details, pitfalls, and avoidances. Neurosurg Rev. 2004;27(4):267–73.
15. Spetzler RF, Zabramski JM, Krisht AF, et al. Preservation of olfaction in anterior craniofacial approaches. J Neurosurg. 1993;79:48–52.
16. Saito K, Takahashi M, Fukuta K, Tachibana E, Yoshida J. Recovery of olfactory function after an anterior craniofacial approach. Skull Base Surg. 1999;9(3):201–6.

The Pterional Approach

4

4.1 Introduction

Throughout the twentieth century, pterional craniotomy was developed by pioneers of neurosurgery that were initially general surgeons interested in cranial surgery. However, in the 1970s, Yasargil published a detailed description of the approach, emphasizing the exposure of the Sylvian fissure at the apex of a triangular region between the frontal and temporal lobes while minimizing brain retraction. It is important to note that a significant amount of brain retraction during a neurosurgical procedure occurs not just during deep dissection but also at the stage of craniotomy, as the brain is exposed and access to the target region is established. By refining the pterional craniotomy, access to the Sylvian fissure was significantly improved, along with exposure to natural cisternal spaces, such as the opticocarotid and oculomotor cisterns, which can be reached directly through the Sylvian fissure [1, 2].

The primary craniometric landmark for this approach is the pterion [3], near which the first burr hole is placed (the keyhole, for the pterional craniotomy. Additional burr holes may be created at the extremities of the craniotomy, corresponding to the frontal and temporal lobes, depending on the surgeon's experience, available instrumentation, and the degree of dura mater adherence to the bone.

Due to its versatility in providing access to the Sylvian fissure, the apices of the temporal and frontal lobes, and structures within the circle of Willis, pterional craniotomy is widely performed. Over time, this technique has evolved, and minimally invasive variants have been developed. Among the alternative approaches derived from pterional craniotomy, the most notable are supra-orbital and mini-pterional craniotomy.

Supplementary Information The online version contains supplementary material available at https://doi.org/10.1007/978-3-032-04664-2_4. The videos can be accessed individually by clicking the DOI link in the accompanying figure caption or by scanning this link with the SN More Media App.

H. de Oliveira Manduca Palmiero, E. G. Figueiredo, *Neurosurgical Approaches Video Atlas*, https://doi.org/10.1007/978-3-032-04664-2_4

4.2 Indications for the Approach

Vascular and skull base neurosurgeons extensively use the pterional approach. Once the Sylvian fissure is exposed with minimal brain retraction and under microscopic visualization, the technique allows for aneurysm clipping within the circle of Willis, resection of intra-axial tumors located at the anterior poles of the frontal and temporal lobes, and access to the third ventricle via the lamina terminalis. Additionally, it facilitates the removal of lesions involving the cavernous sinus, optic nerve, and chiasm, clinoid process, and sphenoid plane, as well as surgical access to the basilar apex [2, 4].

4.3 Operative Set-Up

Patient Positioning The patient is positioned in a supine and neutral alignment. Before removing the headrest to secure the head holder, a rolled sheet cushion is placed under the ipsilateral shoulder to the craniotomy. This maneuver helps optimize cranial exposure on the side of interest while reducing cervicobrachial muscle tension and minimizing the risk of brachial plexus injury.

Head Positioning Some surgeons prefer the *Sugita* head holder, which may provide four-point fixation, while others opt for the *Mayfield* head holder, which uses three-point fixation. Regardless of the system used, the head must be secured to place a fixation point on the ipsilateral mastoid. In the case of the *Sugita* head holder, the second ipsilateral fixation point was positioned slightly higher on the occipital bone. The two contralateral fixation points should follow the superior temporal line, avoiding direct pressure on the squamous part of the temporal bone, as excessive force in this region can lead to fracture with potential complications. Once the head holder is secured (whether *Mayfield* or *Sugita*, the final head and neck positioning is achieved through *three specific maneuvers*, as illustrated in Fig. 4.1:

(a) *Elevation:* If additional elevation is required, the entire head section of the surgical table is raised to ensure that there is no traction on the cervical region. After elevating the table, the patient's legs are raised to create a V-shaped position on the surgical table. After elevating the table, the patient is placed during the procedure.
(b) *Rotation:* The head is rotated contralaterally to the side of the craniotomy to enhance the exposure of the target region. The degree of rotation depends on the surgical objective [4]. The authors prefer a slight degree of rotation, nearly 5 degrees, to facilitate the splitting of the Sylvian fissure. After completing this step, additional rotation may be performed by tilting the surgical table, depending on the target to be reached. Proper head rotation ensures a clear surgical corridor and minimizes the need for brain retraction.
(c) *Extension:* The final adjustment is the head extension, positioning the malar eminence at the highest point of the surgical field [4]. This maneuver effectively elevates the frontal and temporal lobes from the microscopic field of view, thereby optimizing access to the basal cisterns. While some studies have described four to five head positioning adjustments, a practical neurosurgical approach considers

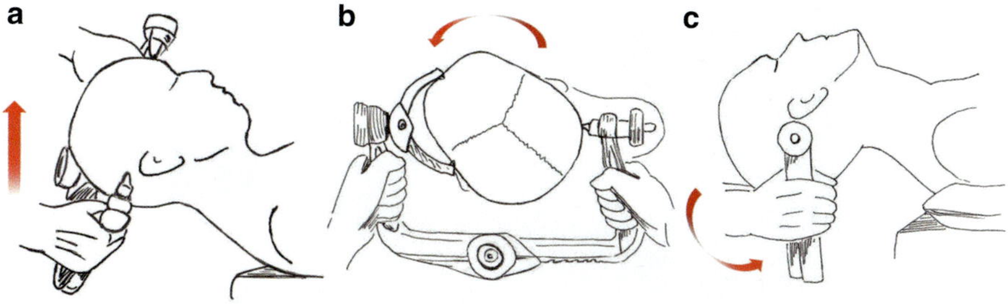

Fig. 4.1 Illustration showing the sequential head movements for positioning: (**a**) Elevation, (**b**) Rotation, (**c**) Extension

only three essential movements—elevation, rotation, and extension—as they provide precise *three-dimensional alignment to expose the target region.*

Skin Preparation At this stage, partial trichotomy is performed to expose the incision site. It is unnecessary to shave the entire scalp because this can have stigmatizing consequences for the patient. According to the literature, it is safe to perform the incision without shaving the hair, provided that the scalp is thoroughly washed with a shampoo solution and chlorhexidine [5, 6]. However, we prefer to shave a narrow strip along the incision line to facilitate hygiene, improve drape adhesion, and optimize wound dressing application.

4.4 Surgical Technique (Video 4.1)

Skin Incision Using a scalpel, we performed the classic arcuate incision, starting at the level of the zygoma, approximately 1 cm anterior to the tragus, and extending toward the midline (Fig. 4.2) [4]. During the incision, we preserve the superficial temporal artery, crucial for vascularizing the temporalis muscle. To minimize the risk of postoperative ischemic skin injury, we did not use Raney clips for scalp hemostasis. Instead, alternative techniques such as gentle bipolar coagulation or suture control are preferred to reduce tissue trauma and optimize wound healing.

Temporal Muscle Flap The temporal branch of the facial nerve travels within the loose areolar tissue (adipose layer) between the superficial layer of the deep temporal and temporoparietal fascia (Fig. 4.3). Thus, the safe dissection of the temporal muscle requires meticulous technique to avoid injury to the facial nerve's temporal branch and preserve muscle function [7, 8].

A vertical incision is made in the superficial fascia of the temporalis muscle, starting 2 cm superior to the orbital rim and extending down to the posterior root of the zygomatic arch, using a scalpel to avoid thermal injury from monopolar electrocautery. Next, a straight incision is made along the superior temporal line, leaving a muscle cuff for later reconstruction, extending posteriorly to the limit of the skin incision. The dissection then proceeds vertically in a straight line, reaching near the auricle.

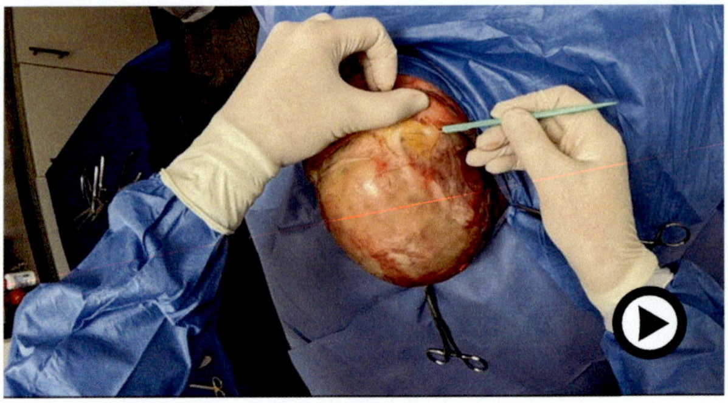

Video 4.1 In this video, we demonstrate the pterional craniotomy step-by-step, emphasizing key anatomical landmarks and technical refinements that improve surgical exposure while reducing complications. This approach provides reliable access to the Sylvian fissure, frontal and temporal lobes, and anterior circulation vessels, remaining a fundamental technique in vascular, oncologic, and skull base neurosurgery (▶ https://doi.org/10.1007/000-hsv)

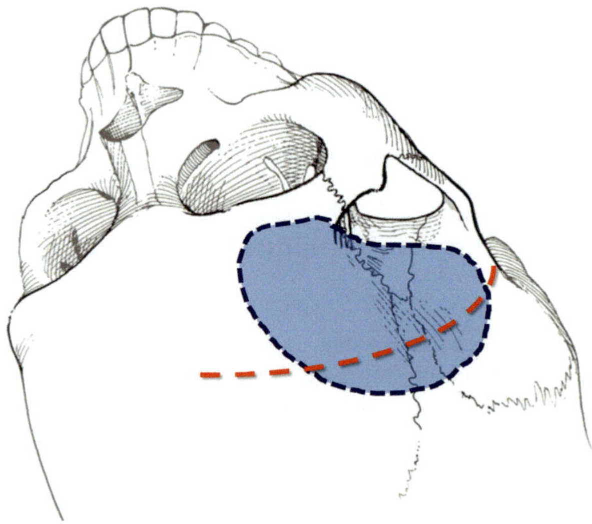

Fig. 4.2 Illustration demonstrating the area of the pterional craniotomy (in blue) and the arc-shaped incision, starting 1 cm anterior to the tragus and extending toward the midline (red dashed line)

At this point, the temporal muscle can be elevated as a single myofascial flap by performing subperiosteal dissection along the bone using a periosteal elevator [4, 9]. Monopolar electrocautery should be avoided because the deep temporal fascia contains branches of the mandibular division of the trigeminal nerve (V3) [9]. Additionally, monopolar use may cause muscle ischemia, increasing the risk of postoperative atrophy and functional deficits.

Craniotomy The craniotomy step in the pterional approach begins with the placement of burr holes. The *keyhole (frontosphenoidal) burr hole* is created just posterior to and superior to the frontozygomatic suture near the pterion. In some cases,

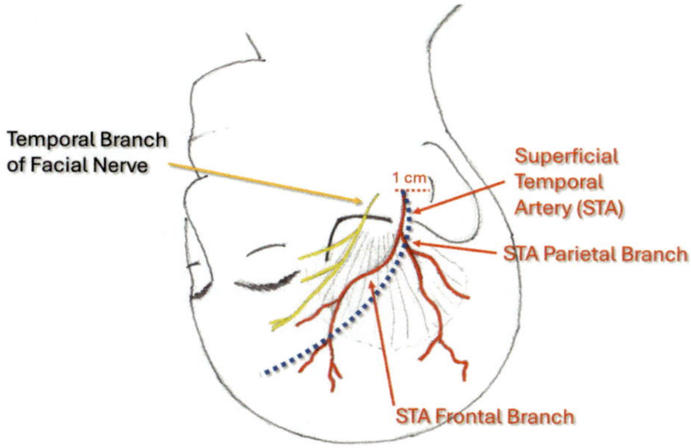

Fig. 4.3 Anatomical illustration based on literature showing the Superficial Temporal Artery (STA) and the temporal branch of the facial nerve. Observe the anatomical relationships between the artery and the nerve, as starting the incision 1 cm anterior to the tragus reduces the risk of nerve injury and allows for early identification of the artery. In this illustration, it is also possible to see the relationship between the arciform incision (blue dashed line), the STA, and the temporal branch of the facial nerve. Note why it is more common to ligate the STA's parietal branch due to its relationship with the arciform incision [4]

an additional posterior burr hole is placed at the inferior temporal line to facilitate the elevation of the bone flap [2, 4, 9].

After creating the burr holes, the craniotomy outline is defined using a craniotome with a footplate. The first cut extends posteriorly along the frontal bone, starting from the keyhole. The second cut runs inferiorly through the temporal bone, extending down to the zygomatic root. The final cut completes the craniotomy along the sphenoid wing, ensuring thin bone removal to enhance the exposure of the skull base and optimize the surgical corridor [2, 4, 9].

After craniotomy, the bone flap is carefully elevated using an elevator to avoid dural tears. The exposed area consists of approximately two-thirds of the frontal lobe and one-third of the temporal lobe (Fig. 4.4). To optimize anterior and lateral exposure of the skull base, a rongeur or high-speed drill is used to thin and remove the sphenoid ridge [4, 9] (Fig. 4.5). This additional bone removal allows for better access to the frontal and temporal lobes, reducing the need for excessive brain retraction and improving the surgical corridor for vascular and skull base procedures.

Dural Opening Before opening the dura mater, we perform dural anchoring using 4-0 Ethibond sutures, for example, to prevent postoperative epidural collection. Although anchoring can be performed at the end of the procedure, intraoperative dural retraction may occur, making it preferable to include this step as part of the surgical approach. The dural edges should be covered with gauze before incision to minimize blood contamination of the brain surface. Once secured, blue surgical drapes should be positioned around the gauze to maintain a clean and controlled operative field and to avoid reflection of the microscope light (Fig. 4.6).

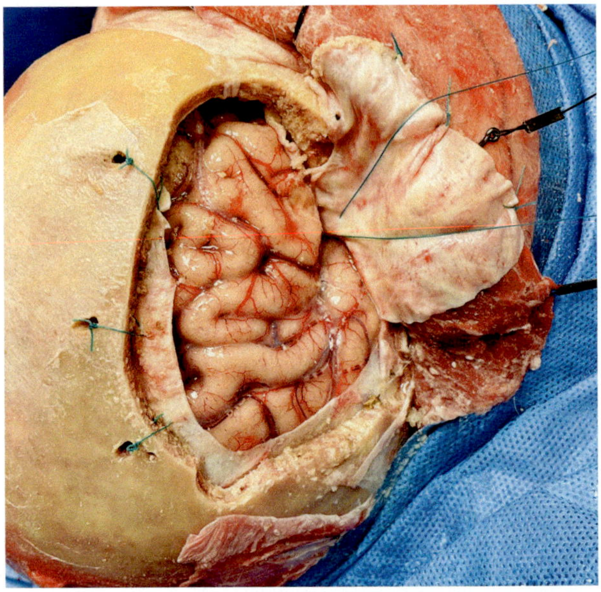

Fig. 4.4 Photograph showing the pterional craniotomy with the dura mater opened and reflected anteroinferiorly

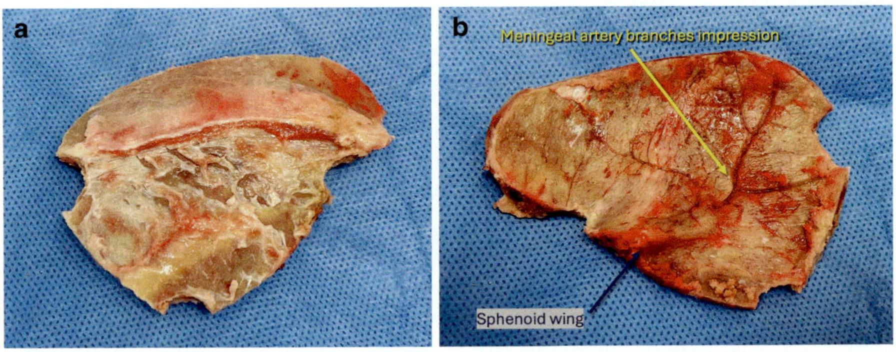

Fig. 4.5 Photographs showing the bone flap viewed externally in **a** and internally in **b**. Note the sphenoid wing and the impression of the middle meningeal artery with its branches

Once dural anchoring is completed and the gauze and blue surgical drapes are in place, the dura is opened toward the Sylvian fissure in a curvilinear or C-shaped fashion (Fig. 4.7). The dural incision started at the frontal vertex of the craniotomy, extending posterior and laterally until the impression of the sphenoid wing in the dura was reached. At this point, it extends almost straight until the meningo-orbital cleft. In addition, an incision of 1.5–2.0 cm is performed in the temporal dura. The edges of the dura were retracted with *Prolene* 4-0 to maintain a blood-free operative field. To facilitate closure, avoid making a midline incision; instead, use a folding maneuver. The dural flap should be reflected anteriorly using sutures, such as 4-0 *Ethibond*, to ensure stability and adequate exposure.

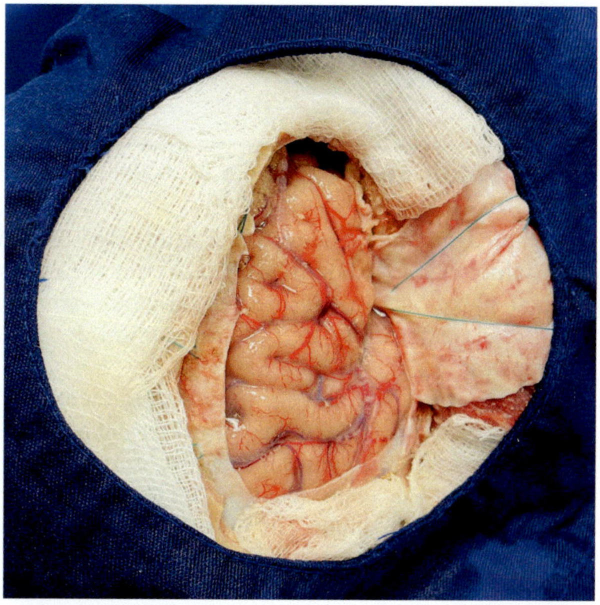

Fig. 4.6 Photograph showing the pterional craniotomy with the blue and white drapes positioned and set up for microsurgery

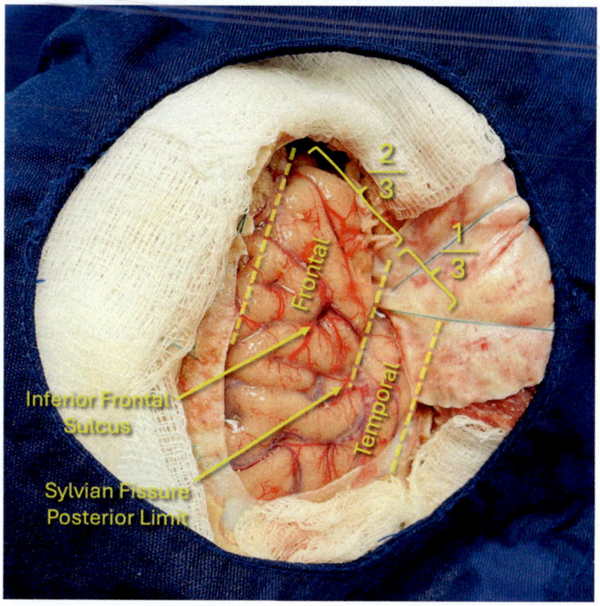

Fig. 4.7 In this photograph, we can identify the extent of exposure of the frontal lobe (2/3) and temporal lobe (1/3) through the pterional craniotomy. The inferior frontal sulcus assists us in recognizing the exposure of the middle and inferior frontal gyri. The posterior limit of the Sylvian fissure, defined by the postcentral and supramarginal gyri, is likewise exposed in the pterional craniotomy

Closure It is commonly said among experienced neurosurgeons that closure begins during the opening. The closure process is significantly easier if the technical steps are followed correctly. We avoid using *Raney* clips to optimize wound healing and structural integrity because they can cause skin damage. In addition, the muscle cuff is preserved along the superior temporal line to facilitate muscle reconstruction.

The dura mater was anchored to prevent retraction, and we avoid making additional dural incisions, limiting the opening to a C-shaped configuration for optimal brain closure and protection.

4.5 Pearls and Pitfalls

- *Patient Positioning:* elevate the head ~15° to improve venous return, and a shoulder cushion should be used to enhance exposure while minimizing brachial plexus strain. Ensure proper *three-axis head positioning (elevation, rotation, extension)* to minimize brain retraction and improve surgical exposure.
- *Skin and Muscle Handling:* to protect the temporal branch of the facial nerve, preserve the superficial temporal artery, and perform subfascial dissection. Avoid *using Raney* clips to prevent skin necrosis.
- *Craniotomy Execution:* place the keyhole burr hole posterior and superior to the frontozygomatic suture. The sphenoid ridge is thinned with a high-speed drill to improve skull base access and minimize brain retraction.
- *Dural opening:* the dura *is pre-anchored* with 4-0 *Ethibond* sutures. A C-shaped incision is made anterior to the dural flap anteriorly with sutures to ensure stable exposure.
- *Closure:* The temporalis muscle cuff is preserved for better function and cosmesis. Secure the bone flap, ensure layered closure, and prevent CSF leakage.

4.6 Alternative Approaches

After detailing the pterional craniotomy technique, its indications, and technical details, it is important to discuss alternative approaches derived from it. We selected the *supra-orbital* approach, as both are widely described in the literature and represent a specialized surgical niche for certain neurosurgeons.

Mini-Pterional With the advancement of surgical techniques, some authors have developed reduced versions of the pterional craniotomy, still centered on the pterion but with a smaller surface area, allowing it to be completely covered by the temporal muscle once closed [10] (*see Chapter about the Mini-Pterional Approach*).

Supraorbital As Reisch described, supraorbital craniotomy has emerged as a minimally invasive approach for accessing the Sylvian fissure, uncus, and mesial temporal lobe. This technique provides direct access to the Sylvian fissure by minimizing cortical retraction and preserving critical vascular and neural structures [11]. It was later modified to extend laterally to the zygoma [12] (*see Chapter about the Supraorbital and Supraorbital Zygomatic Approaches*).

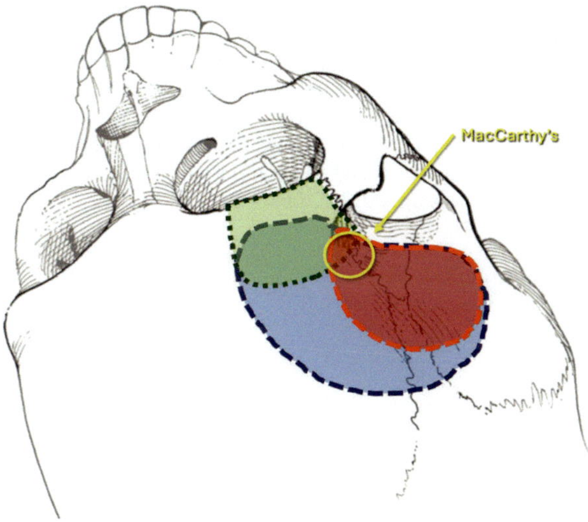

Fig. 4.8 Illustration showing the areas of the pterional craniotomy (blue area) and its variants: supraorbital (green area) and mini-pterional (red area). It is also noted that all share MacCarthy's point (yellow circle)

In comparison, these minimally invasive approaches should be indicated for selected patients with favorable anatomy because they involve less temporal muscle manipulation and less brain retraction. Due to its location, which provides different viewing angles for the surgeon, *supra-orbital zygomatic* craniotomy offers better visualization of contralateral structures [13] (Fig. 4.8).

References

1. Rubio RR, Martinez E, Carceller F, et al. Immersive surgical anatomy of the pterional approach. Cureus. 2019;11(7):e5216.
2. Yasargil MG. Microneurosurgery, vol. 1. Stuttgart: Georg Thieme Verlag; 1984. p. 215–33.
3. Gusmão S, Silveira RL, Arantes A. Pontos referenciais nos acessos cranianos. Arq Neuropsiquiatr. 2003;61(2-A):305–8.
4. Vishteh AG, Spetzler RF, Lawton MT, et al. The pterional approach. Oper Tech Neurosurg. 1998;1(1):39–49.
5. Bekar A, Doğan S, Yilmazlar S, et al. The effect of hair on infection after cranial surgery. Acta Neurochir. 2001;143:533–7.
6. Kretschmer T, Braun V, Richter HP. Neurosurgery without shaving: indications and results. Br J Neurosurg. 2000;14(4):341–4.
7. Yasargil MG, Reichman MV, Kubik S. Preservation of the frontotemporal branch of the facial nerve using the interfascial temporalis flap for pterional craniotomy. J Neurosurg. 1987;67:463–6.
8. Babakurban ST, Serel S, Turhan-Haktanir N, et al. Temporal branch of the facial nerve and its relationship to fascial layers. Arch Facial Plast Surg. 2010;12(1):16–23.
9. Chaddad Neto F, Ribas GC, Oliveira E. A craniotomia pterional. Arq Neuropsiquiatr. 2007;65(1):101–6.
10. Veldeman M, Niemelä M, Hernesniemi J. How I do it – Helsinki style mini-pterional craniotomy for clipping of middle cerebral artery bifurcation aneurysms. Acta Neurochir. 2023;165:489–93.

11. Reisch R, Perneczky A, Tschabitscher M. Surgical technique of the supraorbital keyhole craniotomy. Surg Neurol. 2003;59:223–7.
12. Figueiredo EG, Deshmukh P, Zabramski JM, et al. An anatomical evaluation of the mini-supraorbital approach and comparison with standard craniotomies. Neurosurgery. 2006;59(ONS Suppl 4):212–20.
13. Yagmurlu K, Hicdonmez T, Baca B, et al. Quantitative anatomical analysis and clinical experience with mini-pterional and mini-orbitozygomatic approaches for intracranial aneurysm surgery. J Neurosurg. 2017;127:646–59.

Minimally Invasive Approaches: The Mini-pterional

5

5.1 Introduction

Minipterional craniotomy is a less-invasive modification of the traditional pterional approach. The device is designed to provide adequate exposure to lesions in the anterior and middle cranial fossae while minimizing soft tissue disruption. This technique involves a smaller incision and craniotomy, thereby reducing operative time, blood loss, and postoperative complications, such as temporal muscle atrophy. It is particularly useful for accessing aneurysms in the anterior circulation, tumors of the parasellar and suprasellar regions, and other deep-seated intracranial pathologies. By preserving more of the temporalis muscle and utilizing optimal exposure principles, the mini-pterional approach enhances recovery and cosmetic outcomes, making it a preferred option in select neurosurgical cases [1–3].

The pterional craniotomy, pioneered by Dandy in the early twentieth century, became the standard method for accessing aneurysms of the anterior circulation, evolving with microsurgical advancements by Yasargil, who popularized and refined it in the modern era by integrating microsurgical techniques and enhancing surgical exposure [4, 5]. Over time, refinements have led to smaller variations, such as mini-pterional craniotomy and the small frontolateral approach, which aim to minimize soft tissue trauma and brain retraction while maintaining adequate exposure [4, 6]. Modifying the standard pterional approach introduced a smaller incision and limited craniectomy to improve cosmesis and reduce postoperative complications [4], while the small frontolateral approach offered a direct and protective route for aneurysm clipping with less need for Sylvian fissure dissection [6]. These advancements reflect the trend toward minimally invasive neurosurgical techniques that balance

Supplementary Information The online version contains supplementary material available at https://doi.org/10.1007/978-3-032-04664-2_5. The videos can be accessed individually by clicking the DOI link in the accompanying figure caption or by scanning this link with the SN More Media App.

H. de Oliveira Manduca Palmiero, E. G. Figueiredo, *Neurosurgical Approaches Video Atlas*, https://doi.org/10.1007/978-3-032-04664-2_5

surgical access with reduced morbidity. Here, we describe the mini-pterional approach, as first described by Figueiredo et al. [7].

Minipterional craniotomy offers significant advantages over the standard pterional approach, particularly in reducing temporalis muscle atrophy and minimizing the risk of injury to the frontal branch of the facial nerve [7, 8]. By using a smaller incision and limiting muscle dissection, the mini-pterional approach preserves more of the temporalis muscle, thereby reducing postoperative atrophy and related functional impairments [4, 7]. Additionally, this technique avoids extensive retraction of the soft tissues over the zygomatic arch, which lowers the likelihood of frontal branch facial nerve injury that can result in brow ptosis and esthetic concerns [4, 6]. These enhancements improve both functional and cosmetic outcomes, making mini-pterional craniotomy a preferred option in selected neurosurgical cases.

5.2 Indications for the Approach

Minipterional craniotomy is indicated for neurosurgical procedures that require access to anterior circulation aneurysms, including those at the internal carotid artery (ICA) bifurcation, middle cerebral artery (MCA) bifurcation, anterior communicating artery (AComA), and posterior communicating artery (PComA) [7]. This approach is particularly beneficial for small to medium-sized aneurysms with well-defined necks, as it provides adequate exposure while minimizing brain retraction and soft tissue trauma [9]. Furthermore, the mini-pterional approach is well-suited for resecting suprasellar, parasellar, and sphenoidal wing tumors, such as meningiomas, craniopharyngiomas, and pituitary adenomas, by offering a direct transsylvian corridor that reduces manipulation of surrounding neural structures [7]. It also serves as an alternative to conventional pterional craniotomy in cases that require a minimally invasive route to the orbitofrontal, insular, or anterior temporal regions, thereby optimizing cosmetic and functional outcomes [9].

5.3 Operative Set-Up [7, 9]

Patient Positioning The patient is positioned supine on the operating table with the ipsilateral shoulder slightly elevated using a gel pad or rolled sheet to enhance surgical access. The body is secured to the table with appropriate padding to prevent pressure injuries, and the arms are positioned at the sides or on arm boards, with the contralateral arm hold.

Head Positioning The head is fixed in a three-pin Mayfield head clamp or Sugita to provide stable positioning during the procedure.

(a) *Elevation.* The optimal head elevation is 15°–20° above the cardiac level to promote venous drainage and reduce intracranial pressure.

(b) *Rotation.* The head is rotated 5°–15° contralaterally, depending on the location of the lesion, to optimize the working trajectory while ensuring adequate frontal lobe relaxation. Additional rotation may be achieved by rotating the surgical table as needed.
(c) *Extension.* A slight extension of 10°–15° is applied to align the sphenoid ridge horizontally, facilitating a direct approach to the Sylvian fissure and basal cisterns.

Skin Preparation The pre-auricular region, forehead, and temporal scalp are shaved as necessary to expose the surgical field while preserving cosmesis. The surgical site is prepared with an antiseptic solution, such as chlorhexidine or povidone-iodine, and shampoo, extending from the midline to the zygomatic arch and posteriorly to the mastoid process. Sterile drapes are applied, leaving a window around the planned incision site, ensuring that the eye is covered with a protective film to prevent corneal injury.

5.4 Surgical Technique [7, 8] (Video 5.1)

Skin Incision A curvilinear incision is made along the anterior temporal hairline, starting 1 cm above the zygomatic arch and extending superiorly toward the midpupillary line. The incision followed the natural contours of the forehead to optimize cosmesis while ensuring sufficient exposure.

Muscle Flap The temporalis muscle is dissected using an interfascial approach to preserve the frontal branch of the facial nerve. The facial nerve's temporal branch runs within the superficial layers of the temporalis fascia. A second incision was made between the superior and inferior temporal lines, extending posteriorly while

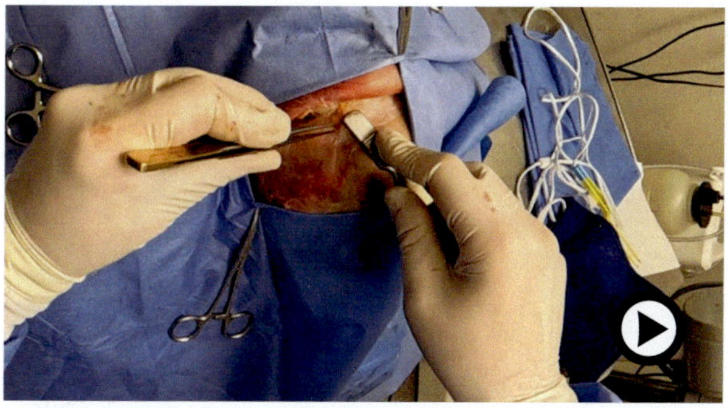

Video 5.1 This video demonstrates the step-by-step execution of the mini-pterional craniotomy using both the standard and Helsinki (lateral supraorbital) techniques, highlighting key technical differences that optimize exposure to anterior circulation aneurysms and skull base lesions while minimizing soft tissue disruption and preserving cosmetic outcomes (▶ https://doi.org/10.1007/000-hsw)

maintaining the temporalis muscle cuff for reconstruction. A single myocutaneous flap is preferred, where the skin and muscle are elevated together and reflected anteriorly using monopolar cautery and blunt dissection. Alternatively, the muscle-splitting technique can be used to minimize muscle atrophy. The sphenoid ridge is exposed, and the muscle is retracted using fishhooks or sutures to maintain tension without excessive trauma.

Craniotomy A single burr is placed at the keyhole region (MacCarthy's point), just above the frontozygomatic suture, ensuring minimal bony removal. A curvilinear craniotomy is performed using a high-speed drill, extending from the frontal bone to the lateral sphenoid wing. The entire craniotomy area was located beneath the temporalis muscle (Figs. 5.1, 5.2, and 5.3). The sphenoid ridge is flattened to improve access to the Sylvian fissure and neurovascular structures. The bone flap is carefully lifted to avoid excessive force on the dura.

5.4.1 The Helsinki Mini-pterional (or Lateral Supraorbital Mini-pterional)

The Helsinki style mini-pterional craniotomy [10] differs from the standard mini-pterional craniotomy [7] in several key aspects, particularly in incision design, temporal muscle cutting, and craniotomy placement. However, both approaches aim to minimize tissue disruption and optimize cosmesis, and both maintain a 3 cm craniotomy centered over the Sylvian fissure, allowing sufficient microsurgical working space.

Skin Incision The incision begins 1 cm anterior to the tragus and 3 cm superior to the zygomatic arch, above the eyeglasses framing, and curves frontally behind the hairline, extending near the midline.

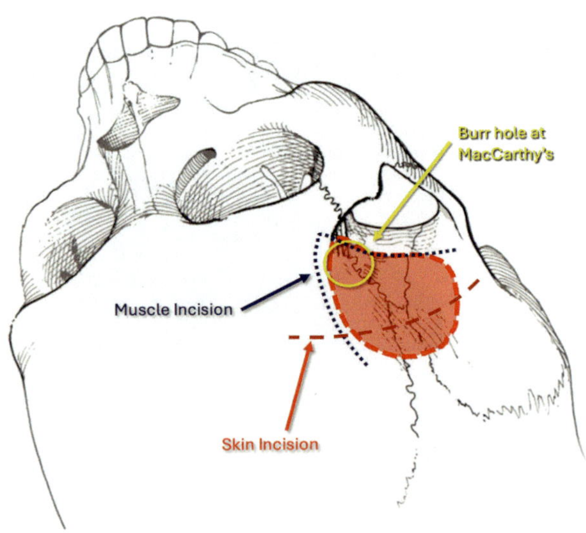

Fig. 5.1 Anatomical illustration showing the skin incision, mini-pterional area (red area), burr hole placement, and its relationship with the temporal muscle incision

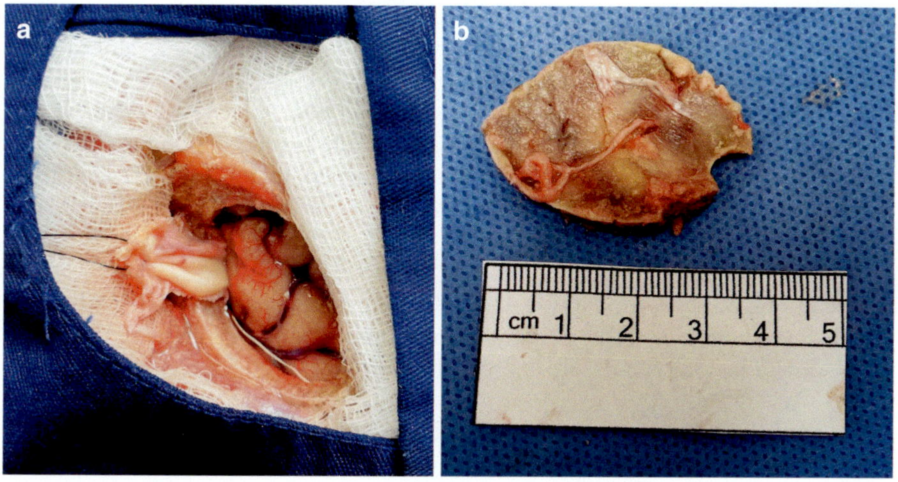

Fig. 5.2 The photograph shows the standard mini-pterional craniotomy (on the left side) in **a** and the bone flap in **b**

Fig. 5.3 Photograph comparing the bone flaps of the pterional craniotomy (above) and the standard mini-pterional craniotomy (below)

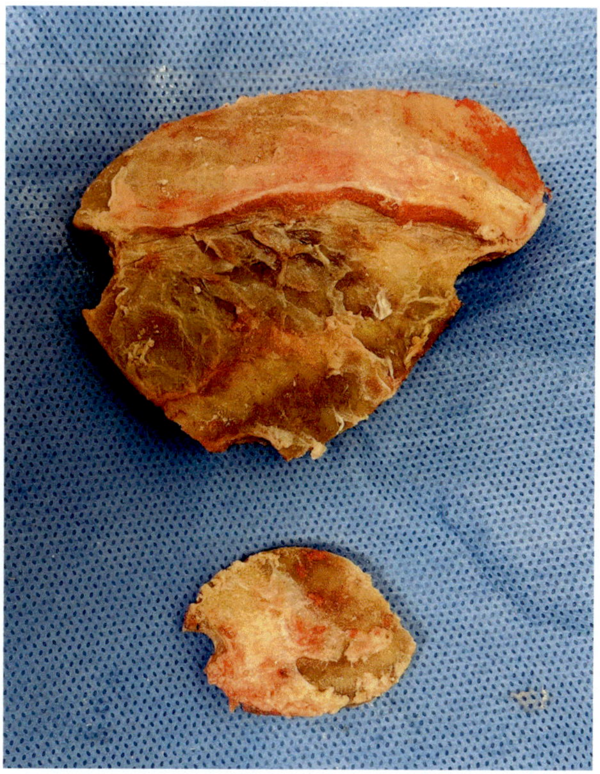

Muscle Flap The temporalis muscle was cut using a V-shaped incision with monopolar cautery, but the periosteal dissection was performed using an elevator to avoid muscle atrophy.

Craniotomy To perform the craniotomy, a burr hole is placed along the posterior edge of the planned craniotomy, the dura is detached, and a 3 cm craniotomy is performed, centered on the Sylvian fissure. The anterior skull base was flattened with minimal drilling (Figs. 5.4 and 5.5).

See in Fig. 5.6 how the Pterional, standard mini-pterional, and Helsinki's mini-pterional craniotomies differ in bony exposure areas while maintaining their relationship with the Sylvian fissure and the pterion.

Dural Opening The dura is incised in a curvilinear or cruciate manner, depending on the surgical target, and is retracted with 4–0 silk sutures or dural tacking stitches. Once the craniotomy is complete, the microsurgical phase begins: the Sylvian fissure is dissected under a microscope to expose the anterior circulation arteries or skull base structures, and cortical retraction is minimized by utilizing CSF drainage through a lumbar drain or by opening the cisterns.

Closure The dura was sutured watertight using either running or interrupted 4–0 nylon sutures, and duraplasty was performed as needed. The bone flap is secured with titanium plates and screws, and any gaps are filled with hydroxyapatite cement to prevent temporal hollowing. The temporalis muscle is dissected to the frontal periosteum using nonabsorbable sutures to minimize postoperative atrophy. The skin is closed in layers using subcuticular absorbable sutures to achieve optimal cosmetic outcomes.

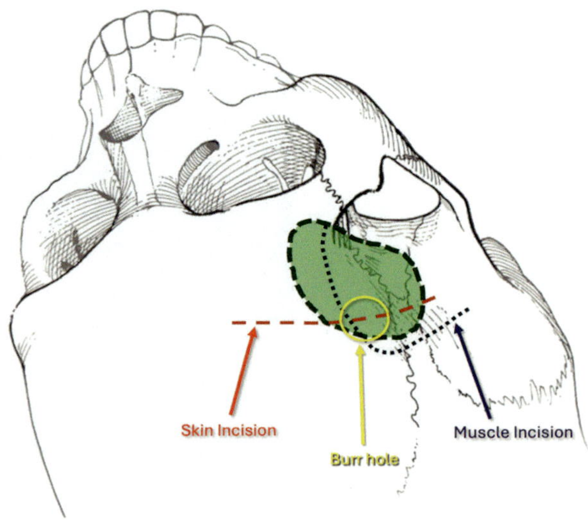

Fig. 5.4 Anatomical illustration of the Helsinki style mini-pterional (or Lateral Supraorbital mini-pterional) showing the skin incision, mini-pterional area (green area), burr hole placement, and its relationship with the temporal muscle incision

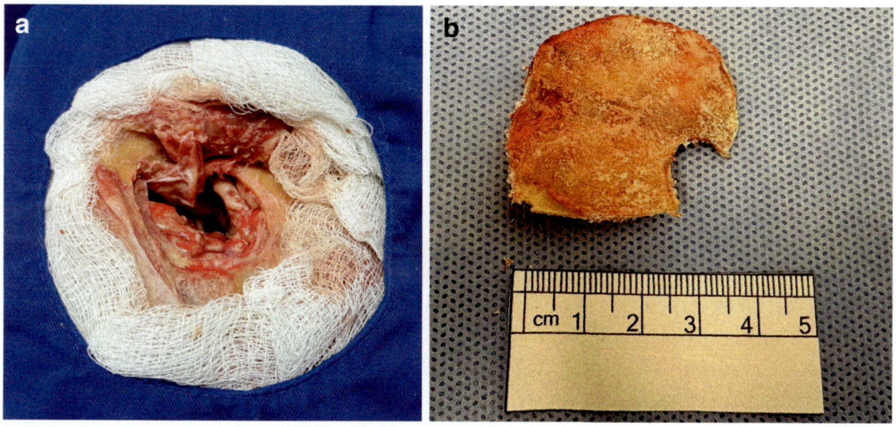

Fig. 5.5 Photographs showing Helsinki's style mini-pterional (on the right side) after the microsurgery in **a** and the bone flap in **b**

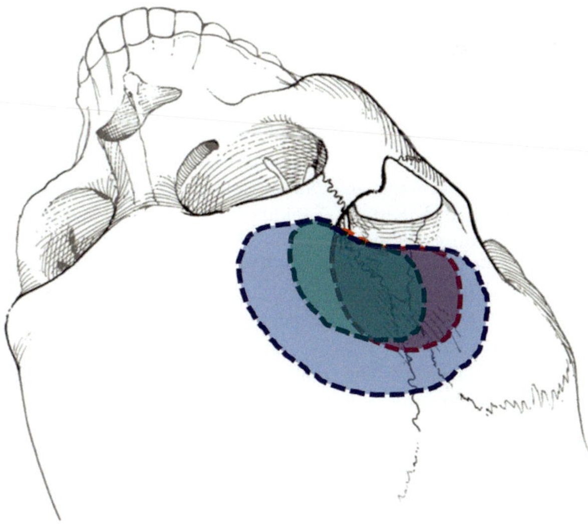

Fig. 5.6 Illustration showing the comparative areas between the pterional (blue area), mini-pterional standard (red area), and Helsinki's mini-pterional style (green area)

5.5 Pearls and Pitfalls

- *Standard mini-pterional: The* incision *starts* 1 cm above the zygomatic arch and extends superiorly toward the midpupillary line; use the interfascial muscle dissection technique and a second cut posteriorly between the temporal lines; place the single burr hole is placed at MacCarthy's point, and a 3 cm craniotomy is performed to ensure adequate working space while minimizing soft tissue disruption.

- *Helsinki's mini-pterional style:* The skin incision will be 1 cm anterior to the tragus and 3 cm above the zygomatic arch in a curvilinear fashion to the midline; cut the temporal muscle in a V-shaped with monopolar; place the burr hole at the posterior edge of the planned craniotomy, and complete the craniotomy Sylvian-centered.
- *Sphenoid Ridge Flattening:* Minimal drilling is performed to enhance exposure to the Sylvian fissure while avoiding excessive bone removal.
- *Dural opening: A* curvilinear or cruciate incision with tenting sutures is used to prevent epidural venous oozing.
- *Microsurgical Exposure:* Visualization is optimized by opening basal cisterns for CSF drainage to enhance brain relaxation.
- *Closure Technique:* Perform watertight dural closure; reapproximate the temporalis muscle to the frontal periosteum to prevent postoperative hollowing; use titanium plates and hydroxyapatite cement to restore the skull contour and improve cosmesis.

References

1. Figueiredo J, Vaz-Guimarães F, Ribas GC, et al. The minipterional craniotomy: indications, technical aspects, and surgical results. Neurosurg Rev. 2020;43(3):907–15.
2. Reisch R, Perneczky A. Ten-year experience with the supraorbital subfrontal approach through an eyebrow skin incision. Neurosurgery. 2005;57(4 Suppl):242–55.
3. Zabramski JM, Kiris T, Sankhla SK, Cabiol J, Spetzler RF. Orbitozygomatic craniotomy. Neurosurgery. 1998;42(5):1205–13.
4. Harland SP, Hussein A, Gullan RW. Modification of the standard pterional approach for aneurysms of the anterior circle of Willis. Br J Neurosurg. 1996;10(2):149–53.
5. Yasargil MG, Fox JL. The microsurgical approach to intracranial aneurysms. Surg Neurol. 1975;3:7–14.
6. Brock M, Dietz H. The small frontolateral approach for the microsurgical treatment of intracranial aneurysms. Neurochirurgia. 1978;21:185–91.
7. Figueiredo EG, et al. The minipterional craniotomy: technical description and anatomic assessment. Neurosurgery. 2007;61(ONS Suppl 2):ONS256–65.
8. Tsunoda S, et al. Comparison of postoperative temporalis muscle atrophy between the muscle-preserving pterional approach and the mini-pterional approach in the treatment of unruptured intracranial aneurysms. Neurosurg Rev. 2022;45(1):507–15.
9. Jägersberg M, Brodard J, Qiu J, et al. Quantification of working volumes, exposure and target-specific maneuverability of the pterional craniotomy and its minimally invasive variants. World Neurosurg. 2017;101:710–717.e2.
10. Veldeman M, et al. How I do it – Helsinki style mini-pterional craniotomy for clipping of middle cerebral artery bifurcation aneurysms. Acta Neurochir. 2023;165:489–93.

Minimally Invasive Approaches: Supraorbital and Supraorbital-Zygomatic

6

6.1 Introduction

Minimally invasive cranial approaches have emerged as alternatives to traditional craniotomies that reduce surgical morbidity while maintaining effective access to intracranial targets. Techniques such as mini-pterional and supraorbital craniotomies, often referred to as key-hole approaches, offer less soft tissue disruption, smaller working volumes, and comparable deep exposure to standard pterional craniotomies. These methods have been quantitatively evaluated using navigation-based imaging to assess their exposure and maneuverability, demonstrating their feasibility for various anterior and middle cranial fossa pathologies [1, 2].

Minimally invasive cranial approaches follow the key-hole surgery concept, aiming to access intracranial structures through the smallest possible openings while preserving surrounding tissues and reducing patient morbidity. In line with this goal, these approaches were developed to minimize temporal muscle and fat pad atrophy, reduce skin incision, and promote fast operative recovery. Despite their benefits, complications such as transient facial nerve palsy, supraorbital hyperesthesia, and periorbital edema must be considered when selecting an approach [1–3].

Pterional craniotomy evolved throughout the twentieth century, and it was pioneered by neurosurgeons who were originally general surgeons who had an interest in cranial surgery. However, in the 1970s, Yasargil provided a detailed modern description of the approach, emphasizing its effectiveness in exposing the Sylvian fissure at the apex of a triangular region between the frontal and temporal lobes while minimizing brain retraction [4, 5]. This refinement has established pterional

Supplementary Information The online version contains supplementary material available at https://doi.org/10.1007/978-3-032-04664-2_6. The videos can be accessed individually by clicking the DOI link in the accompanying figure caption or by scanning this link with the SN More Media App.

H. de Oliveira Manduca Palmiero, E. G. Figueiredo, *Neurosurgical Approaches Video Atlas*, https://doi.org/10.1007/978-3-032-04664-2_6

craniotomy as the gold standard for treating anterior circulation aneurysms and skull base tumors. Over time, further modifications led to the development of minimally invasive variants, such as mini-pterional craniotomy, which retains the benefits of the traditional technique while reducing surgical trauma and enhancing postoperative recovery [2]

Supraorbital craniotomy, performed through a curvilinear incision behind the hairline or through an eyebrow incision, is a minimally invasive key-hole approach that provides access to the anterior cranial fossa, sellar, and parasellar regions while minimizing brain retraction and preserving cosmetic outcomes [6]. This approach has been used to effectively treat aneurysms and tumors in the supra- and parasellar areas [6]. A variation, the supraorbital-zygomatic approach extends by incorporating the zygomatic bone and lateral orbital wall, thereby enhancing access to deep skull base structures while maintaining the principles of minimal invasiveness [7] (Fig. 6.1).

Minimally invasive approaches have been increasingly used for the surgical treatment of both unruptured and ruptured intracranial aneurysms, resulting in reduced surgical morbidity and faster recovery. For elective surgeries, key-hole techniques, such as supraorbital, supraorbital-zygomatic, and mini-pterional craniotomies, provide adequate exposure for aneurysm clipping while minimizing brain retraction, soft tissue dissection, and postoperative complications [8]. In cases of ruptured aneurysms, minimally invasive strategies aim to balance effective aneurysm obliteration with minimal disruption to surrounding structures, often incorporating early cerebrospinal fluid drainage and brain relaxation techniques to optimize the surgical corridor [8]. Compared with conventional craniotomies, these approaches have similar aneurysm occlusion rates and superior cosmetic and functional outcomes [9].

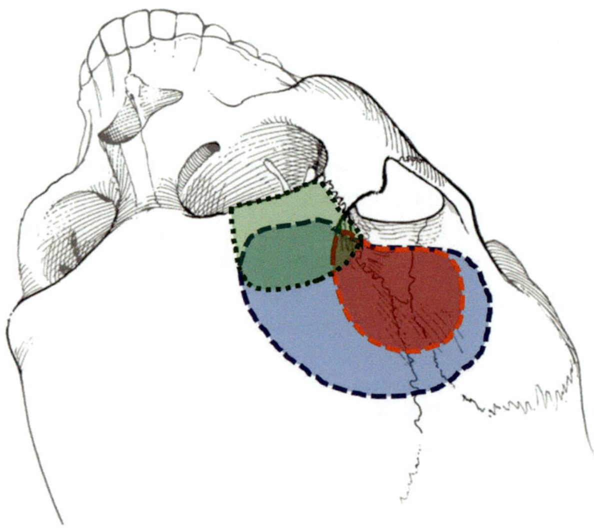

Fig. 6.1 Anatomical illustration showing the pterional, supraorbital, and mini-pterional areas

6.2 Indications for the Approach

The supraorbital and supraorbital-zygomatic approaches are minimally invasive techniques for lesions in the anterior cranial fossa, sellar, and parasellar regions, as well as selected aneurysms of the anterior circulation. The supraorbital approach, performed through an eyebrow incision, is particularly useful for anterior communicating artery aneurysms, internal carotid artery aneurysms, and tumors involving the suprasellar and orbital regions, allowing access with minimal soft tissue disruption and excellent cosmetic outcomes [6]. The supraorbital-zygomatic approach extends this exposure by incorporating the zygomatic bone and lateral orbital wall, making it advantageous for larger skull base tumors, complex aneurysms, and lesions requiring greater lateral access, such as those at the middle fossa (mesial temporal lobe, e.g., selective amygdalo-hippocampectomy) or cavernous sinus [7]. These approaches reduce brain retraction, improve surgical angles, and enhance the visualization of deep-seated structures while maintaining minimally invasive neurosurgery.

6.3 Operative Set-Up [6, 7]

Patient Positioning The patient is in the supine position on the operating table, ensuring proper alignment for optimal surgical access. A Mayfield three-pin or Sugita head holder is used to stabilize the head for precise positioning.

Head Positioning

(a) *Elevation.* The head is elevated approximately 15°–20° above the cardiac level to facilitate venous drainage and minimize intracranial pressure.

(b) *Rotation.* The head is rotated 10°–30° contralaterally, depending on the target lesion, with more rotation required for anterior communicating artery aneurysms and less for parasellar lesions.

(c) *Extension.* The head is extended 10°–15° to promote gravity-assisted frontal lobe retraction, optimizing exposure of the surgical corridor while avoiding excessive tension on the bridging veins.

Skin Preparation The surgical field is sterilized from the forehead to the upper neck, including the periorbital region. The eyebrow and surrounding or frontotemporal skin (depending on the incision) are cleansed with an antiseptic solution (shampoo and chlorhexidine or povidone-iodine) while ensuring ocular surface protection. Draping is performed to expose the supraorbital region while maintaining a sterile environment while preserving anatomical landmarks for precise incision placement.

6.4 Surgical Technique [6, 7] (Video 6.1)

Skin Incision The incision was made using the following procedure:

(a) *Eyebrow Incision:* A curved incision is made along the lateral two-thirds of the eyebrow, preserving the supraorbital nerve when possible. This provides access to the supraorbital key-hole without significant cosmetic impact.
(b) *Frontotemporal Incision:* A short curvilinear incision behind the hairline extends from 1 cm above the zygomatic arch toward the midline, allowing a more lateral exposure for the supraorbital-zygomatic modification or the supraorbital depending on the neurosurgeon's choice.

Muscle Flap The frontal belly of the occipitofrontalis and orbicularis oculi muscles is carefully dissected to avoid injury to the frontalis branch of the facial nerve. In the frontotemporal incision, the temporalis muscle is elevated subperiosteally and retracted posteriorly to expose the orbital rim and key-hole region.

Craniotomy A single burr hole is placed just behind the superior temporal line, followed by a small (approximately 2.5 × 1.5 cm) supraorbital craniotomy using a high-speed drill. The inner aspect of the orbital rim can be drilled to enhance the visualization of deep structures, especially in the supraorbital-zygomatic approach. For the supraorbital-zygomatic approach, a burr hole can be placed at the frontozygomatic suture (Figs. 6.2, 6.3, and 6.4).

Dural Opening The dura is opened curvilinearly or C-shaped, with the base toward the supraorbital rim to allow maximum exposure. Cerebrospinal fluid drainage from the basal cisterns facilitates brain relaxation, minimizing the need for retraction.

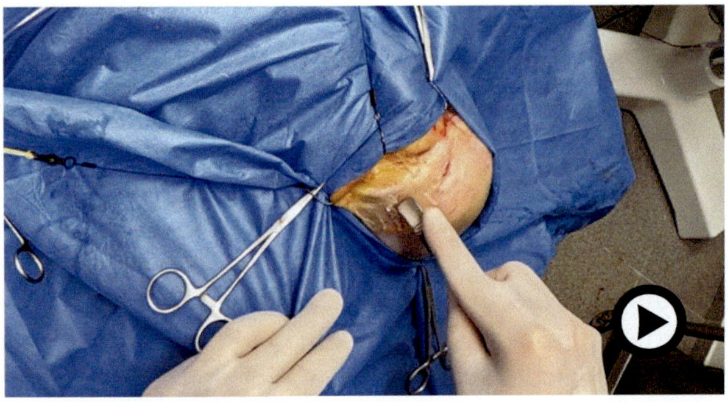

Video 6.1 In this video, we demonstrate the supraorbital craniotomy step-by-step, emphasizing key technical details and anatomical landmarks that enable safe and effective access to anterior cranial fossa and parasellar lesions through a minimally invasive corridor (▶ https://doi.org/10.1007/000-hsx)

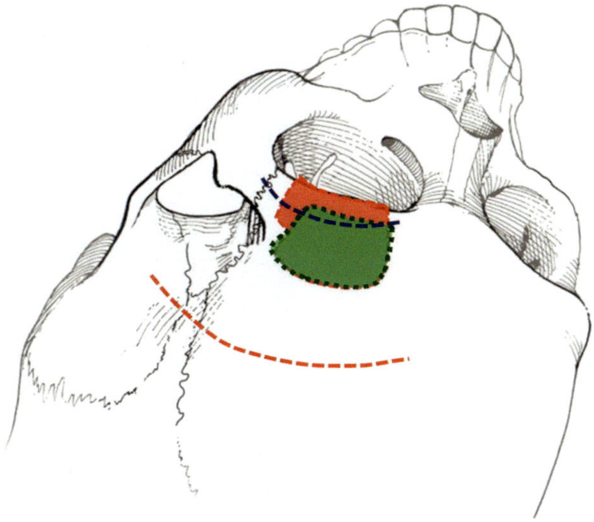

Fig. 6.2 Illustration showing the areas of the supraorbital (green area) and supraorbital-zygomatic (green and red areas combined) craniotomies and eyebrow (blue dashed line) and frontotemporal incisions (red dashed line)

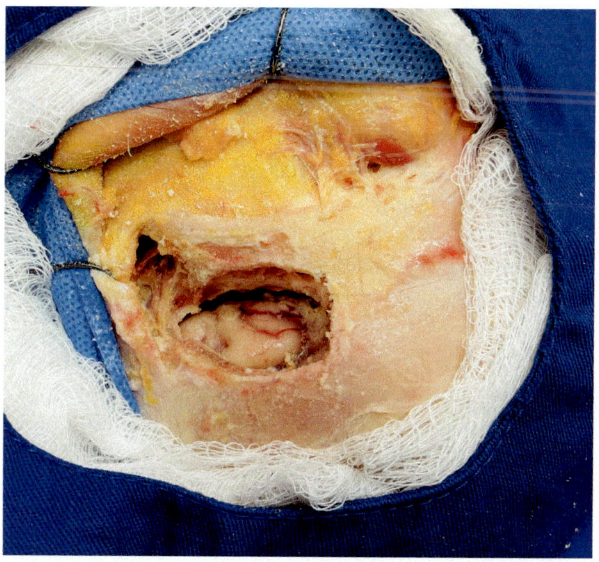

Fig. 6.3 Photograph depicting a supraorbital craniotomy with gauzes and a blue fenestrated drape

Closure The dura was closed in a watertight fashion to prevent cerebrospinal fluid leakage. The bone flap is secured using titanium plates or sutures. The muscle and soft tissues are reapproximated with interrupted sutures, and the skin is closed with absorbable sutures or adhesive glue to optimize cosmetic results.

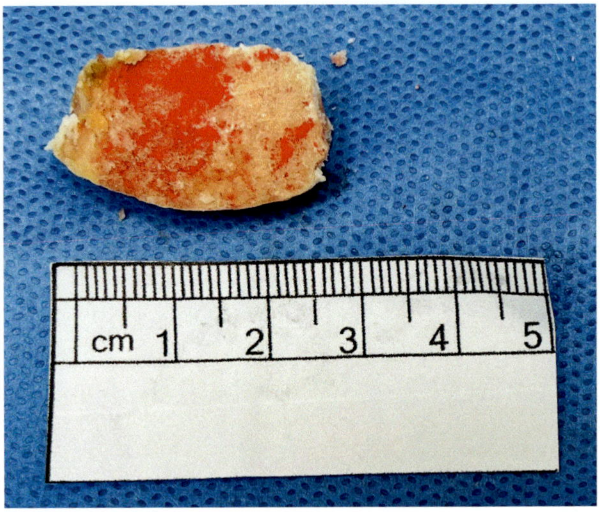

Fig. 6.4 Photograph showing the bone flap with an approximate diameter of 2.5 cm

6.5 Pearls and Pitfalls

- *Minimal Invasiveness:* This technique reduces soft tissue dissection, brain retraction, and postoperative morbidity while maintaining adequate exposure. It is also associated with a faster recovery and shorter hospital stay compared with traditional craniotomies.
- *Cosmetic Advantage:* Eyebrow incision offers excellent esthetic outcomes with minimal visible scarring.
- *Versatility:* Use for anterior circulation aneurysms, skull base tumors, and parasellar lesions.
- *Orbital Rim Drilling:* Enhances visualization of deep-seated structures, particularly in the supraorbital-zygomatic approach.
- *Neuronavigation:* Useful for precise planning and minimizing craniotomy size while maximizing exposure.
- *Early CSF Drainage:* Facilitates brain relaxation, reducing the need for excessive retraction.
- *Limited Working Space:* Requires precise microsurgical skills due to restricted maneuverability.
- *Inadequate exposure for deep lesions: This approach may* not be optimal for lesions requiring extensive lateral or posterior access.
- *Risk of Supraorbital Nerve Injury:* If not carefully preserved, it may cause transient or permanent hypesthesia.
- *Facial nerve considerations:* There is a risk of temporary or permanent frontalis weakness if the incision is improperly placed.

References

1. Jägersberg M, Brodard J, Qiu J, et al. Quantification of working volumes, exposure, and target-specific maneuverability of the pterional craniotomy and its minimally invasive variants. World Neurosurg. 2017;101:710–7.
2. Rychen J, Croci D, Roethlisberger M, et al. Minimally invasive alternative approaches to pterional craniotomy: a systematic review. World Neurosurg. 2018;113:163–79.
3. Figueiredo J, Vaz-Guimarães F, Ribas GC, et al. The minipterional craniotomy: indications, technical aspects, and surgical results. Neurosurg Rev. 2020;43(3):907–15.
4. Rubio RR, Martinez E, Carceller F, et al. Immersive surgical anatomy of the pterional approach. Cureus. 2019;11(7):e5216.
5. Yasargil MG. Microneurosurgery, vol. 1. Stuttgart: Georg Thieme Verlag; 1984. p. 215–33.
6. Reisch R, Perneczky A, Filippi R. Surgical technique of the supraorbital keyhole craniotomy. Surg Neurol. 2003;59:223–7.
7. Figueiredo EG, Deshmukh V, Nakaji P, et al. An anatomical evaluation of the mini-supraorbital approach and comparison with standard craniotomies. Neurosurgery. 2006;59(ONS Suppl 4):ONS-212–20.
8. Karadimas S, Shakil H, Almeida JP, et al. Minimally invasive and outpatient aneurysm surgery: new concepts. Neurosurg Clin N Am. 2022;33:371–82.
9. Xia Z, Wu X, Li J, et al. Minimally invasive surgery is superior to conventional craniotomy in patients with spontaneous supratentorial intracerebral hemorrhage: a systematic review and meta-analysis. World Neurosurg. 2018;115:266–73.

The Frontotemporal-Orbito-Zygomatic Approach

7

7.1 Introduction

Frontotemporal orbitozygomatic (FtOZ) craniotomy evolved from the pterional approach. In the pterional approach, following frontotemporal craniotomy and sphenoid bone drilling, access is gained to the Sylvian fissure, a natural corridor between the frontal and temporal lobes, and from there to the circle of Willis. This approach can be conceived as a skull base extension of the pterional approach. Since the early twentieth century, studies have described the supraorbital approach [1]. However, during the 1980s, some neurosurgeons began publishing a modified approach derived from pterional craniotomy, expanding it to the orbital and zygomatic regions. This modification enabled broader skull base access while minimizing brain retraction [2–6].

Al-Mefty demonstrated that skull base structures can be accessed with minimal brain retraction. Additionally, FtOZ craniotomy provides multiple angles of visualization of the skull base through subfrontal, transsylvian, and subtemporal corridors within the same surgical procedure [6, 7]. After decades of refinement, the FtOZ approach has remained fundamentally unchanged despite the development of minimally invasive variations, such as the supraorbital-zygomatic approach, which also offers subfrontal, transsylvian, and subtemporal perspectives [8]. Moreover, the integrated use of the endoscope has become an additional tool to enhance visualization for the skull base surgeon.

FtOZ in One, Two, and Three-Piece Approaches Technically, the FtOZ approach evolved by incorporating the orbital region into the frontotemporal craniotomy (pterional approach) [3], leading to the frontotemporal-orbital craniotomy.

Supplementary Information The online version contains supplementary material available at https://doi.org/10.1007/978-3-032-04664-2_7. The videos can be accessed individually by clicking the DOI link in the accompanying figure caption or by scanning this link with the SN More Media App.

H. de Oliveira Manduca Palmiero, E. G. Figueiredo, *Neurosurgical Approaches Video Atlas*, https://doi.org/10.1007/978-3-032-04664-2_7

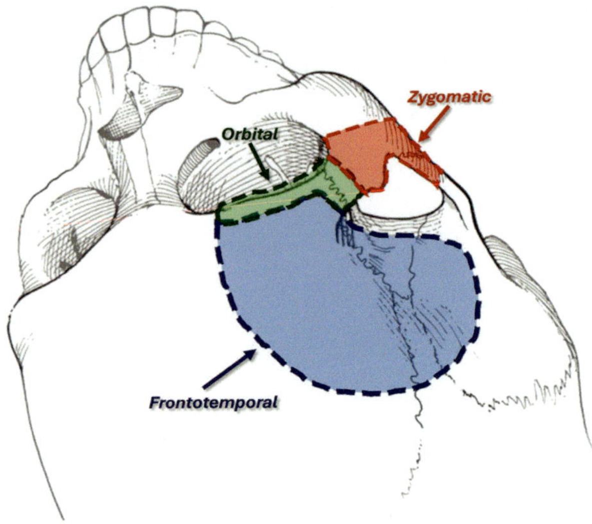

Fig. 7.1 Illustration showing the three FtOZ pieces: (**a**) frontotemporal (blue), (**b**) orbital (green), (**c**) zygomatic (red)

Subsequently, a further modification was made to the zygomatic region [4, 5]. Thus, from an anatomical perspective, the FtOZ craniotomy consists of three osseous components: (a) The frontotemporal segment, (b) The orbital segment, and (c) The zygomatic segment (Fig. 7.1).

7.2 Indications for the Approach

Frontotemporal-orbitozygomatic (FtOZ) craniotomy allows access to lesions such as spheno-orbital meningiomas [2], midline suprasellar masses (including tuberculum sellae meningiomas, craniopharyngiomas, pituitary tumors, and lesions of the anterior third ventricle region), optic-carotid region tumors, osseous lesions such as fibrous dysplasia [1], and pathologies involving the interpeduncular cistern and upper paraclival region [2]. Additionally, it is utilized in vascular procedures, including clipping of anterior communicating artery and basilar tip aneurysms [2].

7.3 Operative Set-Up

Patient Positioning The patient is positioned supine, with the head secured in a Mayfield or Sugita head holder [2, 9, 10]. Al-Mefty recommends using a lumbar drain to regulate CSF drainage, facilitate brain relaxation, and minimize the need for brain retraction. We do not recommend its use because the cerebrospinal fluid may be rapidly released from the cisterns.

Head Positioning Once the *Mayfield* or *Sugita* head holder is secured, head positioning follows the following principles:

(a) *Elevation:* the head is elevated approximately 15° above the thoracic level to facilitate venous return. Additionally, the head of the surgical table may be raised depending on the patient's anatomy and cervical mobility. It is crucial to elevate the lower limbs when adjusting the table's head position to prevent patient slippage during surgery.
(b) *Rotation:* the head is rotated contralaterally to the craniotomy side, typically between 15° and 60°, depending on the anatomical location of the pathology [2, 9].
(c) *Extension:* the head is slightly extended, positioning the malar eminence at the highest point of the surgical field. This maneuver facilitates posterior displacement of the frontal lobe, thereby widening the surgical corridor [2].

Skin Preparation The scalp was cleansed with shampoo and chlorhexidine, followed by trichotomy, creating a 2-cm strip along the incision line. Trichotomy enhances surgical site hygiene, improves drape adherence, and optimizes wound dressing application [10].

7.4 Surgical Technique (Video 7.1)

Skin Incision A curvilinear incision is made starting 1 cm anterior to the tragus at the level of the zygomatic arch, following the hairline, and extending toward the contralateral pupil region [2, 9, 10] (Fig. 7.2). A cold scalpel was used to avoid monopolar electrocautery, with only the bleeding vessels coagulated using bipolar electrocautery. *Raney* clips are not recommended because they can compromise the cutaneous vascular supply. The superficial temporal artery is carefully preserved, with selective coagulation and transection of the posterior branch only if it is large-caliber and interferes with flap mobilization.

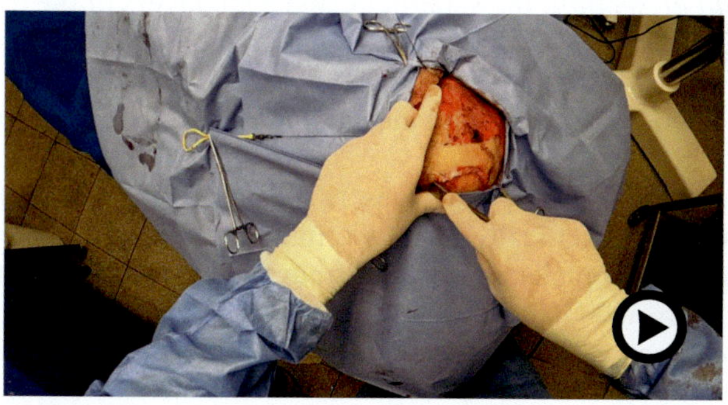

Video 7.1 In this cadaveric surgical video, we demonstrate the two-piece frontotemporal-orbitozygomatic (FtOZ) approach, emphasizing key anatomical landmarks and technical steps that enable extensive skull base exposure while preserving structural integrity for reconstruction (▶ https://doi.org/10.1007/000-hsy)

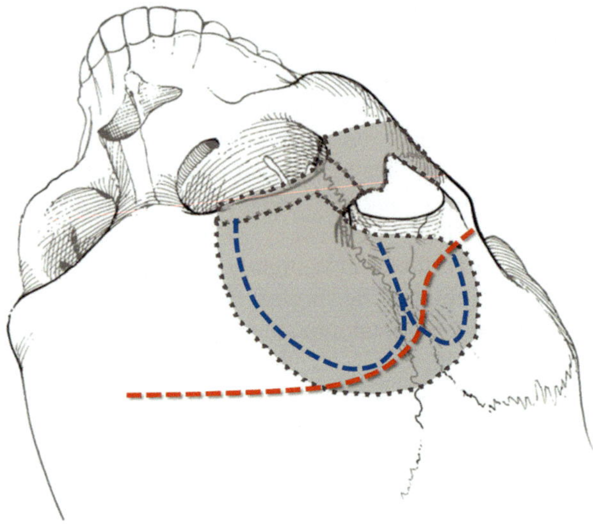

Fig. 7.2 Illustration showing the curvilinear incision, starting 1 cm anterior to the tragus at the level of the zygomatic arch, maintained 1 cm behind the hairline, and extending to the contralateral pupil region (dashed red line). The entire three-piece craniotomy area is also highlighted (shaded in gray), and the light blue represents the dural opening

Muscle Flap We perform the temporal muscle dissection using the Yasargil technique [11] while preserving the facial nerve and freeing the periorbita following these steps [2, 10]:

(a) *A vertical incision* is made in the superficial fascia of the temporalis muscle, starting 2 cm superior to the orbital rim and extending down to the zygomatic arch, using a scalpel to avoid thermal injury from monopolar electrocautery. Next, a straight incision is made along the superior temporal line, leaving a muscle cuff for later reconstruction, extending posteriorly to the limit of the skin incision. The dissection proceeds vertically in a straight line, reaching near the auricle, similar to pterional craniotomy.
(b) *Interfascial dissection:* the superficial and deep layers of the temporalis fascia are carefully separated along the interfascial plane to protect the frontotemporal branch of the facial nerve. The nerve runs within the loose areolar tissue between these layers and must be preserved to prevent frontalis muscle palsy.
(c) *Muscle elevation:* the temporalis muscle is detached in a Yasargil-like manner, meaning it is split vertically along the muscle fibers and retracted inferiorly rather than being completely detached from the bone. This treatment preserves vascular supply and facilitates repositioning.
(d) *Muscle mobilization:* the muscle is reflected inferiorly by subperiosteal dissection, keeping it attached to the zygomatic arch. Alternatively, if a three-piece orbitozygomatic osteotomy is performed, the muscle is mobilized while keeping its tendinous insertion intact.
(e) *Hemostasis and retraction:* bipolar coagulation is used minimally to preserve muscle viability, and retraction is performed using rubber bands or sutures to prevent ischemia.

This technique ensures effective exposure while minimizing postoperative muscle atrophy and facial nerve injury.

The periorbita is dissected from the orbital rim using a dissector, performing delicate yet precise movements toward the bony surface to avoid periorbital injury. If the periorbita is damaged, periorbital fat tissue becomes visible.

Craniotomy To perform craniotomy, we follow these steps based on whether one-piece, two-piece, or three-piece craniotomy is required.

7.4.1 One-Piece OZ Craniotomy [2]

First burr hole (MacCarty's Point): placed at the keyhole region, just posterior to the frontozygomatic suture, anterior to the superior temporal line [12]. Alternatively, two additional burr holes can be used. The second burr hole was located at the pterion, just above the superior temporal line, facilitating the basal cut. A third burr bole can be placed at the posterior temporal region to facilitate posterior disconnection of the temporal bone.

Craniotomy cut: the bone flap is elevated in a single piece, including the frontal, temporal, orbital roof, and zygomatic components. Finally, the lateral orbital rim is osteotomized using a reciprocating saw. The orbital roof is disconnected along the frontal base.

7.4.2 Two-Piece OZ Craniotomy [13]

Frontotemporal craniotomy: the initial burr holes and cuts are the same as above.

Separate Orbital-Zygomatic Osteotomy: the orbital rim and zygomatic arch are cut and removed as a second piece. The temporalis muscle remains partially attached to the zygomatic arch (Figs. 7.3, 7.4, and 7.5).

7.4.3 Three-Piece OZ Craniotomy

To perform the FtOZ craniotomy in three parts [10], we first create the burr holes as follows: first at MacCarty's Point, second at the posterior, and third burr hole at the posterior temporal. Sequentially for the bone removal: (a) Frontotemporal craniotomy (first piece); (b) Orbital bar removal (second piece): cutting the lateral orbital rim and roof; (c) Zygomatic arch removal (third piece): the zygoma is osteotomized to allow better access to the middle fossa.

Dural Opening The craniotomy was completed with wide frontotemporal exposure. The dural opening can be C-shaped, with its base directed anteriorly and

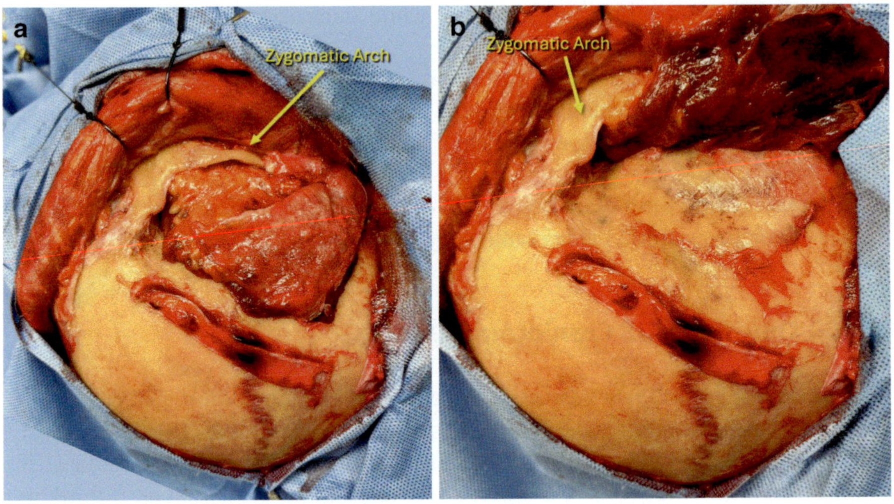

Fig. 7.3 Photographs showing the temporalis muscle over the temporal bone before (**a**) and after being everted inferiorly (**b**). The temporalis muscle is related to the zygomatic arch, requiring dissection down to its base on the temporal bone to remove the orbito-zygomatic piece

Fig. 7.4 Photograph illustrating the frontotemporal-orbitozygomatic craniotomy before being covered by gauze and the blue fenestrated drape

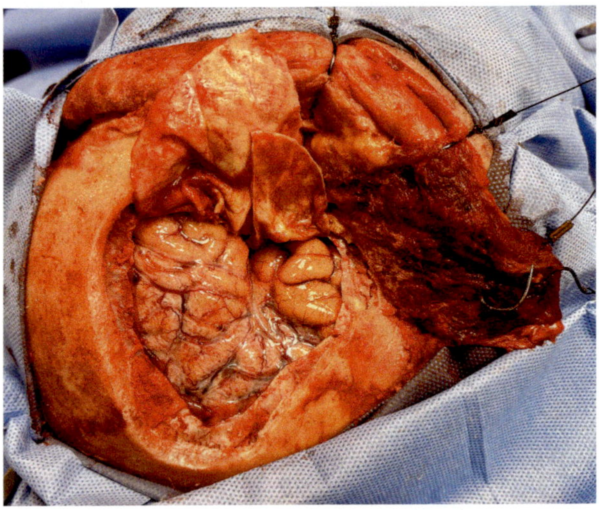

folded in half using Ethibond sutures. However, as described in the literature and routinely practiced, we prefer an M-shaped or S-shaped dural opening [10]. In this approach, the first part of the "M" corresponds to the frontal region, with its base directed posteriorly, while the second part of the "M" corresponds to the temporal region, with its base directed anteriorly (Figs. 7.2 and 7.6). This configuration optimizes basal exposure of the frontal and temporal lobe. We recommend anchoring the dura to elevate the dural edges, improve access, and minimize retraction (Fig. 7.7) [2].

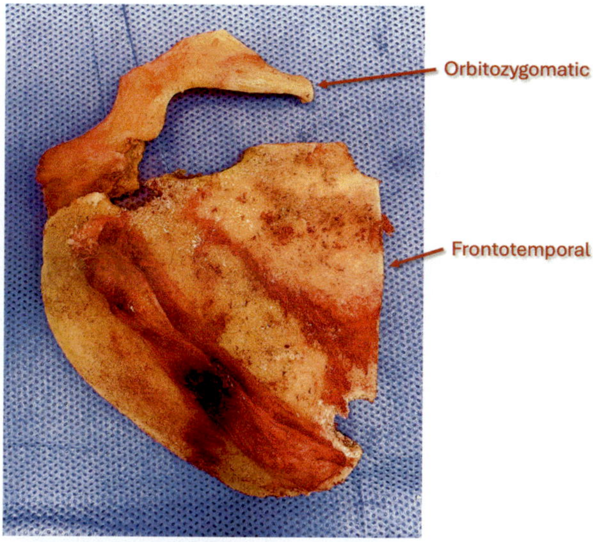

Fig. 7.5 See in this photograph the two bone fragments corresponding to the piece from the frontotemporal craniotomy and the piece from the orbitozygomatic region

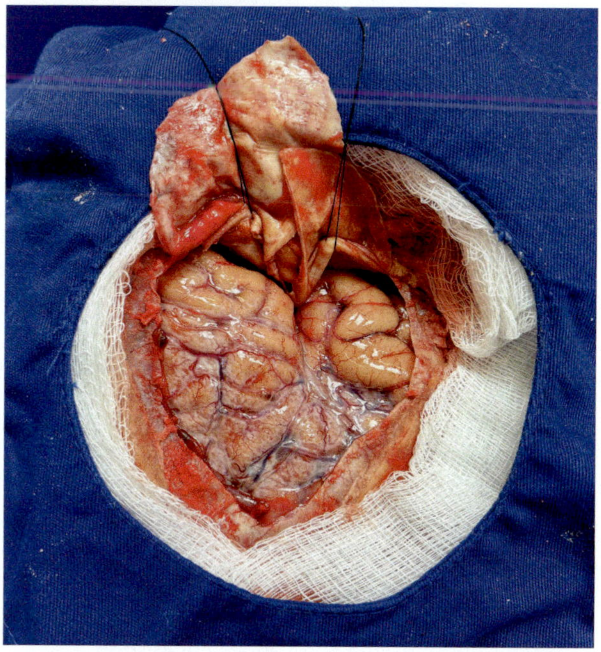

Fig. 7.6 In this photograph, we see the frontotemporal-orbitozygomatic craniotomy with gauze and the blue fenestrated drape; the dura mater opened and ready for microsurgery

Closure A major distinction between the One-, Two-, and Three-Piece craniotomies lies in the reconstruction process. We achieve esthetic and functional bone segment restoration using mini-plates. The orbital fragment, which constitutes the roof of the orbit, must be precisely repositioned to prevent ocular movement impairment or enophthalmos [14]. Similarly, the zygomatic fragment is closely related to

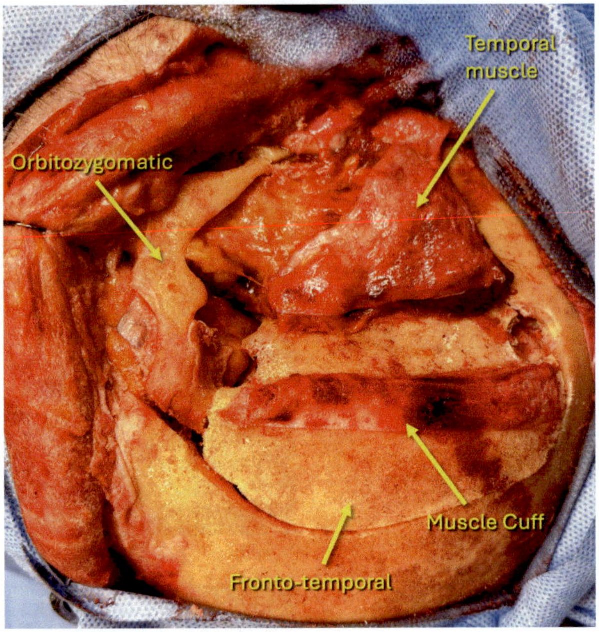

Fig. 7.7 See in this photograph the repositioned bone fragments (orbitozygomatic and fronto-temporal pieces); the temporalis muscle is reflected and should be reapproximated to the muscle cuff

the temporalis muscle and plays a crucial role in facial esthetics and temporomandibular joint dysfunction [15].

Bone Flap Repositioning Depending on the craniotomy technique, the bone flap is reattached as follows: One-Piece: reattached using mini plates and screws; Two-Piece: orbital-zygomatic segment fixed first, then the craniotomy; Three-Piece: zygomatic arch, orbital roof, and cranial bone are repositioned in sequential order.

The dural closure must be watertight and may require the use of fascia and adipose tissue grafts, as described by Al-Mefty [9]. At the end of the procedure, the temporalis muscle is repositioned using resorbable sutures or burr hole anchoring to minimize atrophy and maintain the esthetic contour.

7.5 Pearls and Pitfalls

- *Rotation of the head:* Excessive contralateral rotation (>60°) may cause jugular venous compression and venous congestion.
- *Interfascial dissection:* The frontotemporal branch of the facial nerve is dissected by carefully separating the superficial and deep layers of the temporalis fascia.
- *Sequential Bone Removal:* In a three-piece craniotomy, the frontotemporal bone, orbital roof, and zygomatic arch are removed to ensure better skull base access.

- *Periorbita Dissection:* Aggressive periorbital dissection risks fat prolapse, potentially affecting ocular function and esthetics. Apply delicate yet precise movements toward the bony surface to avoid periorbital injury.
- *Zygomatic Arch Removal:* Failure to fully mobilize the zygoma limits lateral skull base exposure and increases brain retraction requirements.
- *Dural opening:* An S-shaped dural incision was made to improve the exposure of the basal frontal and temporal lobes.
- *Dural Closure:* Failure to achieve a watertight seal increases the risk of CSF leakage and infection. If necessary, fascial lata and adipose grafts can be used for dural closure.
- *Reconstruction with miniplates:* Stable bone fixation to prevent cosmetic deformity, diplopia, enophthalmos, restriction of extraocular movement, temporalis muscle atrophy, and temporomandibular joint dysfunction.

References

1. Al-Mefty O, Smith RR. Tailoring the cranio-orbital approach. Keio J Med. 1990;39(4):217–24.
2. El Ahmadieh TY, Cavallo C, Syed HR, et al. Frontotemporal-orbitozygomatic approach and its variants: technical nuances and video illustration. Oper Neurosurg. 2022;23(6):441–8.
3. Jane JA, Park TS, Becker DP. The supraorbital approach: technical note. Neurosurgery. 1982;11:537–42.
4. Pellerin P, Lesoin F, Dhellemmes P, et al. Usefulness of the orbitofrontomalar approach associated with bone reconstruction for frontotemporosphenoid meningiomas. Neurosurgery. 1984;15(5):715–8.
5. Hakuba A, Kawai S, Katsuyama J, et al. The orbitozygomatic infratemporal approach: a new surgical technique. Surg Neurol. 1986;26:271–6.
6. Al-Mefty O. Supraorbital-pterional approach to skull base lesions. Neurosurgery. 1987;21(4):474–7.
7. Al-Mefty O, Anand VK. Zygomatic approach to skull-base lesions. J Neurosurg. 1990;73:668–73.
8. Figueiredo EG, Deshmukh P, Nakaji P, et al. An anatomical evaluation of the mini-supraorbital approach and comparison with standard craniotomies. Neurosurgery. 2006;59(ONS Suppl 4):ONS-212–20.
9. Sindou M. Practical handbook of neurosurgery: chapter how to perform cranio-orbital zygomatic approaches by Al-Mefty O. New York: Springer Wien; 2009.
10. Chaddad-Neto F, Rassi-Neto A, Oliveira E. Orbitozygomatic craniotomy in three pieces: tips and tricks. Arq Neuropsiquiatr. 2016;74(3):228–34.
11. Yasargil MG. Microneurosurgery, vol. 1. Stuttgart: Georg Thieme Verlag; 1984. p. 215–33.
12. Abdel Aziz KM, Sanan A, van Loveren HR, et al. The one-piece orbitozygomatic approach: the MacCarty burr hole and the inferior orbital fissure as keys to technique and application. Acta Neurochir. 2002;144:15–24.
13. Tanriover N, Ulm AJ, Rhoton AL Jr, et al. One-piece versus two-piece orbitozygomatic craniotomy: quantitative and qualitative considerations. Oper Neurosurg. 2006;2(58):ONS-229–37.
14. Zabramski JM, Kiris T, Sankhla SK, et al. Orbitozygomatic craniotomy: technical note. J Neurosurg. 1998;89:336–41.
15. van Furth WR, Agur AM, Delashaw JB, et al. The orbitozygomatic approach. Neurosurgery. 2005;58(ONS Suppl 1):ONS-103–7.

Extradural and Intradural Clinoidectomy

8

8.1 Introduction

The anterior clinoid process is a bony projection of the sphenoid bone at the junction of the lesser wing and the sphenoid body. As a bridge, the optic strut connects the lesser sphenoid wing to the sphenoid body [1, 2]. It is situated near critical structures, such as the optic nerve, internal carotid artery, and ophthalmic artery, making it a significant landmark in neurosurgical procedures [1] (Fig. 8.1).

Anterior clinoidectomy is performed to enhance surgical access to critical structures in the parasellar and paraclinoid regions of the skull base. By removing the anterior clinoid process, surgeons can better visualize and manage lesions such as paraclinoid aneurysms and parasellar tumors, including meningiomas, located near vital structures such as the internal carotid artery and optic nerve. This procedure facilitates safer dissection and manipulation of these areas, thereby reducing the risk of injury to adjacent neurovascular structures [3].

Dolenc in the 1980s described extradural anterior clinoidectomy as a surgical step for clipping ophthalmic artery aneurysms of the internal carotid artery [4, 5] and gaining access to cavernous sinus lesions [6]. The rationale for the extradural approach to the anterior clinoid is the protection provided by the dura mater to intracranial structures [7]. The intradural method allows for *en bloc* removal of the clinoid process, thereby minimizing bone dust dispersion and reducing operative time. However, this procedure requires meticulous handling to protect the surrounding neurovascular structures [2, 3].

Supplementary Information The online version contains supplementary material available at https://doi.org/10.1007/978-3-032-04664-2_8. The videos can be accessed individually by clicking the DOI link in the accompanying figure caption or by scanning this link with the SN More Media App.

H. de Oliveira Manduca Palmiero, E. G. Figueiredo, *Neurosurgical Approaches Video Atlas*, https://doi.org/10.1007/978-3-032-04664-2_8

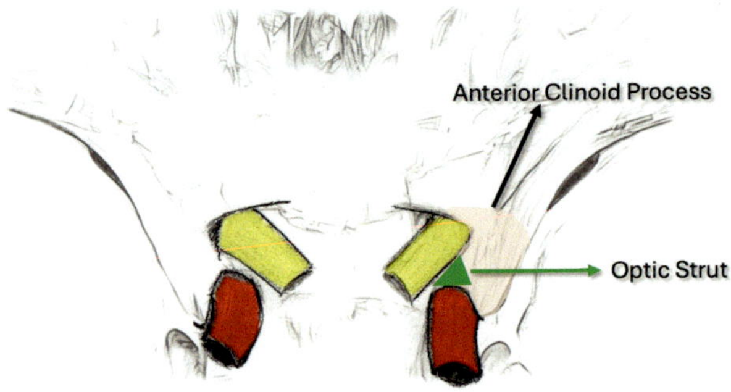

Fig. 8.1 Illustration showing the anterior clinoid process and the optic strut (green triangle), the optic nerves (highlighted in yellow), and the internal carotid arteries (highlighted in red)

8.2 Indications

Anterior clinoidectomy is indicated for the surgical management of vascular and neoplastic lesions in the paraclinoid and parasellar regions. Vascular indications primarily include aneurysms of the internal carotid artery, particularly those involving the ophthalmic and clinoidal segments, where removal of the anterior clinoid process facilitates proximal control and clipping of the aneurysm, and skull base tumors. In terms of neoplastic conditions, clinoidectomy is often performed for meningiomas originating from or extending into the anterior clinoid process, as well as other tumors such as pituitary adenomas and craniopharyngiomas that encroach upon the optic nerve or internal carotid artery. By resecting the anterior clinoid process (ACP), surgeons can better expose and access these critical structures, thereby enhancing the safety and efficacy of the procedure [8–10]. Anterior clinoidectomy improves exposure for treating ophthalmic artery aneurysms and medial sphenoid wing lesions, such as meningiomas [7].

8.3 Operative Set-Up

To perform anterior clinoidectomy using either the extradural or intradural technique, the classic craniotomy approach that provides access to the anterior clinoid is the pterional approach. The pterional approach is a suitable alternative. Variants of the pterional approach, such as the minipterional, supraorbital, or even the frontotemporal-orbitozygomatic approach, also allow for clinoidectomy. The following steps should be standardized across these approaches to ensure proper positioning and access to the ACP:

Patient Positioning The patient is placed in the supine position, and a rolled sheet cushion is placed under the ipsilateral shoulder to the craniotomy, thereby reducing the brachial plexus strain.

Head Positioning The head is fixed using Sugita or Mayfield head holders.

Elevate the head ~15° to improve venous return.

The craniotomy side *is rotated contralaterally* to enhance the exposure of the target region. For anterior clinoidectomy, a 45° view is preferred for better exposure of the clinoid [2].

Extension is needed to position the malar eminence at the highest position in the surgical field. This maneuver positions the anterior clinoid in front of the surgeon's field of view.

Skin Preparation Partial trichotomy is performed to expose the incision site. Use shampoo and chlorhexidine to clean the skin.

8.4 Surgical Technique (Video 8.1)

Skin Incision Using a scalpel, we performed the classic arcuate incision, starting at the level of the zygoma, approximately 1 cm anterior to the tragus, and extending toward the midline. During the incision, try to preserve the superficial temporal

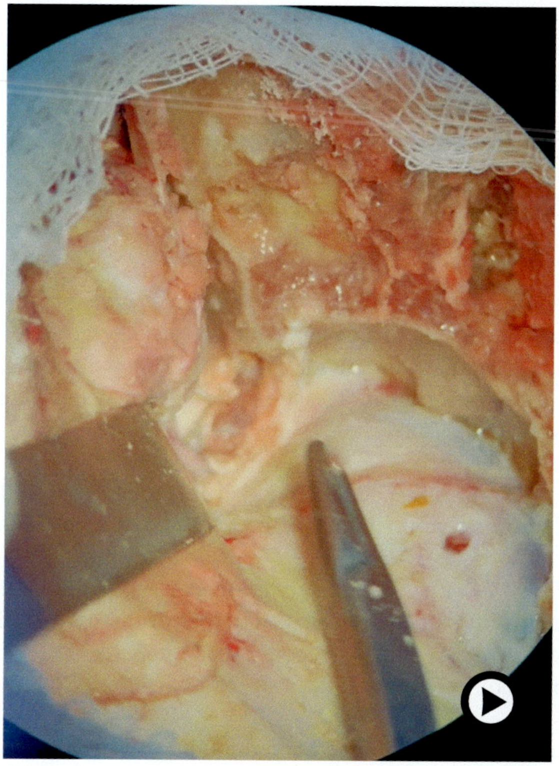

Video 8.1 In this video, we demonstrate anterior clinoidectomy using both extradural and intradural techniques, outlining the step-by-step microsurgical strategies to safely access the parasellar and paraclinoid regions while preserving critical neurovascular structures (▶ https://doi.org/10.1007/000-hsz)

artery [11, 12]. Avoid using *Raney* clips for scalp hemostasis. Use gentle bipolar coagulation instead of monopolar.

Muscle Flap Proceed with the interfascial dissection anteriorly to preserve the facial nerve branch and elevate the muscle after subperiosteal dissection using a periosteal elevator [13]. The dissection of the temporalis muscle follows the principles of straight incisions: first starting 2 cm superior to the orbital rim and extending down to the zygomatic arch; a straight incision along the superior temporal line, leaving a muscle cuff for later reconstruction; and vertically proceeding in a straight line, reaching near the auricle [11–13].

Craniotomy Proceed with the craniotomy following the specific steps for each technique. Considering the pterional craniotomy, the first burr hole will be placed at the keyhole (frontosphenoidal) and, if necessary, at the temporal bone. Dissectors and a periosteal elevator are used to carefully lift the bone flap.

Sphenoid Ridge Drilling: a rongeur or high-speed drill is used to flatten the sphenoid ridge, which facilitates access to the superior orbital fissure and the lateral aspect of the anterior clinoid process [11, 12].

8.4.1 Extradural Anterior Clinoidectomy [7, 14]

Once the sphenoid ridge is flattened and the dura mater remains intact, we proceed with the extradural clinoidectomy as follows:

(a) *Identification and coagulation of the meningo-orbital band*: This dural fold connects the dura mater to the periorbita at the lateral edge of the superior orbital fissure. Coagulate and divide the band to allow further dissection.
(b) *Peeling of the temporal dura:* The temporal dura mater is gently peeled from the lateral wall of the cavernous sinus, exposing the ACP and the proximal optic nerve.
(c) *Drilling the ACP:* A high-speed diamond drill is used to carefully drill the anterior clinoid process while taking care to avoid thermal injury to adjacent structures.
(d) *Removal of the ACP:* once adequately thinned, remove the anterior clinoid process using micro-instruments, ensuring complete removal to optimize exposure.
(e) *Unroofing of the optic canal:* if necessary, the optic canal is decompressed by drilling into its bony covering to improve visualization.

After extradural anterior clinoidectomy, dural anchoring is performed, followed by a C-shaped opening and subsequent microsurgical steps (Fig. 8.2).

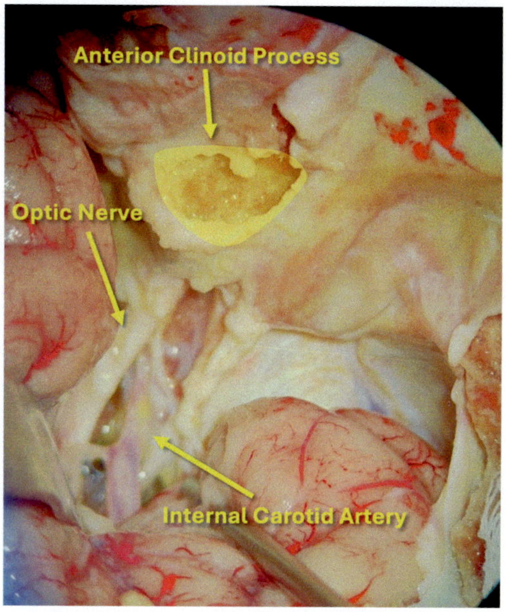

Fig. 8.2 In this picture, by using an intradural microscopic view, we see the area related to the anterior clinoid process once the extradural clinoidectomy is performed, as well as the optic nerve and the internal carotid artery

8.4.2 Intradural Anterior Clinoidectomy [1, 12, 15, 16]

After drilling the sphenoid bone and performing dural anchoring, we performed a C-shaped dural opening using delicate Metzenbaum scissors. This grants access to the intradural space, and we follow the steps:

(a) *Sylvian fissure dissection:* the Sylvian fissure is carefully dissected to expose the optic nerve and internal carotid artery.
(b) *Identification of key structures:* the optic nerve, internal carotid artery, and anterior clinoid process are covered by the dura mater.
(c) *Clinoid dural opening* is a fundamental step in intradural clinoidectomy: during intradural clinoidectomy, the dura is first coagulated from medial to lateral, creating a line intersecting the anterior clinoid process from its free edge to the meningo-orbital band. The coagulated dura is then incised with a no. 11 blade, following the same medial to lateral sequence to minimize vascular and nerve injury. Using *Rhoton* microdissectors, the delineated dura is carefully elevated, including the inferior aspect of the lateral anterior clinoid process edge, which forms the cavernous sinus roof. Finally, the dural flap is reflected posteriorly, excised with microscissors and microforceps, and removed. At this point, the optic strut, a bony ridge connecting the ACP to the sphenoid bone, is also located.
(d) *Drilling the ACP:* A high-speed diamond drill (1–3 mm) is used to carefully drill the ACP, following the same dural coagulation line for *en bloc* removal. However, clinoid drilling can also be performed without *en bloc* extraction.

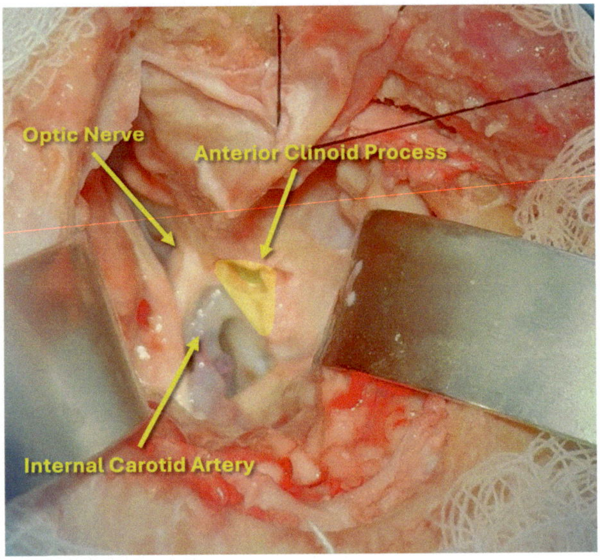

Fig. 8.3 In this picture, we see the area related to the anterior clinoid process once the intradural clinoidectomy is performed, as well as the optic nerve and the internal carotid artery

Maintaining the dissected dura mater helps the surgeon protect the surrounding neurovascular structures. The drilling was performed in a controlled manner with abundant saline irrigation to avoid thermal injuries [3].

(e) *Removal of the ACP:* once adequately thinned, the remaining ACP bone is removed, providing enhanced exposure to the paraclinoid region (Fig. 8.3).
(f) *Optic canal unroofing:* if necessary, the optic canal is unroofed by removing its bony covering to decompress the optic nerve. In addition, we fenestrated the optic nerve sheath to better expose the ophthalmic artery.

Depending on the pneumatization of the clinoid, its removal—whether *en bloc* or partial—may result in communication with the paranasal sinuses. Intraoperative management is recommended after identifying any such connection to prevent postoperative cerebrospinal fluid rhinorrhea. This can be achieved using a fragment of the temporalis muscle and biological glue to seal the defect. Careful manipulation to remove the ACP is mandatory to avoid third nerve injury. Preoperative planning should include a thorough review of CT imaging to assess the degree of clinoid pneumatization [6].

8.5 Pearls and Pitfalls

- *Patient Positioning:* elevating the head by ~15° improves venous return, and a 45° head rotation optimizes anterior clinoid exposure.
- *Surgical Exposure:* flattening the sphenoid ridge with a drill before proceeding with clinoidectomy enhances visualization.

- *Extradural Clinoidectomy:* performing clinoidectomy before dural opening allows protection of intracranial structures.
- *Clinoid Pneumatization:* preoperative CT evaluation helps assess pneumatization to anticipate possible communication with the paranasal sinuses. If the paranasal sinus is opened, sealing with a temporalis muscle graft and biological glue can reduce the risk of postoperative CSF rhinorrhea.
- *Optic Nerve Injury:* excessive retraction or aggressive drilling near the optic canal may cause optic nerve ischemia or visual deficits.
- *Cavernous Sinus Bleeding:* aggressive drilling of the lateral anterior clinoid process may lead to venous bleeding because of its relationship with the roof of the cavernous sinus. This can occur with both extradural and intradural anterior clinoidectomy.

References

1. Ye C, Yang X, Li Z, et al. Anterior clinoid process and the surrounding structures. J Craniofac Surg. 2013;24(6):2098–102.
2. Lehmberg J, Krieg SM, Meyer B. Anterior clinoidectomy. Acta Neurochir. 2014;156:415–9.
3. Alejandro SA, Yagmurlu K, Chaddad-Neto F, et al. Anterior clinoidectomy: intradural step-by-step en bloc removal technique. World Neurosurg. 2021;146:217–31.
4. Dolenc VV. A combined epi- and subdural direct approach to carotid-ophthalmic artery aneurysms. J Neurosurg. 1985;62:667–72.
5. Dolenc V. Direct microsurgical repair of intracavernous vascular lesions. J Neurosurg. 1983;58:824–31.
6. Mikami T, Minamida Y, Koyama J, et al. Anatomical variations in pneumatization of the anterior clinoid process. J Neurosurg. 2007;106:170–4.
7. Jean WC. How I do it: extradural clinoidectomy. Acta Neurochir. 2019;161:2583.
8. Pacheco Junior MG, dos Santos F, Panigassi ACC, et al. Tailored anterior clinoidectomy: beyond the intradural and extradural concepts. Cureus. 2021;13(5):e14874.
9. Kulwin C, Tubbs S, Cohen-Gadol AA. Anterior clinoidectomy: description of an alternative hybrid method and a review of the current techniques with an emphasis on complication avoidance. Surg Neurol Int. 2011;2:140.
10. Yonekawa Y, Ogata N, Imhof HG, et al. Selective extradural anterior clinoidectomy for supra- and parasellar process: technical note. Neurosurg Focus. 1997;87(4):636–42.
11. Vishteh AG, Spetzler RF, Lawton MT, et al. The pterional approach. Oper Tech Neurosurg. 1998;1(1):39–49.
12. Chaddad Neto F, Ribas GC, Oliveira E. A craniotomia pterional. Arq Neuropsiquiatr. 2007;65(1):101–6.
13. Yasargil MG. Microneurosurgery, vol. 1. Stuttgart: Georg Thieme Verlag; 1984. p. 215–33.
14. Mishra S, Leão B, Rosito DM. Extradural anterior clinoidectomy: technical nuances from a learner's perspective. Asian J Neurosurg. 2017;12:189–93.
15. Meybodi AT, Benet A, Rassi-Neto A, et al. Anterior clinoidectomy using an extradural and intradural 2-step hybrid technique. J Neurosurg. 2019;130:238–47.
16. Auricchio AM, Calvanese F, Lehecka M. Exoscopic extradural anterior clinoidectomy. Neurosurg Focus Video. 2024;10(1):V4.

The Interhemispheric Approach

9

9.1 Introduction

The interhemispheric approach is a surgical technique that provides access to deep midline brain structures by navigating through the interhemispheric fissure. This method is particularly useful for reaching the parafalcine and paraventricular regions and contralateral approaches through the midline [1]. The first descriptions referred to Dandy's posterior approach to the pineal region, and progressively, new anterior approaches were published [1]. Yasargil described the interhemispheric approach for the resection of frontoparietal AVM [2]. The interhemispheric approach can also include access to the sellar and suprasellar regions via the interfrontal route [1, 3].

The interhemispheric approach is closely associated with the superior sagittal sinus. Anatomical studies have shown that the superior sagittal sinus can deviate laterally from the midline, with a tendency to be slightly positioned to the right of the sagittal suture in many individuals. The lateral displacement can be up to 1 cm [4]. This anatomical particularity is important because the superior sagittal sinus tends to be located toward the right. Thus, craniotomy should be performed more lateral to the right on this side. Furthermore, when performing the dural opening on the left side, we can open closer to the midline, whereas on the right side, we must be more cautious due to the risk of "premature" opening of the superior sagittal sinus, which may require suturing for repair.

The superior sagittal sinus is typically divided into three-thirds based on anatomical and surgical references [5]:

Supplementary Information The online version contains supplementary material available at https://doi.org/10.1007/978-3-032-04664-2_9. The videos can be accessed individually by clicking the DOI link in the accompanying figure caption or by scanning this link with the SN More Media App.

H. de Oliveira Manduca Palmiero, E. G. Figueiredo, *Neurosurgical Approaches Video Atlas*, https://doi.org/10.1007/978-3-032-04664-2_9

(a) *Anterior third (frontal third)*: extends from the foramen cecum (near the crista galli) to the coronal suture; offers less risk of venous injury when accessing the frontal interhemispheric fissure.
(b) *Middle third (parietal third)*: extends from the coronal suture to the lambda (near the parietal-occipital junction); there is a high risk of venous injury, and careful dissection is needed to preserve the bridging veins.
(c) Posterior third (occipital third): extends from the lambda to the confluence of sinuses (torcular Herophili); injury to this segment can cause catastrophic venous infarction or hemorrhage.

Another anatomical landmark for the interhemispheric approach is the corpus callosum at the depth of the access. Accessing the ventricular system through the interhemispheric approach often involves a transcallosal route, which requires careful consideration of the corpus callosum's anatomy to minimize potential complications. The extent and location of the callosotomy (surgical incision of the corpus callosum) are critical factors affecting surgical outcomes. Although sectioning the anterior part of the corpus callosum may not be associated with severe distinct symptoms, it can cause a decrease in the spontaneity of speech, ranging from mild slowness in initiating speech to mutism. In contrast, division of the posterior corpus callosum and splenium may cause a broad range of behavioral abnormalities. Therefore, the extent of the commissural section should be limited to the extent of surgical necessity [1].

9.2 Indications for the Approach

The interhemispheric approach is indicated for lesions in the midline and deep brain structures, with specific access routes depending on the lesion's location [1]:

(a) *The anterior* interhemispheric approach is used for lesions in the frontal midline region, including anterior third ventricular tumors, anterior corpus callosum lesions, anterior parafalcine meningiomas, anterior communicating artery aneurysms with superior projection, and sellar and suprasellar lesions.
(b) *The median interfrontal (transcallosal)* approach provides access to the lateral and third ventricles for resecting intraventricular tumors such as colloid cysts, craniopharyngiomas, and central neurocytomas. The interhemispheric-transcallosal approach is also essential for ventricular surgeries, including tumor resection and the management of obstructive hydrocephalus. Additionally, corpus callosotomy, a surgical procedure for drug-resistant epilepsy, is performed via the interhemispheric route to sever interhemispheric connections and reduce seizure propagation.
(c) *The posterior interhemispheric (interparieto-occipital)* approach is used for pineal region tumors, posterior trigone ventricular lesions [6], and deep-seated arteriovenous malformations.

9.3 Operative Set-Up

To perform the interhemispheric approach, whether anterior, middle, or posterior, we follow the following surgical steps [7, 8]:

Patient Positioning The patient is then placed in the supine position on the operating table. A gel pad or rolled sheet bolster is placed under the shoulders to optimize positioning and reduce the need for flexion between the head and cervical region, which compresses the jugular veins. A *Mayfield* or *Sugita* head holder was used to stabilize the head. The arms are tucked along the body (Fig. 9.1).

Head Positioning

(a) *Elevation.* The head is elevated by approximately 15° to facilitate venous drainage and reduce intracranial pressure. We achieved additional elevation using the back shoulders pack.

(b) *Rotation.* Minimal or no rotation is required to maintain the midline trajectory, ensuring a perpendicular approach to the falx and corpus callosum.

(c) *Extension.* The head is slightly flexed or kept neutral to align the interhemispheric fissure with the surgeon's line of vision while avoiding excessive tension on the bridging veins. Here is an important point: it is not uncommon for the neurosurgeon to overestimate the access, believing it is anterior when, in fact, it is shifting toward the end of the middle and posterior thirds. Therefore, we recommend following anatomical landmarks, such as the coronal suture and lambda, and encouraging neuronavigation.

Skin Preparation The entire scalp was prepared using an antiseptic solution (shampoo and chlorhexidine, or povidone-iodine). The surgical field should extend from the glabella to the occiput to ensure sterility during craniotomy and dural exposure. The face and ears were protected with sterile drapes, providing an adequate window for microscope positioning.

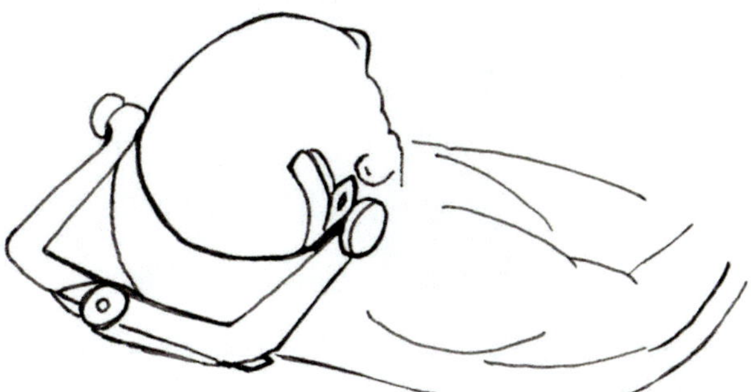

Fig. 9.1 Illustration showing the patient in a supine position, with the head fixed in a Mayfield and flexed by tilting the head over the cervical region and elevating the headrest

9.4 Surgical Technique [3, 7, 8] (Video 9.1)

Skin Incision We recommend a straight or transverse curvilinear incision crossing the midline, depending on the specific interhemispheric approach (anterior, median, or posterior). The incision must be centered on the preplanned craniotomy and preferably guided by imaging (CT, or MRI) and neuronavigation. Care should be taken to preserve the vascular supply of the scalp using a blade, with caution to avoid monopolar cautery.

Muscle Flap A myocutaneous flap is elevated in the subperiosteal plane to minimize bleeding and preserve periosteal integrity for closure. Generally, the incision does not extend laterally to the superior temporal line.

Craniotomy A unilateral frontal, parietal, or occipital craniotomy is performed, depending on the target area. The location of the superior sagittal sinus was carefully evaluated using preoperative imaging to guide the extent and lateralization of the craniotomy. We recommend placing two burr holes along the midline over the superior sagittal sinus to facilitate dural detachment. A third or fourth burr hole is placed at the extremities of the craniotomy. The dura was carefully detached using a periosteal elevator, avoiding injury to the sinus (Figs. 9.2 and 9.3).

Dural Opening A U-shaped dural incision was made using the approach (Fig. 9.4). The dural flap is reflected toward the superior sagittal sinus to control sinus retraction. The bridging veins draining into the superior sagittal sinus are identified and preserved whenever possible to prevent venous infarction. In cases in which the bridging veins must be sacrificed, temporary venous occlusion techniques may be used before coagulation.

Interhemispheric dissection and access to deep structures: the interhemispheric fissure is carefully dissected using microsurgical techniques, working between the

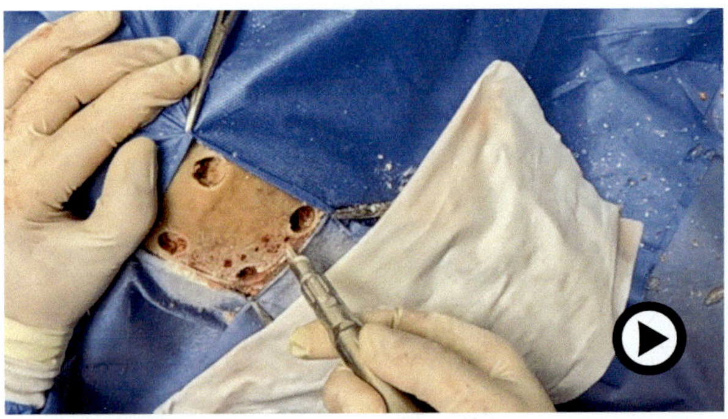

Video 9.1 This video illustrates the interhemispheric approach through a detailed cadaveric dissection, showcasing key steps, anatomical landmarks, and technical nuances essential for safe access to deep midline and ventricular lesions (▶ https://doi.org/10.1007/000-ht0)

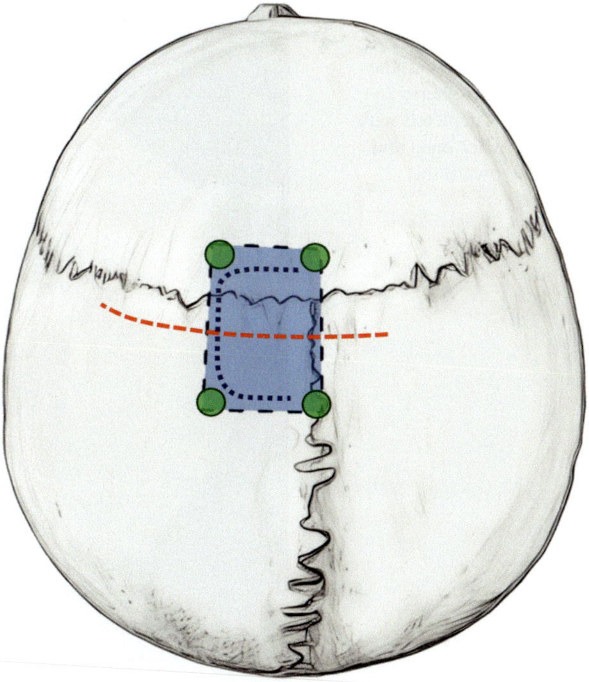

Fig. 9.2 Illustration showing an example of unilateral craniotomy for the interhemispheric approach with trephination points (green circles) and an example of a straight incision (red dashed line). The U-shaped dural opening is represented in navy blue

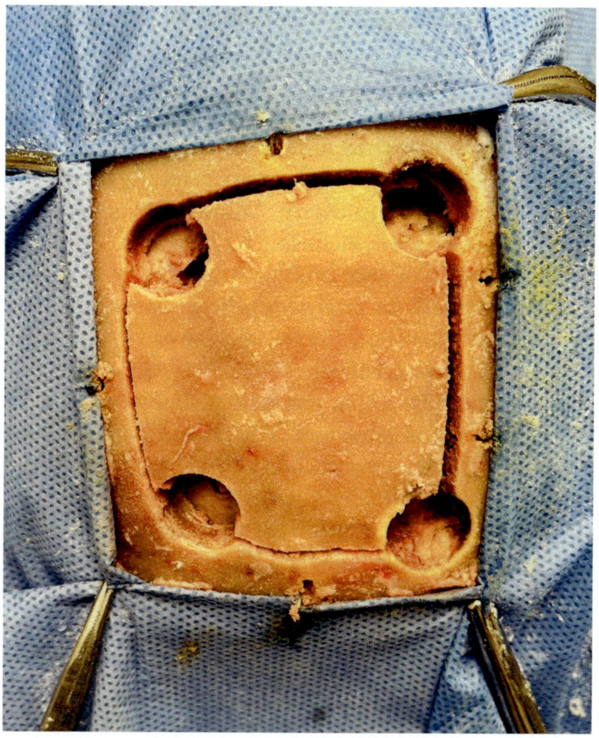

Fig. 9.3 Craniotomy was performed on the left side near the midline

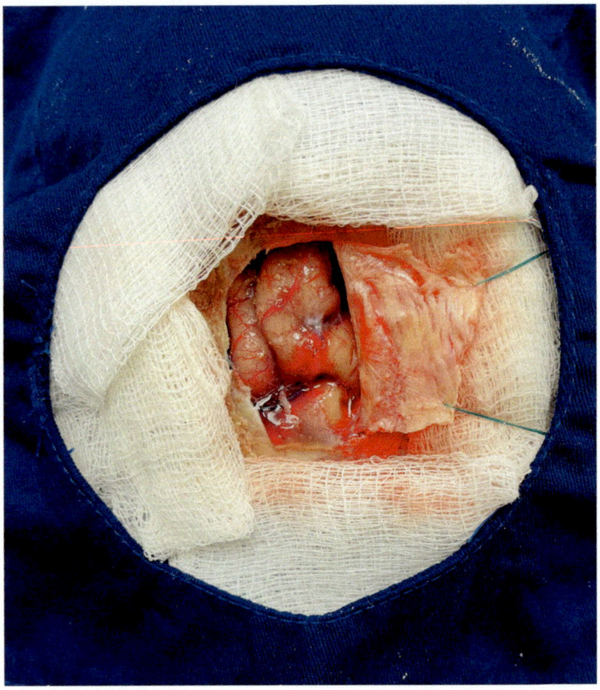

Fig. 9.4 In this photograph from the cadaveric dissection, the left interhemispheric approach is depicted with the dura mater open and reflected toward the midline

cerebral hemispheres. The falx cerebri is a key anatomical landmark for deep dissection. Cerebrospinal fluid drainage via lumbar puncture or intraoperative ventricular tap facilitates brain relaxation, facilitating retraction-free dissection. We used a cotton patch that was gradually inserted into the interhemispheric space to assist the opening of the interhemispheric fissure. This patch helps with dissection and hemostasis. Arachnoid adhesions and veins were carefully managed using bipolar coagulation and sharp dissection. If necessary, callosotomy is performed using microsurgical techniques to preserve interhemispheric fibers. Preserving bridging veins while maximizing the exposure of deep midline structures minimizes morbidity.

The contralateral interhemispheric approach is a microsurgical technique that optimizes access to deep-seated midline and lateral ventricular lesions while minimizing brain retraction. This method uses gravity-assisted retraction, allowing the contralateral hemisphere to fall naturally, thereby enhancing the surgical corridor without the need for fixed retractors. The patient is positioned supine, with the lesion side down, and the head turned laterally so that the sagittal midline is nearly horizontal, optimizing the line of sight into the interhemispheric fissure and ventricle. A contralateral craniotomy is performed, exposing the superior sagittal sinus and the falx, followed by a carefully planned dural opening to preserve the bridging veins. For transcallosal access, a 2-cm callosotomy is typically performed to enter the ipsilateral ventricle while maintaining the integrity of the corpus callosum. This approach avoids cortical incisions, reduces retraction-related injury, and provides a more lateral angle, which is particularly beneficial for tumors, arteriovenous malformations, and cavernous malformations. Additionally, image guidance and neuronavigation are crucial for precise skin incision placement, craniotomy planning, and falx incision alignment over the lesion. The transfalcine variant further extends this method by creating a falx window, enabling direct access to contralateral parasagittal and medial subcortical lesions while preserving healthy brain tissue. This technique is particularly effective in the presence of perilesional edema and represents a refined surgical approach for deep-seated lesions with reduced morbidity [9, 10].

Closure The dura is closed with continuous suturing and the use of autologous pericranium or dural substitutes, if needed. The bone flap is secured with miniplates and screws or Nylon sutures, ensuring anatomical repositioning. The muscle, if dissected, is reapproximated using absorbable sutures, and the skin is closed with either staples or nonabsorbable sutures. A subgaleal or epidural drain may be placed if there is a risk of significant bleeding.

9.5 Pearls and Pitfalls

- *Patient Positioning*: To promote venous drainage and reduce intracranial pressure, maintain a neutral or slightly flexed head position with 15° elevation.
- *Craniotomy Planning*: Preoperative imaging (CT/MRI) and neuronavigation are used to direct craniotomy lateralization, particularly because the superior sagittal sinus (SSS) often deviates to the right.
- *Bridging Vein Preservation*: Identify and preserve critical bridging veins during dural opening to prevent venous infarction. If sacrifice is necessary, temporary occlusion should be considered before coagulation.
- *Cotton Patch Technique for Fissure Opening*: Small cotton patches are inserted incrementally into the interhemispheric fissure to facilitate dissection. This technique performs a gentle separation and minimizes forceful retraction.
- *Controlled CSF Drainage*: A lumbar drain or ventricular tap can relax the brain and reduce the need for excessive retraction.
- *Contralateral Approach*: A transfalcine corridor can enhance the visualization of contralateral lesions while avoiding unnecessary cortical retraction. Gravity-assisted retraction reduces the need for mechanical retractors.
- *Overestimating the Access Location*: Neurosurgeons often misjudge anterior positioning, leading to an approach that shifts toward the middle or posterior third. To ensure precision, follow landmarks (coronal suture, lambda) and use neuronavigation.

References

1. Anetsberger SA, Marbacher S, Fandino J, et al. Interhemispheric approach. Acta Biomed. 2021;92(Suppl 4):e2021351.
2. Yasargil MG. Microneurosurgery, vol. IIIA. Stuttgart: Georg Thieme Verlag; 1987.

3. Aftahy AK, Albers J, Bertalanffy H, et al. The interhemispheric fissure – surgical outcome of interhemispheric approaches. Neurosurg Rev. 2021;44:2099–110.
4. Ghosh A, Chi J, Holsgrove D. Neuroanatomy, superior sagittal sinus. In: StatPearls [Internet]. Treasure Island: StatPearls Publishing; 2023.
5. Patchana T, Branstetter BF, Kim LJ, et al. Superior sagittal sinus: a review of the history, surgical considerations, and pathology. Cureus. 2019;11(5):e4597.
6. Zanini MA, de Aguiar PH, Leal AG, et al. Trigone ventricular meningiomas: surgical approaches. Arq Neuropsiquiatr. 2011;69(4):670–5.
7. Meyer FB. Atlas de Neurocirurgia: Acessos Básicos ao Crânio e Procedimentos Vascular. Rio de Janeiro: DiLivros; 2005. p. 83–123.
8. Fossett DT, Caputy AJ. Operative neurosurgical anatomy. New York and Stuttgart: Thieme; 2001. p. 27–31. Chapter 6.
9. Lawton MT, Golfinos JG, Spetzler RF. The contralateral transcallosal approach: experience with 32 patients. Neurosurgery. 1996;39(4):729–34.
10. Ferroli P, Acerbi F, Tringali G, et al. Gravity-aided transfalcine removal of a contralateral subcortical ependymoma: neurosurgical technique. Acta Neurochir. 2007;149:1147–50.

The Pretemporal and Transcavernous Approach (Dolenc's)

10

10.1 Introduction

The pretemporal approach is a neurosurgical technique that combines elements of the pterional, subtemporal, and temporopolar approaches to provide comprehensive access to deep-seated brain regions, such as the interpeduncular and petroclival areas. This method involves frontotemporal craniotomy, allowing surgeons to navigate through the Sylvian fissure and temporal lobe to reach target areas with minimal brain retraction. The approach is particularly beneficial for treating complex aneurysms and tumors located in challenging regions [1–3]. Moreover, the pretemporal approach slightly expands craniotomy to the temporal bone while maintaining an approximately 1:1 ratio between frontal and temporal bone exposure (Fig. 10.1). This balanced exposure optimizes surgical access to the interpeduncular and petroclival regions while minimizing brain retraction.

However, it is essential to clarify that while this approach provides broad access to the temporal lobe and adjacent structures, it does not necessarily expose all of the temporal lobe entirely but rather the areas relevant to the surgical corridor. In addition, orbozygomatic osteotomy may be performed to optimize skull base exposure.

Additionally, using the same pretemporal craniotomy technique allows us to approach the cavernous sinus through a combined epidural–intradural technique, as developed by Dolenc. The Dolenc approach to the cavernous sinus is a combined extradural and intradural method that is specifically designed to provide comprehensive access to this intricate neurovascular area. As described by Vinko Dolenc, this technique enables direct surgical exposure while minimizing damage to critical structures. The procedure is performed through frontotemporal craniotomy, which includes extradural removal of the anterior clinoid process,

Supplementary Information The online version contains supplementary material available at https://doi.org/10.1007/978-3-032-04664-2_10. The videos can be accessed individually by clicking the DOI link in the accompanying figure caption or by scanning this link with the SN More Media App.

H. de Oliveira Manduca Palmiero, E. G. Figueiredo, *Neurosurgical Approaches Video Atlas*, https://doi.org/10.1007/978-3-032-04664-2_10

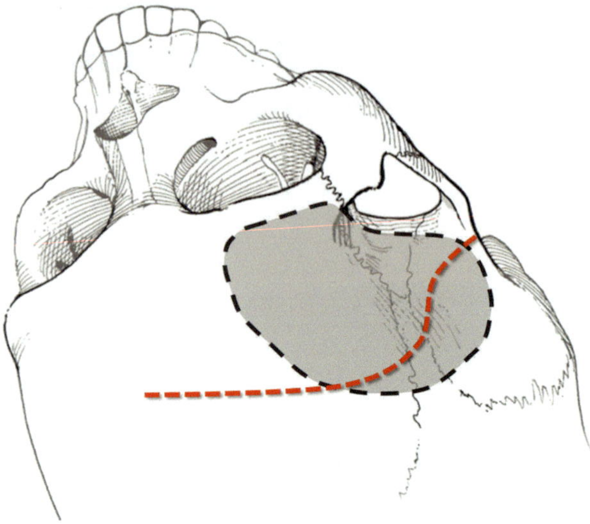

Fig. 10.1 Illustration showing the arcuate incision to perform the pretemporal craniotomy identified by the gray area

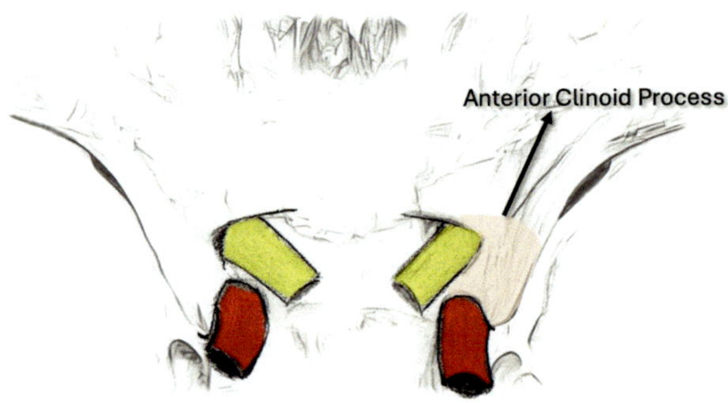

Fig. 10.2 Illustration of the epidural approach to the anterior clinoid process and its laterality in relation to the cavernous sinus (green area)

unroofing of the optic canal, and opening of the of the cavernous sinus to mobilize the internal carotid artery and adjacent cranial nerves. The dura is then incised to facilitate intradural dissection, allowing for safe manipulation of vascular lesions, tumors, and aneurysms within the cavernous sinus. This technique has transformed skull base surgery by enhancing accessibility and reducing morbidity [4–6].

The cavernous sinus is a complex venous structure at the skull base that houses critical neurovascular elements, including the internal carotid artery, cranial nerves III, IV, V (V1, V2), and VI, and extensive venous connections (Fig. 10.2). Considering its deep location and vital structures, surgical access to this region has historically been challenging. The Dolenc's approach, which builds upon a pretemporal craniotomy, provides a safe and effective route to the cavernous sinus by incorporating both extradural and intradural dissection. By removing the anterior clinoid process, unroofing the optic canal, and opening the cavernous sinus, surgeons gain direct access to the internal carotid artery and surrounding cranial nerves. This approach, initially developed for carotid-ophthalmic aneurysms, has since become a cornerstone technique in skull base surgery, demonstrating the versatility and effectiveness of the pretemporal corridor in neurosurgical practice [1, 4–6].

10.2 Indications for the Approach

The pretemporal approach is indicated for lesions located in the interpeduncular, petroclival, and cavernous sinus regions and for complex aneurysms of the internal carotid artery (ICA), basilar apex, and posterior circulation. This approach offers a broad surgical corridor with minimal brain retraction by using frontotemporal craniotomy, opening the Sylvian fissure, and performing extradural modifications, such as anterior clinoidectomy and optic canal unroofing. It is especially beneficial in vascular neurosurgery, including the treatment of carotid-ophthalmic aneurysms and basilar tip aneurysms, as outlined by Dolenc. Additionally, its application extends to skull base tumors, particularly those involving the cavernous sinus, where a combined epidural and intradural approach facilitates safe dissection of neurovascular structures. The pretemporal route, when integrated with the Dolenc approach, enhances surgical exposure, allowing precise manipulation of tumors, vascular lesions, and nerve compressions while reducing morbidity [4–8].

10.3 Operative Set-Up [1, 9]

Following the induction of general anesthesia, considering the pretemporal approach both for access to the Sylvian fissure, pretemporal region, oculomotor nerve, internal carotid artery, basilar artery apex, and interpeduncular cistern via the intradural route, as well as for the combined extra- and intradural access to the cavernous sinus for the treatment of lesions affecting the surrounding neurovascular structures, we proceed with the following steps:

Patient Positioning The patient is positioned supine on the surgical table, with the shoulder at the edge of the table to facilitate optimal head positioning. The head is secured using a skull fixation device (*Mayfield* or *Sugita* frame) to ensure stability during the procedure. The patient's torso is slightly elevated to promote venous drainage and reduce intracranial pressure.

Head Positioning

(a) *Elevation.* The head is elevated above the right atrium (15°) to facilitate venous return and prevent brain swelling.

(b) *Rotation.* The surgical trajectory is then rotated contralaterally by 30°–45°, depending on the side of the lesion, to align the surgical trajectory with the Sylvian fissure.

(c) *Extension.* A slight extension of the head is performed to increase the working angle and facilitate access to the anterior clinoid process and cavernous sinus. Additionally, the malar prominence should be positioned as the highest point to improve exposure.

Skin Preparation The scalp is shaved in a limited fashion (approximately 2 cm from the incision line) to maintain sterility while ensuring proper adhesion of the surgical drapes. The incision area is marked from the superior rim of the zygomatic arch to the contralateral pupillary line, ensuring adequate exposure while preserving the frontal branch of the facial nerve. The skin is disinfected using shampoo and chlorhexidine, or povidone-iodine. Benzoin can improve the adherence of sterile drapes.

10.4 Surgical Technique [1, 9]

Skin Incision A curvilinear frontotemporal incision is made with a blade, starting approximately 1 cm anterior to the tragus and extending superiorly toward the contralateral mid pupillary line, ensuring adequate exposure of the frontotemporal region and Sylvian fissure. The incision is carried through the subcutaneous tissue and galea to expose the temporalis muscle.

Muscle Flap The temporal branch of the facial nerve travels within the loose areolar tissue (adipose layer) between the superficial layer of the deep temporal and temporoparietal fascia. Thus, the safe dissection of the temporal muscle requires meticulous technique to avoid injury to the facial nerve's temporal branch and preserve muscle function [10, 11]. A vertical incision is made in the superficial fascia of the temporalis muscle, starting 2 cm superior to the orbital rim and extending down to the posterior root of the zygomatic arch, using a scalpel to avoid thermal injury from monopolar electrocautery. Next, a straight incision is made along the superior temporal line, leaving a muscle cuff for later reconstruction, extending posteriorly to the limit of the skin incision. The dissection then proceeds vertically in a straight line, reaching near the auricle. The temporalis muscle is dissected using a rugine, detaching it from the temporal bone, and then retracted laterally or in a pedicled fashion to preserve its vascularization. Hemostasis is achieved using bipolar coagulation, and retractors are placed to maintain exposure.

Craniotomy The frontotemporal craniotomy is performed using three burr holes: one at the keyhole region (MacCarthy's keyhole), one at the posterior aspect of the superior temporal line, and one at the squamous part of the temporal bone. The bone flap is removed, and the sphenoid wing is drilled to flatten the skull base, reducing the need for brain retraction (Figs. 10.3 and 10.4).

10.4.1 The Intradural Pretemporal Approach [1, 2]

First, if necessary, the anterior clinoid process is removed (clinoidectomy) using an extradural or intradural technique to expose the internal carotid artery and optic nerve (Video 10.1).

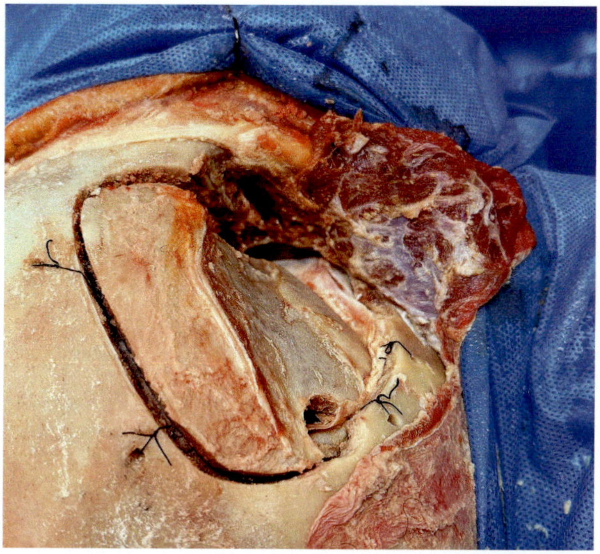

Fig. 10.3 In this picture, the bone flap over the frontotemporal craniotomy area extends to the temporal region, characterizing the craniotomy for the pretemporal approach

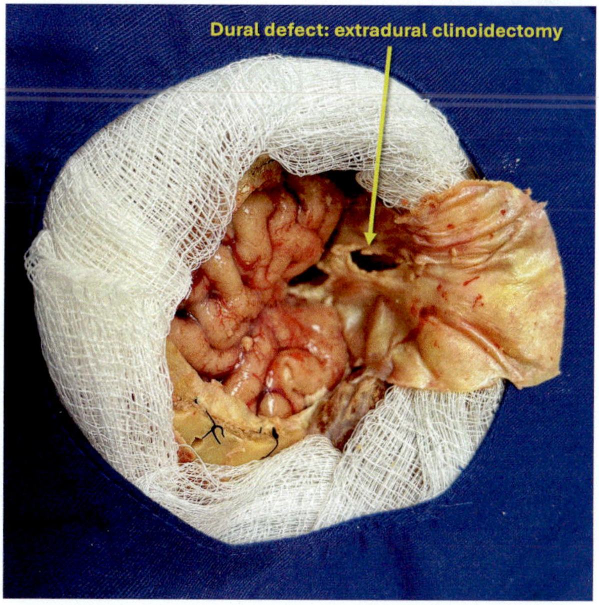

Fig. 10.4 In this photograph, we see the dural opening with a defect extending toward the Sylvian fissure, corresponding to the extradural clinoidectomy performed through the Dolenc approach

Dural Opening The dura is opened in an S-shaped or curvilinear manner, with the convex portion directed toward the Sylvian fissure. This allows adequate exposure of the frontal and temporal lobes, the Sylvian fissure, and deep neurovascular structures. The Sylvian fissure is dissected to facilitate access to the internal carotid artery, basilar artery apex, and cavernous sinus when needed. Cerebrospinal fluid is drained from the Sylvian and basal cisterns to allow brain relaxation (Fig. 10.4).

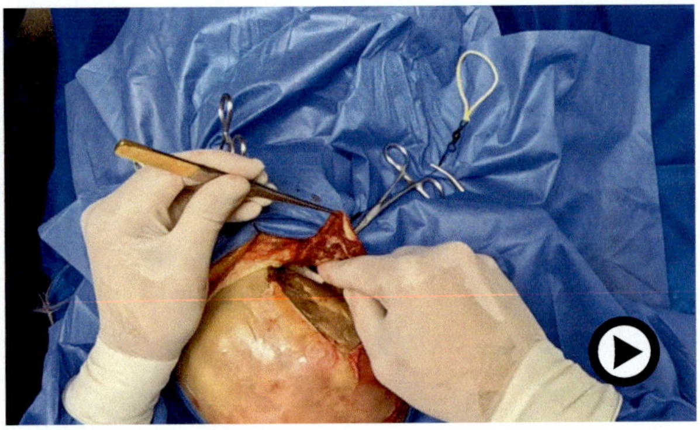

Video 10.1 In this video, we demonstrate the pretemporal approach, detailing the extradural and intradural steps (including Dolenc's technique) to access the cavernous sinus, anterior clinoid, and critical neurovascular structures of the anterior and middle cranial fossae (▶ https://doi.org/10.1007/000-ht1)

10.4.2 For Dolenc's Approach [4, 6, 9, 12–14]

The Dolenc approach is a combined extradural and intradural technique designed to provide access to the cavernous sinus and surrounding neurovascular structures, including the internal carotid artery (ICA), oculomotor nerve, trochlear nerve, trigeminal nerve, and abducens nerve. We followed these steps as described in the literature (Fig. 10.5):

Extradural Stage This phase focuses on removing bone structures and unroofing key neurovascular corridors.

(a) Orbital Roof and Optic Canal: the posterior two-thirds of the orbital roof are removed using a high-speed drill and rongeurs; the optic canal is unroofed using a diamond burr, allowing mobilization of the optic nerve while avoiding injury.
(b) Extradural Anterior Clinoidectomy: the anterior clinoid process is removed using a drill and Kerrison rongeur; the optic strut is drilled away to detach the clinoid fully; this step decompresses the optic nerve and exposes the clinoidal segment of the ICA, allowing better proximal vascular control.
(c) Superior Orbital Fissure and Meningo-Orbital Band: the superior orbital fissure is opened, removing the lateral bony wall to expose the cavernous sinus wall; the meningo-orbital band is cut, facilitating further temporal dura peeling and mobilization.
(d) Foramen Rotundum and Foramen Ovale: the bony rim of the foramen rotundum is removed, mobilizing the maxillary division (V2) of the trigeminal nerve; similarly, the foramen ovale is widened, allowing the mandibular division (V3) of the trigeminal nerve to be exposed.

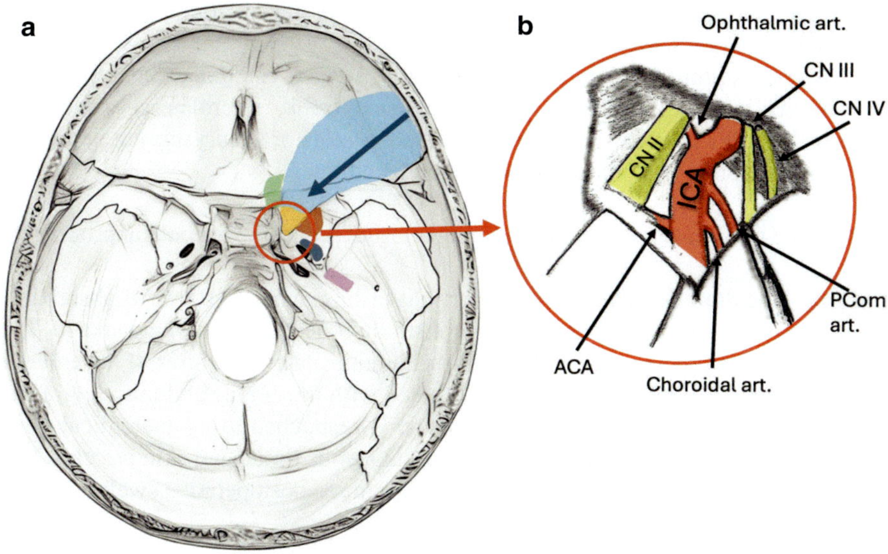

Fig. 10.5 Anatomical illustration of the Dolenc approach. On the left (**a**), the intracranial representation shows the main corridor of the Dolenc approach for the extradural stage (blue area and blue arrow); the anterior clinoidectomy region (yellow area); the roof of the optic canal (green area); laterally, the cavernous sinus region, corresponding to the lateral bony wall of the superior orbital fissure (orange area); and adjacent regions that can also be accessed: the bony rim of the foramen ovale (navy blue area) and the bony region of Glasscock's triangle (purple area). On the right (**b**), the achieved exposure through the Dolenc approach is shown, revealing the optic nerve, the carotid artery, and its branches (ophthalmic artery, posterior communicating artery, and anterior choroidal artery), as well as the oculomotor and trochlear nerves [4]

(e) Glasscock's triangle and Petrous Internal Carotid Artery (ICA): The Glasscock's triangle is drilled to expose the petrous segment of the ICA; this provides proximal control in cases requiring vascular reconstruction or aneurysm management.

Intradural Stage The dura is then opened to access the cavernous sinus and its contents (Fig. 10.5).

(a) Dural Opening: a curvilinear or S-shaped dural incision is made along the Sylvian fissure, which extends medially to the optic nerve and laterally across the temporal lobe.
(b) Sectioning the Carotid Rings: the proximal and distal dural rings surrounding the clinoidal ICA are identified and carefully incised; this step mobilizes the ICA, providing access to paraclinoid aneurysms and cavernous sinus lesions.
(c) Cranial Nerve Dissection: the oculomotor nerve is identified at the tentorial edge, and its dural sheath is incised; the trochlear nerve is identified posterior to the oculomotor nerve, with careful dissection to prevent injury; the ophthalmic division (V1) is dissected, exposing Meckel's cave and enabling access to

trigeminal schwannomas; the abducens nerve is traced from Dorello's canal, ensuring its preservation.

(d) Cavernous Sinus Exploration: the cavernous sinus is entered, exposing the ICA and its branches; the meningohypophyseal trunk, inferolateral trunk, and McConnell's capsular artery are preserved; tumors or aneurysms are addressed using clipping, coagulation, or resection techniques.

We resume from this point using a common closure procedure for both approaches:

Closure The dura was closed in a watertight fashion using 4–0 or 5–0 absorbable sutures, with reinforcement using dural substitute if needed to prevent leakage. The bone flap is then repositioned and secured with mini-plates or sutures. If the anterior clinoid process is removed, the defect is sealed with fibrin glue and muscle graft to prevent CSF leakage. The temporalis muscle is reattached to its anatomical position, ensuring cosmetic restoration. The subcutaneous tissue and skin are closed in layers, and a pressure dressing is applied to minimize postoperative swelling.

10.5 Pearls and Pitfalls

- *The Pretemporal and Dolenc Approaches* require precise execution to optimize exposure while minimizing complications. Proper head positioning with 15° elevation and 30°–45° contralateral rotation aligns the Sylvian fissure, improving access and reducing brain retraction.
- *During Sylvian fissure dissection,* proximal-to-distal exposure of the ICA and oculomotor nerve is essential. CSF drainage from basal cisterns aids brain relaxation.
- *The extradural anterior clinoidectomy* provides access to the clinoidal ICA and cavernous sinus. Removing the optic strut and anterior clinoid process ensures vascular control. Continuous irrigation prevents thermal injury to the optic nerve, and careful incision of the dural rings allows for safe ICA mobilization.
- *Exposure of the cavernous sinus requires precise extradural and intradural dissection.* Opening the superior orbital fissure and incising the meningo-orbital band facilitate temporal dura mobilization.
- *Watertight dural closure* and repair with fibrin glue and muscle, if necessary, to prevent CSF leaks during closure. Venous congestion, ICA rupture, and nerve injury are major complications requiring meticulous technique. The mastery of these approaches ensures safe and effective outcomes.

References

1. Chaddad-Neto F, Rassi-Neto A, Oliveira E, et al. Pretemporal craniotomy. Arq Neuropsiquiatr. 2014;72(2):145–51.
2. Oliveira E, Tedeschi H, Wen HT, et al. The pretemporal approach to the interpeduncular and petroclival regions. Acta Neurochir. 1995;136:204–11.

3. Figueiredo EG. Joining the masters: the Dolenc-Kawase approach – letters to the Editor. J Neurosurg. 2016;124:1543.
4. Dolenc VV. A combined epi- and subdural direct approach to carotid-ophthalmic artery aneurysms. J Neurosurg. 1985;62(5):667–72.
5. Tedeschi H, de Oliveira E, Tzu WH, Rhoton AL Jr. Acesso cirúrgico ao seio cavernoso. Temas Atuais de Neurocirurgia. 2004.
6. Van Loveren HR, Keller JT, El-Kalliny M, Scodary DJ, Tew JM Jr. The Dolenc technique for cavernous sinus exploration: cadaveric prosection. J Neurosurg. 1991;74(5):837–44.
7. Rutkowski MJ. Pretemporal transcavernous approach for resection of an orbito-cavernous oculomotor schwannoma. J Neurol Surg B Skull Base. 2022;83(Suppl S3):e621–2.
8. Huang M, Su J, Xiao Q, Ma Q, Long W, Liu Q. Pretemporal transcavernous approach for resection of non-meningeal tumors of the cavernous sinus: single-center experience. Front Surg. 2022;9:810606.
9. Bhaisora KS, Singh G, Das KK, Srivastava AK. How I do it—Dolenc approach for clipping of ventral wall paraclinoid ICA aneurysm. Acta Neurochir. 2024;166:406.
10. Yasargil MG, Reichman MV, Kubik S. Preservation of the frontotemporal branch of the facial nerve using the interfascial temporalis flap for pterional craniotomy. J Neurosurg. 1987;67:463–6.
11. Babakurban ST, Serel S, Turhan-Haktanir N, et al. Temporal branch of the facial nerve and its relationship to fascial layers. Arch Facial Plast Surg. 2010;12(1):16–23.
12. Labib M, Youssef AS. The cavernous sinus: surgical approaches, open and endoscopic. In: Youssef AS, editor. Contemporary skull base surgery: a comprehensive guide to functional preservation. Springer Nature: Berlin, Heidelberg, Germany; 2022. p. 331–46.
13. Figueiredo EG, Tavares WM, Rhoton AL Jr, de Oliveira E. Nuances and technique of the pretemporal transcavernous approach to treat low-lying basilar artery aneurysms. Neurosurg Rev. 2010;33(2):129–35.
14. Liao CH, Lin CF, Wang JT, Wang WH, Chen SC, Hsu SPC. The learning curve for cavernous sinus surgery illustrated by symptomatic intracavernous aneurysm clipping through a pretemporal transcavernous approach. J Neurosurg. 2024;183–93.

Subtemporal and Subtemporal and Anterior-Transpetrous Approaches (Kawase's)

11

11.1 Introduction

The subtemporal approach is a surgical technique used in neurosurgery to access lesions in the middle cranial fossa, upper brainstem, and posterior circulation. It can be performed *extradurally*, where the temporal dura is elevated to expose the middle fossa structures, often used for petroclival lesions and cavernous sinus pathology, or *intradurally*, where the dura is opened to access the mesial temporal lobe, cranial nerves III and IV, basilar tip, superior cerebellar artery, and ambient cistern [1–4].

The *intradural subtemporal* approach is also a technique for accessing the mesial temporal lobe, including the hippocampus, parahippocampal gyrus, and amygdala, in the surgical management of medically refractory temporal lobe epilepsy and select neoplasms. This approach involves low temporal craniotomy, followed by gentle retraction of the temporal lobe to expose the fusiform gyrus and collateral sulcus, allowing for a transsylvian or transventricular route to the mesial structures. The vein of Labbé must be preserved to prevent venous infarction, and excessive retraction should be avoided to minimize postoperative cognitive deficits [5–7].

From the temporal craniotomy, the subtemporal intradural and subtemporal extradural approaches can be used to access the middle cranial fossa (Fig. 11.1a). The *subtemporal intradural* approach extends this exposure by retracting the temporal lobe to reach the ambient cistern, superior cerebellar artery, and basilar apex, commonly used for vascular and deep-seated tumor surgery. The *subtemporal extradural* approach differs in that it involves dissection beneath the dura, often elevating the middle fossa dura to access the cavernous sinus, Meckel's cave, and petroclival region without directly manipulating the brain.

Supplementary Information The online version contains supplementary material available at https://doi.org/10.1007/978-3-032-04664-2_11. The videos can be accessed individually by clicking the DOI link in the accompanying figure caption or by scanning this link with the SN More Media App.

H. de Oliveira Manduca Palmiero, E. G. Figueiredo, *Neurosurgical Approaches Video Atlas*, https://doi.org/10.1007/978-3-032-04664-2_11

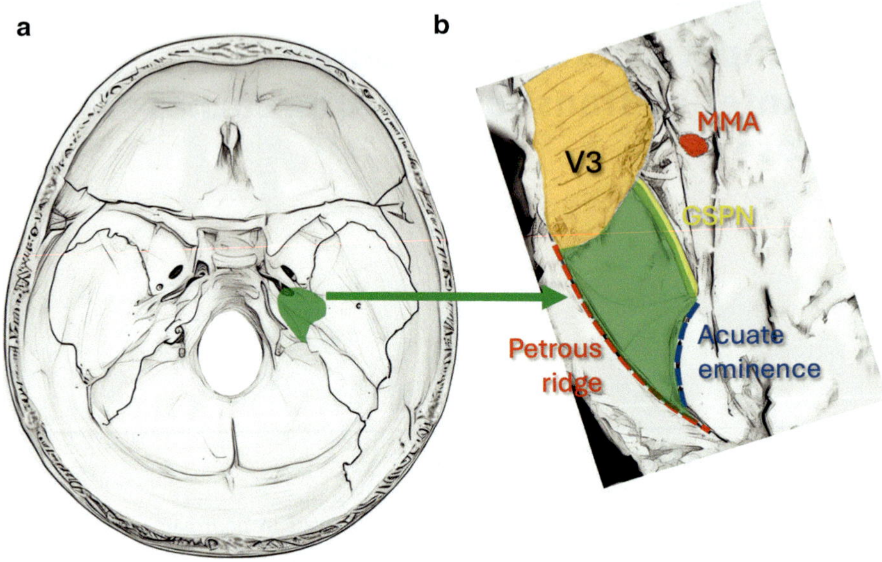

Fig. 11.1 Anatomical illustration of the Kawase approach. On the left (**a**), the petrous apex, the target of Kawase's anterior petrosectomy, is shown. On the right (**b**), the anatomical landmarks of Kawase's triangle are depicted with its boundaries: anterior—trigeminal impression, posterior—arcuate eminence, lateral—greater superficial petrosal nerve (GSPN), and medial—petrous ridge

Petrosectomy is a broader term referring to the surgical removal of a portion of petrous temporal bone. The subtemporal-medial-transpetrous approach (Kawase's) is a specific type of anterior petrosectomy. Petrosectomy can be partial (anterior, posterior, or subtotal) or complete, depending on the extent of bone removal. The Kawase approach (also called anterior petrosectomy) involves removal of the petrous apex anterior to the internal auditory canal, specifically targeting Kawase's quadrilateral area, to access the upper clivus, ventral brainstem, and basilar artery. Other types of petrosectomy include posterior petrosectomy (used in translabyrinthine or transcochlear approaches) [8, 9].

The *Kawase's approach* shares initial steps with the subtemporal craniotomy and extradural approach until the petroclival region is reached. Both procedures began with temporal craniotomy and elevation of the middle fossa dura in the extradural plane, with careful identification and protection of the greater superficial petrosal nerve (GSPN) and middle meningeal artery. The key distinction occurs when the Kawase approach proceeds with drilling the Kawase quadrangle, a bony area at the petrous apex bordered by the trigeminal impression (Anterior), arcuate eminence (Posterior), the GSPN (Lateral), and petrous ridge (Medial) (Fig. 11.1b). This drilling creates an anteromedial corridor to the posterior fossa without the need for significant brain retraction, enabling access to the petroclival meningiomas, upper clivus, ventral brainstem, and basilar artery perforators [10–13] (Fig. 11.1a, b).

11.2 Indications for the Approach

The subtemporal intradural, subtemporal extradural, and Kawase approaches are indicated for lesions in the middle cranial fossa, petroclival region, and upper posterior fossa, each selected based on the pathology's location and extent. The *subtemporal intradural* approach is primarily used to detect basilar tip aneurysms, superior cerebellar artery aneurysms, and pontine cavernous malformations. It is also used for mesial temporal tumors because it provides a direct corridor to the ambient cistern and interpeduncular fossa. In contrast, the *subtemporal extradural* approach is indicated for cavernous sinus tumors, trigeminal schwannomas, Meckel's cave lesions, and petroclival meningiomas because it allows extradural elevation of the temporal dura to expose the middle fossa floor and skull-base structures while minimizing brain retraction. The *Kawase's approach*, a modification of the *subtemporal extradural technique*, is specifically used for petroclival meningiomas, ventral brainstem tumors, mid- and lower basilar trunk aneurysms, and anterior pontine lesions because it provides a ventral, extradural route to the posterior fossa by drilling the petrous apex, avoiding cerebellar retraction. The proper selection of these approaches depends on the lesion's location, extension into the posterior fossa, as well as the need to minimize brain manipulation [8, 9, 14].

11.3 Operative Set-Up [15–17]

At this moment, we focus on the temporal and subtemporal approaches for performing *temporal craniotomy.*

Patient Positioning The patient is then placed in the supine position on the operating table. The head is fixed using Mayfield or Sugita, ensuring stability and minimizing the pressure points.

Head Positioning

(a) *Elevation.* The head is elevated 15°–30° above the heart level to promote venous drainage and reduce intracranial pressure. The head of the surgical table should be tilted to help elevate the table and minimize cervical traction.

(b) *Rotation.* The head is rotated 10°–30° contralateral to the side of the craniotomy to enhance the surgical working angle.

(c) *Extension.* A slight extension (chin up) is applied to facilitate access to the middle cranial fossa. However, excessive extension should be avoided to prevent jugular vein compression.

Skin Preparation The scalp and ear were prepared using shampoo and antiseptic solution (chlorhexidine or povidone-iodine). The hair in the incision area may be shaved or separated to maintain sterility while preserving cosmesis. The surgical side is draped to expose the zygomatic arch to the superior temporal line. Local epinephrine infiltration can reduce scalp bleeding.

11.4 Surgical Technique (Video 11.1)

Skin Incision A horseshoe-shaped (U-shaped) incision is made in the temporal region, with the base directed inferiorly to facilitate muscle elevation and retraction. The incision extends from just anterior to the tragus, curving superiorly above the zygomatic arch and back toward the posterior temporal region. The superficial temporal artery was preserved to maintain scalp perfusion. The scalp and underlying soft tissues are elevated as a single flap and retracted anteriorly to expose the temporalis muscle.

Muscle Flap The temporalis muscle can be separated from the skin flap using delicate Metzenbaum scissors or preserved as a single myocutaneous flap. After making the skin incision with a scalpel and coagulating any bleeding vessels with bipolar cautery, the muscle is cut using monopolar cautery but is dissected from the bone tissue with a periosteal elevator (rugine) to preserve vascularization. Following the direction of the skin incision, the temporalis muscle is elevated toward the ear. The temporalis muscle is then dissected and retracted inferiorly, exposing the keyhole and the squamous part of the temporal bone. Care should be taken to minimize muscle devascularization and prevent postoperative atrophy.

Craniotomy A temporal craniotomy is performed, extending from the pterion posteriorly to the squamous temporal bone, typically 4–5 cm in diameter, using four burr holes. The inferior edge of the craniotomy is positioned just above the zygomatic

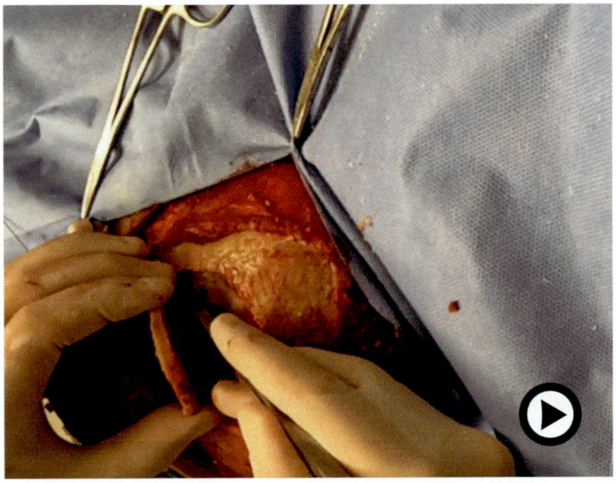

Video 11.1 This video demonstrates the temporal craniotomy followed by the subtemporal approach, including Kawase's anterior petrosectomy, highlighting the key anatomical landmarks, extradural dissection, and drilling techniques essential for accessing the petroclival region with minimal brain retraction (▶ https://doi.org/10.1007/000-ht2)

arch, optimizing the subtemporal working corridor. The sphenoid wing is drilled down to flatten the skull-base, facilitating both the intradural subtemporal and extradural anterior petrosectomy (Kawase) approaches. The middle meningeal artery can be coagulated and divided if necessary using the extradural approach (Figs. 11.2, 11.3, and 11.4).

For the Intradural Approach: Dural Opening: we recommend dural anchoring, and the dura is opened with delicate Metzenbaum scissors in a U-shaped fashion parallel to the temporal bone but reflected toward the ear inferiorly. The microscope is positioned and follows the microsurgical steps.

For the Extradural Approach and Kawase's [8]: once the craniotomy is completed and using the extradural corridor, the sphenoid wing is drilled to flatten the skull base and enhance subtemporal exposure. The procedure is as follows:

(a) *Extradural middle fossa dissection:* the greater superficial petrosal nerve (GSPN) is identified by tracing it from the foramen spinosum toward the geniculate ganglion. Carefully coagulate and divide the middle meningeal artery if necessary. Elevating the middle fossa dura extradurally, exposes the Meckel's cave, the petrous apex and the arcuate eminence.

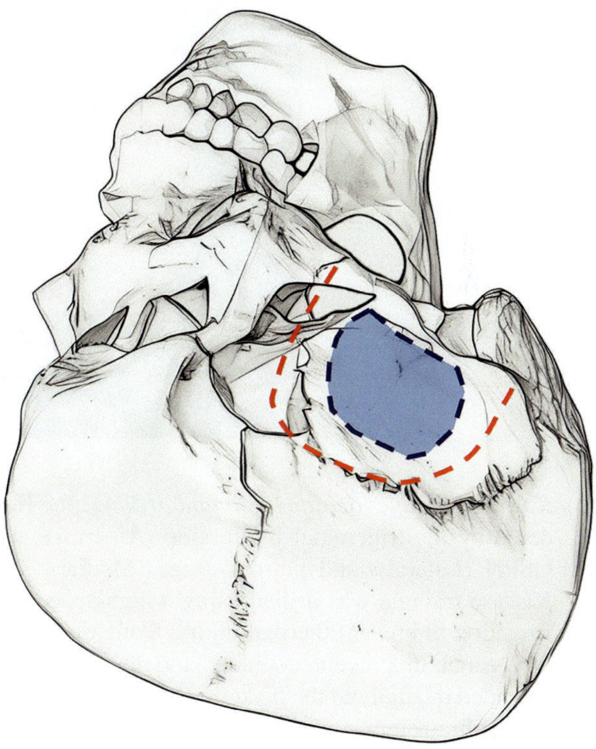

Fig. 11.2 Anatomical illustration showing the subtemporal craniotomy region for the Kawase approach. The red dashed line represents the horseshoe-shaped (U-shaped) incision

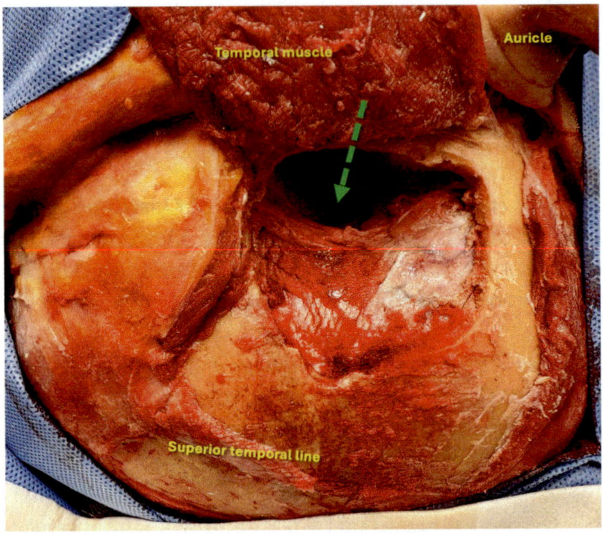

Fig. 11.3 Surgical photograph showing the subtemporal craniotomy area, the temporalis muscle reflected inferiorly, the auricle, and the superior temporal line as anatomical landmarks. The green arrow indicates the direction of the subtemporal corridor toward the petrous apex

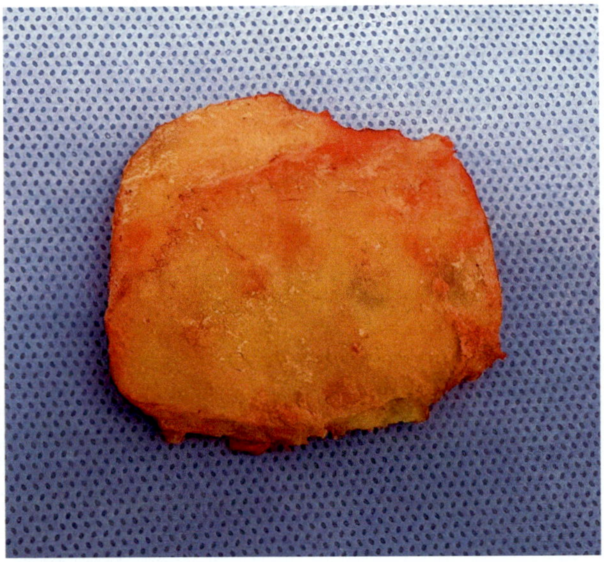

Fig. 11.4 This picture shows the temporal craniotomy bone flap

(b) *Kawase triangle identification and drilling:* the Kawase quadrilateral was bordered by the trigeminal impression (Anterior), arcuate eminence (Posterior), GSPN (Lateral), and petrous ridge (Medial). The petrous apex within the Kawase triangle was drilled using a high-speed diamond burr and continuous irrigation to prevent thermal injury. Skeletonize but preserve the internal auditory canal to prevent cochlear and facial nerve damage. The drilling was extended medially to the posterior fossa, ensuring access to the upper clivus and ventral brainstem.

(c) *Tentorial opening and exposure of the brainstem:* the tentorium is incised parallel to the petrous ridge, preserving the trochlear nerve. Retract the temporal lobe gently, maintain venous drainage, and avoid excessive pressure. Identify and protect the trigeminal, oculomotor, and basilar artery perforators. Ensure optimal exposure of the upper clivus, ventral brainstem, and basilar trunk.

Closure Meticulous hemostasis is achieved, ensuring no CSF leakage. The drilled petrous area is covered with fascia or muscle graft to prevent postoperative CSF fistula. For intradural approaches, the dural closure should be watertight. The dural flap is closed using dural anchoring sutures before closure to prevent retraction-related tension. The temporalis muscle and skin flap are secured to ensure adequate soft tissue coverage. A subcutaneous drain is recommended for fluid collection after surgery.

11.5 Pearls and Pitfalls

- *Minimizing temporal lobe retraction:* excessive pressure increases the risk of venous congestion, ischemia, and postoperative neurological deficits. CSF drainage, head elevation, and mannitol are used to optimize relaxation.
- *Preserving the vein of Labbé:* sacrificing this major venous drainage route can lead to temporal lobe infarction and edema, increasing postoperative morbidity. Identify and protect it early.
- *Identify and protect the GSPN:* this nerve is a key landmark for extradural dissection. Gentle dissection along the route minimizes traction injury and preserves lacrimal gland and facial nerve function.
- *Avoid excessive drilling near the IAC:* aggressive bony removal in this region can damage the cochlea and facial nerve, leading to hearing loss or facial palsy. Maintain a safe margin from the IAC.
- *Use a high-speed diamond burr:* this reduces thermal injury when drilling the petrous apex, preserving the dura and neurovascular structures. Continuous irrigation prevents heat buildup.
- *Preserve the trochlear nerve during tentorial incision:* this delicate nerve runs along the tentorial edge and is easily damaged, leading to postoperative vertical diplopia. Always incise parallel to the petrous ridge.
- *Achieving watertight dural closure:* Devote meticulous suturing and grafting reduce the risk of CSF leakage, which can lead to meningitis and prolonged hospitalization.
- *Monitor for brainstem perforator injury:* small perforators from the basilar artery supply critical midbrain and pontine structures. Even minor damage can lead to neurological impairment.
- *Cover the drilled petrous bone with a fascia or muscle graft.* This creates a barrier against CSF leakage, reinforces the skull-base, and prevents postoperative complications like pseudomeningocele.

References

1. Al-Mefty O, Borba LA. The transzygomatic approach to skull-base lesions. J Neurosurg. 1997;86(5):800–5.
2. Drake CG, Peerless SJ. The subtemporal approach to aneurysms of the basilar artery at the superior cerebellar level. J Neurosurg. 1989;71(3):339–49.
3. González LF, Crawford NR, Horgan MA, et al. Working area and angle of attack in three surgical approaches to the basilar apex. J Neurosurg. 2002;96(5):885–91.
4. Yasargil MG. Microneurosurgery, Vol. IV: Microsurgical anatomy of basal cisterns and vessels of the brain. Stuttgart: Thieme; 1996.
5. Niemeyer P. The transventricular amygdalohippocampectomy in temporal lobe epilepsy. Stereotact Funct Neurosurg. 1958;19(1–3):36–43.
6. Yasargil MG, Türe U, Yasargil DC. Surgical approaches to temporal lobe epilepsy. Neurosurgery. 2004;55(4):935–57.
7. Hori T, Takanashi M, Kurosaki K, et al. Subtemporal selective amygdalohippocampectomy for mesial temporal lobe epilepsy: surgical technique and outcomes. Acta Neurochir. 2019;161(12):2491–500.
8. Kawase T, Shiobara R, Toya S. Anterior transpetrosal-transtentorial approach for sphenopetroclival meningiomas: surgical methods and results. Neurol Med Chir (Tokyo). 1991;31(6):300–11.
9. Tanriover N, Abe H, Rhoton AL Jr. Comparison of surgical exposures to the petroclival region: Kawase versus extended middle fossa approach. Neurosurgery. 2009;64(5 Suppl 2):ONS-205–19.
10. Kawase T, Toya S, Shiobara R, Tanada M. Transpetrosal approach for aneurysms of the lower basilar artery. J Neurosurg. 1985;63(6):857–61.
11. Hitotsumatsu T, Matsushima T, Inoue T, Matsumoto K, Fukui M. Quantitative analysis of the surgical exposure of the petroclival region: subtemporal versus presigmoid approach. J Neurosurg. 1999;91(3):462–8.
12. Labidi M, Watanabe K, Shibao S, et al. The Kawase approach: anatomical study and clinical applications. World Neurosurg. 2016;92:42–51.
13. Andaluz N, Beretta F, Keller JT, Zuccarello M. The Kawase approach: anatomical study of the optimal cutting and drilling angles. Neurosurgery. 2006;58(1 Suppl):ONS-157–64.
14. Hitotsumatsu T, Matsushima T, Inoue T, et al. Surgical approaches to the petroclival region: indications and limitations. J Neurosurg. 1999;91(3):462–8.
15. Rhoton AL Jr. The supratentorial cranial base: microsurgical anatomy and surgical approaches. Neurosurgery. 2000;47(Suppl 3):S3-7–S3-27.
16. Lawton MT, Lang MJ. The operating room setup, surgical positioning, and key steps in cranial approaches. Oper Neurosurg (Hagerstown). 2019;17(Suppl 1):S5–S12.
17. Yasargil MG. Microneurosurgery, Vol. I: Microsurgical anatomy of the basal cisterns and vessels of the brain. Stuttgart: Thieme; 1984.

The Parietal and Occipital Approaches 12

12.1 Introduction

The parietal and occipital surgical approaches are vital in neurosurgery because they allow access to superficial and deep-seated lesions within the parietal and occipital lobes, the atrium of the lateral ventricle, and the posterior fossa. These approaches are especially effective for addressing vascular lesions, tumors, and epilepsy while minimizing disruption to eloquent cortical regions. The parietal approach typically involves a transcortical or transsulcal trajectory, enabling direct access to periventricular structures, whereas the occipital approach utilizes natural anatomic corridors to access lesions in the posterior third ventricle, splenium of the corpus callosum, and calcarine region [1–3].

The occipital craniotomy is guided by the inion (external occipireliedprotuberance) as a midline reference, with the superior nuchal line marking the inferior limit and the lambdoid suture above it, while the asterion (the junction of the lambdoid, parietomastoid, and occipitomastoid sutures) is critical for positioning near the transverse sinus [4, 5].

An appropriate surgical corridor selection depends on lesion location, surrounding critical structures, and the potential for postoperative deficits, particularly in visual function and higher-order processing. Advances in neuronavigation, intraoperative imaging, cortical mapping, and precise anatomical knowledge have refined these techniques, ensuring optimal exposure while avoiding injury to the venous sinuses and eloquent cortex. Understanding the anatomical constraints and optimizing the surgical trajectory are crucial for minimizing morbidity and achieving maximal resection [1–3].

Supplementary Information The online version contains supplementary material available at https://doi.org/10.1007/978-3-032-04664-2_12. The videos can be accessed individually by clicking the DOI link in the accompanying figure caption or by scanning this link with the SN More Media App.

H. de Oliveira Manduca Palmiero, E. G. Figueiredo, *Neurosurgical Approaches Video Atlas*, https://doi.org/10.1007/978-3-032-04664-2_12

Ventricular Access To access the lateral ventricles from the parietal and occipital lobes, whether for CSF drainage to promote brain relaxation or for intraventricular lesion access during surgical approaches, two ventricular entry points are used: Keen's point, located 3 cm lateral to the midline and 3 cm above the inion, which provides posterior ventricular access; and Frazier's point, positioned 2–3 cm lateral to the midline and 4 cm above the external auditory meatus, allowing access to the atrium of the lateral ventricle [6–9].

Atrium The parietal craniotomy approach to the lateral ventricle atrium provides safe access to intraventricular lesions. The transsuperior parietal gyrus route minimizes disruption to the optic radiation and language centers. A parieto-occipital craniotomy is performed, followed by transcortical entry into the ventricle. Neuronavigation and ultrasound aid localization. This approach reduces visual deficits compared with the middle temporal route, which risks optic pathway injury. Careful handling of bridging veins can prevent venous infarction. Postoperative outcomes show improved symptoms and low rates of complications, making it a preferred technique [10].

Transtentorial The transtentorial approach via occipital craniotomy provides a direct route to the posteromedial temporal lobe and pulvinar and parahippocampal regions while minimizing cortical disruption. This supratentorial-infraoccipital approach, also known as the occipitopolar approach, involves an occipital craniotomy extending to the torcular Herophili for optimal exposure of the falco-tentorial junction. Patient positioning in a three-quarter prone (*park-bench*) posture facilitates gravitational retraction of the occipital lobe, thereby reducing the need for mechanical retraction. The approach allows dissection through the transverse fissure, providing a natural corridor to deep structures, including the ambient cistern and branches of the posterior cerebral artery. This technique enhances lesion resection while preserving visual pathways and minimizing vascular injury [11].

12.2 Indications for the Approach

The parietal and occipital approaches are indicated for intraventricular tumors (e.g., meningiomas, gliomas), vascular lesions (arteriovenous malformations, aneurysms), and epilepsy surgery, depending on the location of the tumor and surrounding structures. The parietal approach is preferred for lateral ventricle tumors, allowing safe entry via the superior parietal lobule and avoiding optic radiation injury. The occipital transtentorial approach is optimal for posteromedial temporal lobe, pulvinar, and parahippocampal lesions, using the transverse fissure for direct access while minimizing cortical disruption. Patient-specific factors, such as visual function, venous anatomy, and hemisphere dominance, dictate the choice of approach [7, 8, 11].

12.3 Operative Set-Up [2, 12]

Patient Positioning The patient is then positioned in a prone, lateral, or supine position depending on the surgical target. For parietal craniotomy, the supine or lateral position is commonly used to facilitate access to the superior parietal lobule and ventricular structures. For the occipital and parieto-occipital approaches, the prone or three-quarter prone (park-bench) position is preferred to optimize gravity-assisted brain relaxation and minimize retraction (Fig. 12.1).

Head Positioning

(a) *Elevation.* The head is elevated 10°–15° above the heart to promote venous drainage and reduce intracranial pressure. However, depending on the positioning, especially in the lateral or park-bench positions, the entire surgical table headrest should be elevated, or the inverted Trendelenburg position should be used to keep the head elevated above the heart.

(b) *Rotation.* In midline parietal or occipital craniotomies, the head remains neutral to maintain symmetry. For the lateralized approach, the head is rotated contralateral 20°–30° to expose the ipsilateral surgical corridor.

(c) *Extension.* Minimal extension is performed for superior parietal lesions. Mild to moderate flexion is applied for occipital or transtentorial approaches to align the transverse fissure parallel to the surgical field while avoiding excessive brainstem tension.

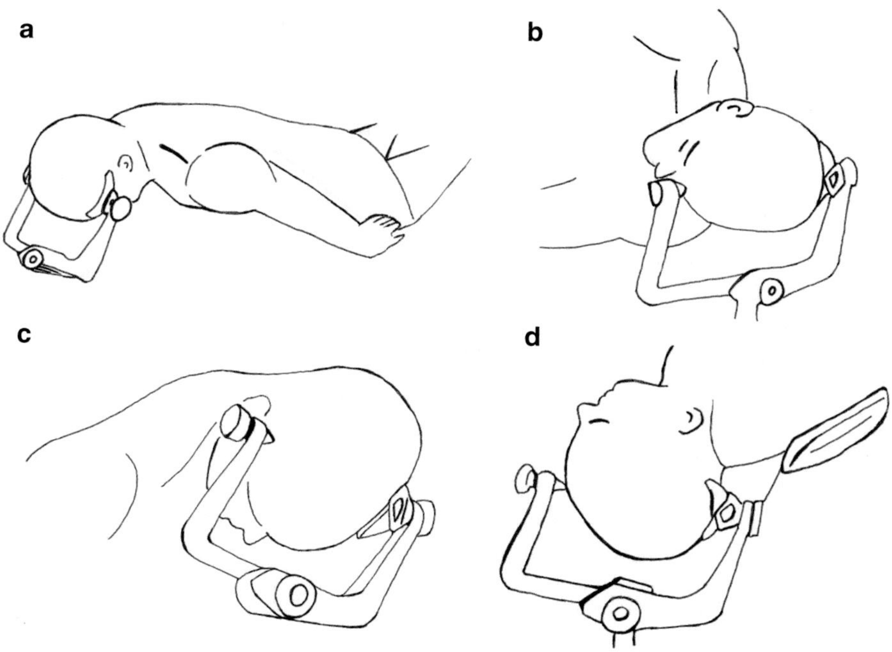

Fig. 12.1 Illustrations showing the positioning for parietal and occipital approaches. In (**a**): prone (or Concord) positioning; in (**b**): lateral positioning with the park bench variation in (**c**); in (**d**): supine positioning for more anterior parietal approaches

Skin Preparation The incision area was marked based on craniometric landmarks to ensure the exposure of key sutures (e.g., lambdoid, sagittal, or coronal). Standard antiseptic preparation (shampoo and chlorhexidine, or povidone-iodine) is performed covering the occipital, parietal, and upper cervical regions in case of extension. The operative field is widely draped, ensuring a sterile margin while allowing access to navigation markers for intraoperative guidance.

12.4 Surgical Technique [2, 12–15] (Video 12.1)

Skin Incision The incision is planned based on craniometric landmarks to optimize the exposure while preserving the vascular supply. A curvilinear, linear, or horseshoe-shaped incision is made, depending on the approach (Fig. 12.2):

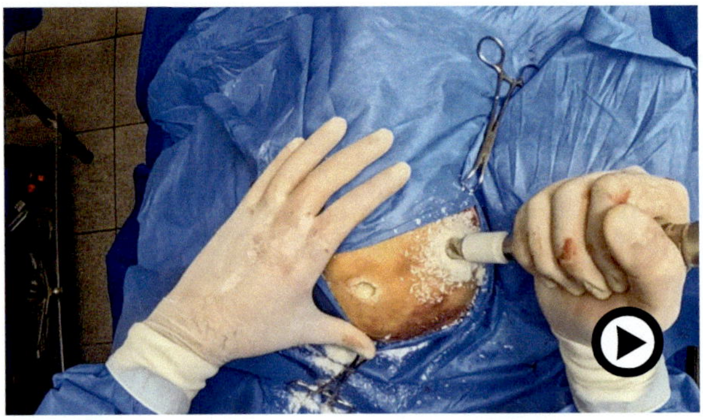

Video 12.1 This video demonstrates the parietal and occipital approaches, highlighting key anatomical landmarks, craniotomy techniques, and microsurgical strategies for accessing deep midline, ventricular, and posterior cortical lesions with minimal disruption to eloquent cortex (▶ https://doi.org/10.1007/000-ht3)

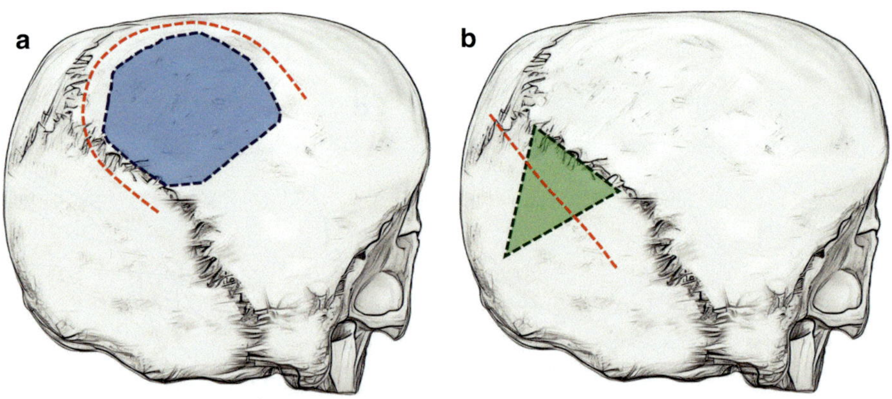

Fig. 12.2 Illustration of the parieto-occipital approach showing the craniotomies. In (**a**), a quadrilateral-shaped parietal craniotomy with a horseshoe-shaped incision (red dashed line) is shown, and in (**b**), a triangular-shaped occipital craniotomy with a linear incision (red dashed line) is depicted

Parietal craniotomy: a linear or horseshoe incision centered around the superior parietal lobule, with respect to the sagittal sinus, when approaching midline lesions.

Occipital craniotomy: a curvilinear incision starting from the lambda and extending to the mastoid based on lesion laterality.

Parieto-occipital craniotomy: a posteriorly curved incision crossing the parietal-occipital junction, avoiding excessive scalp retraction.

Muscle Flap Minimal muscle dissection is required for parieto-occipital craniotomy.

Craniotomy 3 a 4 burr holes were placed strategically at the extremities of the planed craniotomy to expose the underlying dura and avoid sinus injury (Fig. 12.2). A key point is dural detachment with a dissector before cutting, as approaches near the midline or the lambdoid suture carry a higher risk of venous sinus injury:

Parietal approach: burr holes are placed along the superior parietal lobule, avoiding the superior sagittal sinus (Figs. 12.2a, 12.3, and 12.4).

Occipital approach: burr holes are placed near the lambdoid suture, ensuring exposure of the torcular Herophili, if needed (Figs. 12.2b, 12.5, and 12.6).

Parieto-occipital approach: a larger posterior craniotomy extending between the parietal and occipital regions.

The bone flap is elevated using craniotomy cuts while preserving venous sinus integrity.

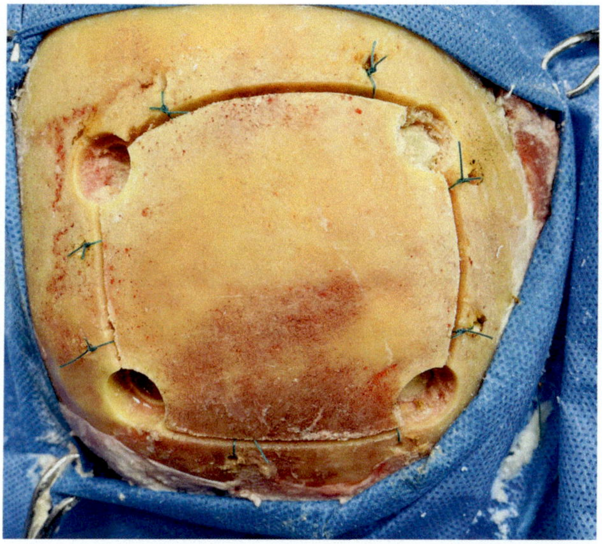

Fig. 12.3 In this picture, pode-se ver the parietal craniotomy com o bone flap

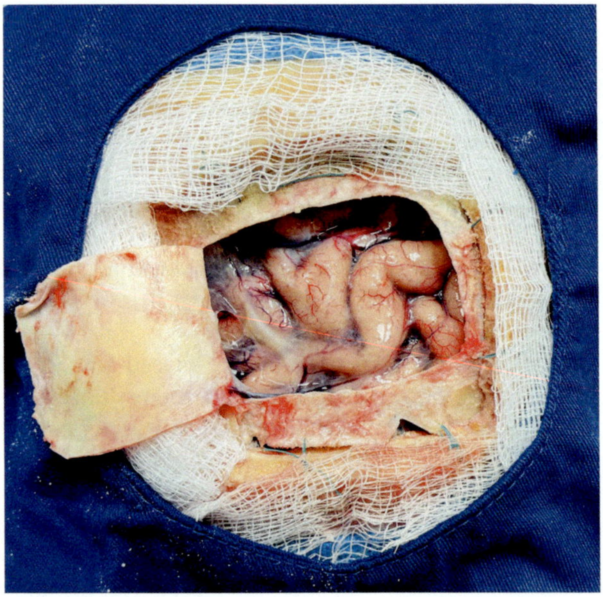

Fig. 12.4 Right parietal craniotomy after dural opening, with gauze and a blue fenestrated drape

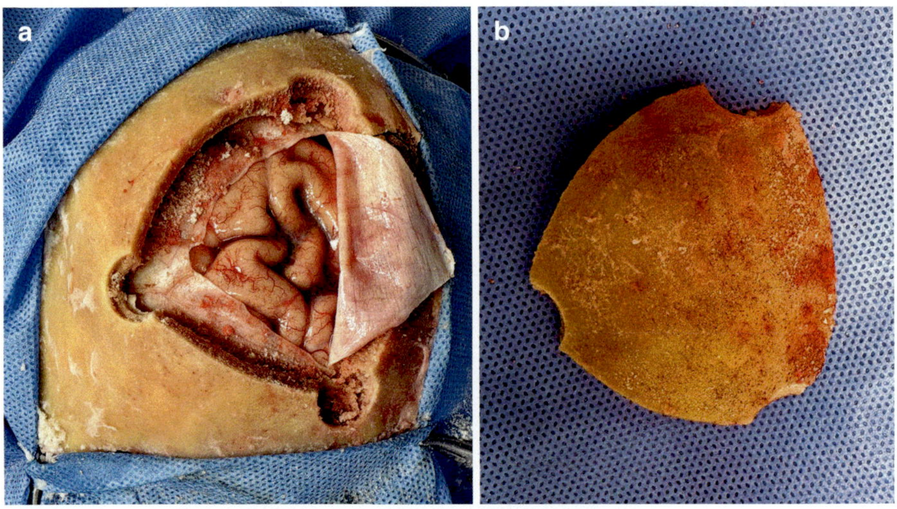

Fig. 12.5 In this photograph, we see the occipital craniotomy with the dura mater everted in (**a**) and the bone flap in (**b**)

Dural Opening The dura is incised in a cruciate or C-shaped manner, depending on the lesion location. For midline or ventricular access, the dura is reflected toward the sagittal sinus. In the occipital transtentorial approach, the dura is incised parallel to the transverse sinus, exposing the tentorium, if required.

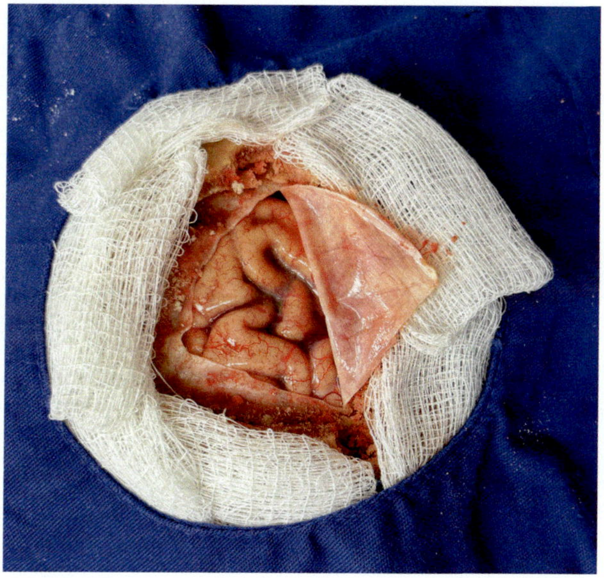

Fig. 12.6 Left occipital craniotomy after dural opening, with gauze and a blue fenestrated drape

Closure Dural closure was performed using a water-tight suture to prevent CSF leakage, and dural substitutes were used if required. The bone flap is then reattached using a miniplate, screws, or sutures. Subcutaneous drain may be placed. Layered closure of the galea and skin is performed, ensuring tension-free adaptation to minimize wound dehiscence.

12.5 Pearls and Pitfalls

- *Patient positioning*: based on the location of the lesion using prone, lateral, or park-bench positioning. Head elevation (10°–15°) improves venous drainage. The inverted Trendelenburg position is used.
- *Neuroanatomy allied with neuronavigation is key*: it guides the precise identification of craniometric and ventricular entry points and localization of lesions and minimizes cortical disruption.
- *Protect the visual pathways*: avoid optic radiation damage, especially in atrial ventricular access; the parieto-occipital approach is safer than the middle temporal route.
- *Sinus awareness*: identify and avoid superior sagittal sinus, transverse sinus, and torcular Herophili; preoperative venous anatomy assessment is crucial.
- *Optimal craniotomy placement*: use burr holes at craniometric landmarks; detach the dura before craniotomy use to prevent dural and venous sinus injury.
- *Gradual brain relaxation*: mannitol or hypertonic saline and CSF drainage (ventricular puncture or lumbar drain) can prevent excessive brain retraction.

- *Tentorial incision risks*: in occipital transtentorial approaches, improper incision can cause injury to deep veins (e.g., vein of Galen, basal vein of Rosenthal).
- *Poor closure technique*: loose closure risks CSF leakage and pseudomeningocele formation.

References

1. Rhoton AL. The cerebral veins. Neurosurgery. 2002;51(4 Suppl):S159–205.
2. Yasargil MG. Microneurosurgery: Vol. IVB. Clinical considerations, surgery of the intracranial aneurysms and results. Stuttgart: Thieme; 1996.
3. Yasuda CL, Centeno M, Vollmar C, et al. The effect of topography and lesion type on parietal lobe functions: a study integrating lesion-symptom mapping and functional connectivity. Neuroimage Clin. 2017;13:291–301.
4. Gusmão S, Silveira RL, Arantes A. Pontos referenciais nos acessos cranianos. Arq Neuropsiquiatr. 2003;61(2-A):305–8.
5. Reis CV, Arantes AA, Nicolato A, Gusmão S. Delimitação dos acessos cranianos. Arq Bras Neurocir. 2012;31(3):135–45.
6. Rhoton AL Jr. The lateral and third ventricles. Neurosurgery. 2002;51(4 Suppl):S207–71.
7. Greenberg MS. Handbook of neurosurgery. 9th ed. New York: Thieme; 2020.
8. Winn HR, Youmans JR. Youmans and Winn neurological surgery. 8th ed. Philadelphia: Elsevier; 2023.
9. Lozier AP, Cohen-Gadol AA. Operative techniques in neurosurgery: neurosurgical operative atlas, vol. 2. New York: Thieme; 2019.
10. Nanda A, Bir SC, Maiti T, Konar S. Intraventricular meningioma: technical nuances in surgical management. World Neurosurg. 2016;88:526–37.
11. Gusmão S, Silveira RL, Oliveira MM. Acesso supratentorial-infraoccipital ou occipitopolar: estudo clínico e anatômico. Arq Neuropsiquiatr. 2005;63(2-A):265–74.
12. Spetzler RF, Smith KA. Supratentorial-infraoccipital approach to posteromedial temporal lobe lesions. J Neurosurg. 1995;82(6):940–4.
13. Siqueira MG. Chapter 6 - Acessos frontal, parietal, occipital e temporal. In: Tratado de Neurocirurgia: volume I. Barueri: Manole; 2016. p. 49–57.
14. Meyer FB. Chapter 4 - Acesso parietal. In: Atlas de Neurocirurgia: Acessos Básicos ao Crânio e Procedimentos Vascular. Rio de Janeiro: DiLivros; 2005. p. 125–62.
15. Fossett DT, Caputy AJ. Chapter 19 - Occipital lobectomy. In: Operative neurosurgical anatomy. New York and Stuttgart: Thieme; 2001. p. 113–4.

The Suboccipital Approach 13

13.1 Introduction

The suboccipital approach through a suboccipital craniotomy remains a cornerstone in neurosurgical access to the posterior fossa, cerebellum, and brainstem, requiring precise anatomical knowledge of the venous sinuses, foramen magnum, and surrounding bony landmarks [1]. The inion, asterion, mastoid processes, digastric points, and foramen magnum define the suboccipital craniotomy limits. The C1 (atlas) becomes relevant when posterior arch removal is needed for additional access to the lower brainstem and foramen magnum decompression [2, 3]. The transverse sinus and torcular Herophili at their confluence with the suboccipital sinus and sigmoid sinus serve as key reference points for planning safe dural incisions [1]. Midline suboccipital craniotomies can preserve structural integrity and reduce postoperative complications [4]. This approach, when executed meticulously, allows for maximal visualization while minimizing complications associated with posterior fossa surgery.

The suboccipital craniotomy provides access to the supracerebellar-infratentorial corridor (Krause's approach), facilitating surgical exposure of the pineal region and thalamus while utilizing the natural cerebellar slope to minimize retraction and brainstem manipulation [1]. In contrast, occipital craniotomy allows direct access to the tentorium and the Poppen approach, a technique primarily used for lesions in the quadrigeminal cistern, posterior third ventricle, and upper brainstem, offering a more direct supratentorial trajectory [3]. Additionally, using suboccipital craniotomy, the fourth ventricle can be exposed through the telovelar and transvermian approaches [5]. Each approach is chosen based on the lesion's location, avoiding unnecessary cortical disruption and optimizing surgical exposure with minimal neurological morbidity [2].

Supplementary Information The online version contains supplementary material available at https://doi.org/10.1007/978-3-032-04664-2_13. The videos can be accessed individually by clicking the DOI link in the accompanying figure caption or by scanning this link with the SN More Media App.

H. de Oliveira Manduca Palmiero, E. G. Figueiredo, *Neurosurgical Approaches Video Atlas*, https://doi.org/10.1007/978-3-032-04664-2_13

The choice between suboccipital craniotomy and craniectomy for posterior fossa surgery is debated due to differences in postoperative outcomes. Craniotomy, which replaces the bone flap, provides structural support and reduces pseudomeningocele (4% vs. 19.2%) and CSF leaks (2% vs. 11.5%) compared with craniectomy [6]. Craniectomy, with permanent bone removal, may relieve brainstem compression but is linked to higher complication rates (32.6% vs. 7%) [7]. Despite the assumption that craniectomy prevents postoperative hydrocephalus, studies have not revealed any significant benefit [7]. Given its lower morbidity, craniotomy is a preferential procedure.

Ventricular drainage using the Dandy or Frazier points is commonly performed during suboccipital procedures to relax the brain and reduce intracranial pressure. Positioned 2–3 cm lateral to the midline and 4 cm above the external auditory meatus, the Frazier point offers a safe trajectory to the frontal horn of the lateral ventricle, facilitating efficient CSF diversion before dural opening. Alternatively, the Dandy point is situated 3 cm above the inion and 2 cm lateral to the midline. This technique helps minimize cerebellar retraction, enhances surgical exposure, and lowers the risk of postoperative complications, such as brain swelling and herniation [4].

13.2 Indications for the Approach

The suboccipital approach is indicated for lesions in the posterior fossa, cerebellum, brainstem, and fourth ventricle, including tumors (medulloblastomas, hemangioblastomas, metastases), vascular lesions (cavernomas, AVMs, aneurysms), and Chiari malformations [6]. It provides access to the supracerebellar-infratentorial corridor (for pineal and thalamic lesions) and the cerebellopontine angle (for vestibular schwannomas and meningiomas) [7]. This approach is also used in foramen magnum decompression for Chiari malformation and vascular decompression for trigeminal neuralgia [6]. The choice between midline and paramedian variations depends on the location of the lesion; midline approaches are preferred for fourth ventricle and vermian tumors and paramedian for supracerebellar-infratentorial approaches [6].

13.3 Operative Set-Up

Patient Positioning The patient is placed in the prone, lateral park-bench, or semi-sitting position, depending on the lesion's location. The prone position is the most commonly used for midline lesions, whereas the park-bench position is preferred for lateralized lesions, such as cerebellopontine angle tumors (Fig. 13.1) [6].

The semi-sitting position is used in neurosurgery for posterior fossa and upper cervical spine procedures and offers enhanced venous drainage, reduced intracranial pressure, improved cerebellar relaxation, and better visualization of

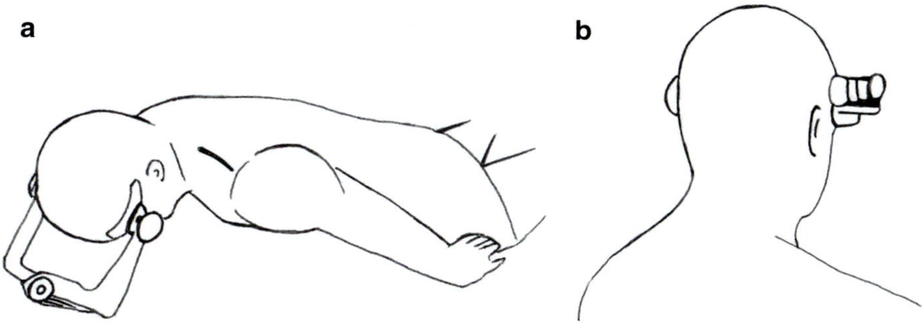

Fig. 13.1 In this illustration, we show two positions for the suboccipital approach: in (**a**), the patient is positioned in Concorde, and (**b**), in a semi-sitting position

midline structures [8]. This position minimizes cerebellar retraction, facilitating supracerebellar-infratentorial approaches to the pineal region and posterior third ventricular tumors [9]. However, it presents challenges, including hypotension, venous air embolism, paradoxical air embolism, and pneumocephalus, necessitating preoperative screening for a patent foramen ovale and intraoperative transesophageal echocardiography (TEE) monitoring to mitigate risks [10]. While its use has declined because of concerns about air embolism and hemodynamic instability, standardized protocols incorporating TEE, fluid management, and controlled positioning have significantly reduced complications, making it a viable option in experienced centers [9].

Head Positioning (Considering the Patient in Prone)

(a) *Elevation.* The head was aligned on the same axis as the cervical spine and chest, and we used the inverted Trendelenburg position. This position is often employed to promote brain relaxation by facilitating venous drainage. The head should be positioned 10°–15° higher than the chest.
(b) *Rotation.* In the lateral approach, minimal rotation may be applied to ensure that the mastoid and occipital bones remain accessible.
(c) *Flexion.* The head is flexed to widen the posterior fossa exposure, aligning the foramen magnum with the surgical field for optimal access to the brainstem and cerebellum [7].

Skin Preparation The scalp, posterior neck, and upper back are prepared with shampoo and antiseptic solution (chlorhexidine or povidone-iodine), extending from the vertex to the shoulders to maintain a sterile field. The ears were protected with sterile drapes, and the incision site was outlined to ensure exposure of the inion, asterion, mastoid region, and foramen magnum as key landmarks for craniotomy [6].

13.4 Surgical Technique (Video 13.1)

Skin Incision A midline or paramedian skin incision is made from the external occipital protuberance (inion) to C2, depending on the surgical approach. The incision extends laterally to expose key landmarks, including the asterion, digastric point, and superior nuchal line. The occipital artery, which can be used for bypass or grafting, should be preserved.

Muscle Using monopolar cautery, the paraspinal and suboccipital muscles are dissected in layers and reflected inferiorly. The splenius capitis, semispinalis capitis, and rectus capitis posterior major muscles are elevated with bipolar coagulation and sharp dissection to avoid excessive thermal injury. The muscles are either retracted laterally or sutured to the periphery for exposure, preserving soft tissue for later closure.

Craniotomy We recommend starting the craniotomy by placing burr holes at the upper extremities, 1 cm above the asterion bilaterally to expose the transverse-sigmoid sinus junction. Additional burr holes should be placed along the superior nuchal line to facilitate craniotomy, thereby ensuring venous sinus avoidance. Dural detachment is fundamental before bone cutting. A high-speed drill was used to complete the craniotomy, removing a bone flap between the transverse sinus superiorly and the foramen magnum inferiorly (Fig. 13.2). If additional space is needed, the posterior arch of C1 is removed, ensuring delicate dissection with Metzenbaum scissors and dissectors, avoiding monopolar cautery near the vertebral arteries. The safe zone to avoid vertebral arteries when dissecting the posterior arch of C1 is 1 cm lateral to the midline. The use of a Kerrison rongeur is recommended for the removal

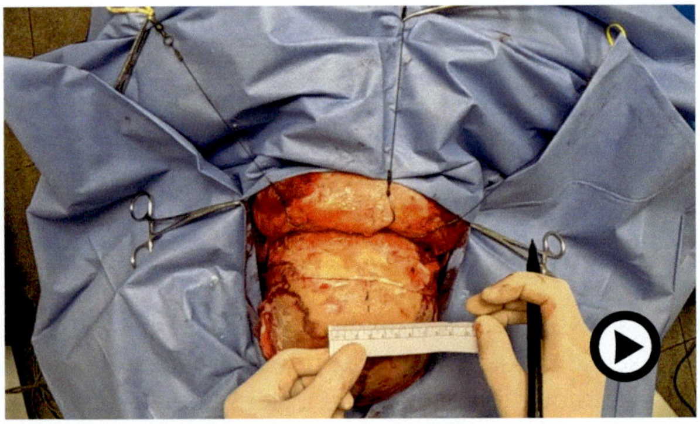

Video 13.1 This video illustrates the suboccipital approach performed in the prone position, detailing the key anatomical landmarks, bone work, and dural opening, and CSF drainage strategies for safe access to posterior fossa and fourth ventricle lesions. It also demonstrates ventricular access through Frazier's and Dandy's points for external ventricular drain (EVD) placement (▶ https://doi.org/10.1007/000-ht4)

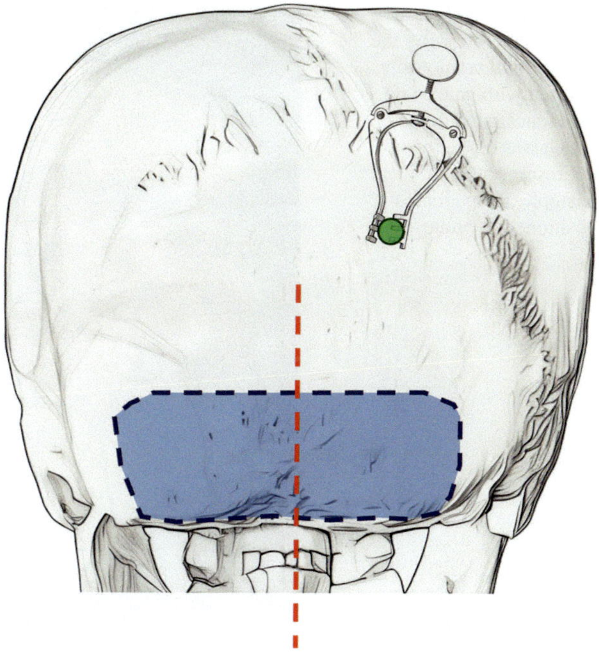

Fig. 13.2 Anatomical illustration of the suboccipital craniotomy showing a burr hole at Dandy's point with a Jansen retractor; the red dashed line corresponds to the midline straight incision. The EVD was placed before craniotomy

of the C1 arch. After craniotomy, venous bleeding from the bone edges is common and can be controlled with *Surgicel*, *Gelfoam*, and moist gauze placement.

Dural Opening The dura was opened using delicate Metzenbaum scissors in a Y- or curvilinear fashion to ensure that the torcular Herophili, transverse, and sigmoid sinuses remained intact (Fig. 13.3).

Brain Relaxation To promote brain relaxation and facilitate surgical access, the following two strategies are recommended:

(a) A ventricular drain (EVD) was placed at the Frazier point before opening to reduce intracranial pressure. We typically begin the procedure by placing the EVD before the craniotomy, keeping the drain closed until the dural opening, at which point CSF drainage is performed for brain relaxation (Figs. 13.4 and 13.5).
(b) Additional CSF drainage is performed from the cerebellum-medullary cistern following dural incision.

Closure A watertight closure was performed using autologous pericranium or dural substitutes reinforced with fibrin glue to minimize CSF leakage. Bone flap replacement: In craniotomy, the bone flap is secured with mini-plates or sutures. If craniectomy is performed, duraplasty-only closure is completed. The muscle layers are reapproximated, and the skin is closed in layers using absorbable sutures for the deep layers and nonabsorbable sutures for the skin.

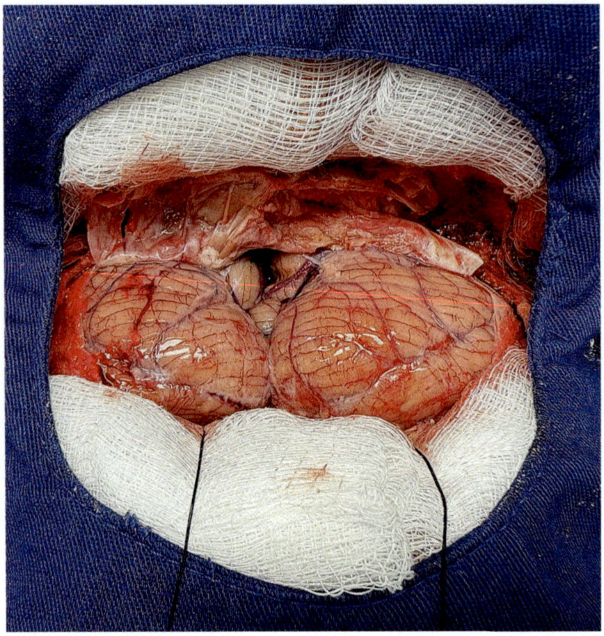

Fig. 13.3 Intraoperative photographs showing the suboccipital craniotomy covered with gauze and a blue fenestrated drape, which was ready for microsurgery. In this example, the patient is positioned in prone

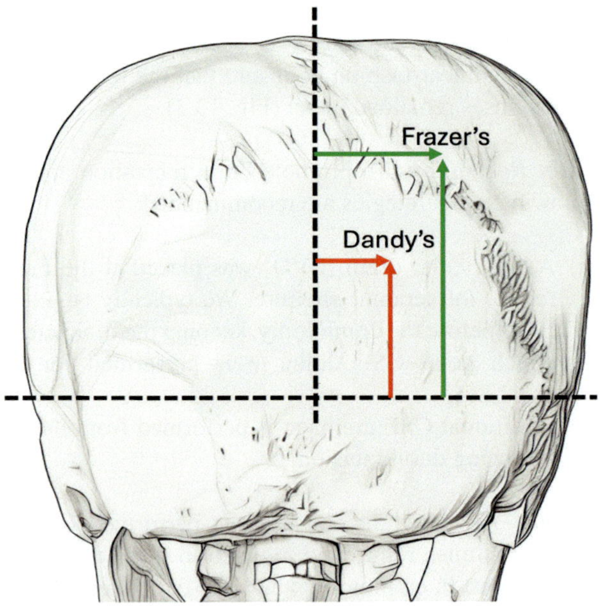

Fig. 13.4 Anatomical illustration showing two possible sites for EVD placement before the suboccipital craniotomy procedure. Frazier's point is 3–4 cm from the midline and 6–7 cm above the inion, and Dandy's point is 3 cm above the inion and 2 cm lateral to the midline

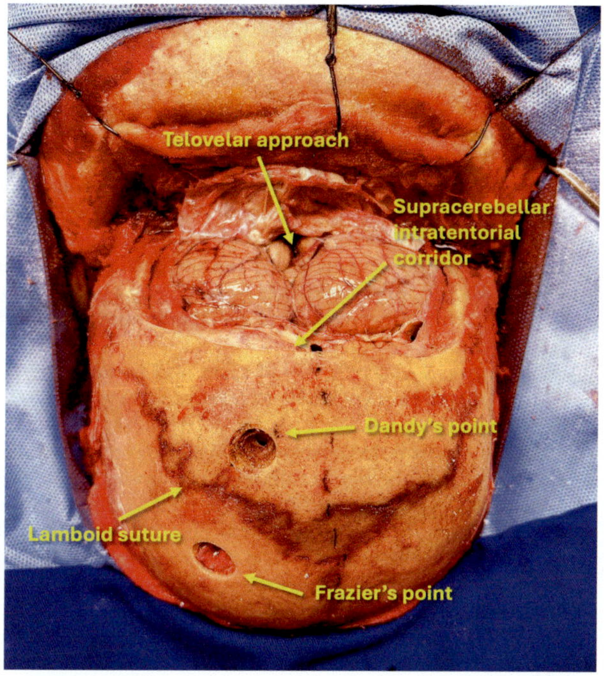

Fig. 13.5 In this image, we can see the Dandy and Frazier points for ventricular puncture and anatomical landmarks such as the sagittal suture. Additionally, the telovelar approach through the cerebellar tonsils is marked, as well as the supracerebellar-infratentorial corridor

13.5 Pearls and Pitfalls

- *Positioning*: Ensure proper prone, park-bench, or semi-sitting positioning with head elevation for venous drainage. If prone, elevate the head by inverted Trendelenburg. Over-rotating the head can impair venous return and increase intracranial pressure.
- *Craniotomy*: Burr holes are placed at the asterion to expose the transverse-sigmoid sinus junction.
- *C1 Removal*: Stay 1 cm lateral to midline to avoid vertebral artery injury; use a Kerrison rongeur.
- *Dural Opening*: A Y- or curvilinear incision is made to preserve the venous sinuses.
- *CSF Drainage*: An EVD is placed at the Dandy or Frazier points, and the CSF is draining at the cisterna magna after opening the dura.
- *Closure*: Ensure watertight dural repair with fibrin glue to prevent CSF leakage. Loose dural suturing increases the risk of CSF leakage and pseudomeningocele.

References

1. Cage T, Benet A, Golfinos J, McDermott MW. A superior cerebellar convexity two-part craniotomy to access the paramedian supra and infratentorial space: technical note. Cureus. 2016;8(6):e664.
2. Ribas GC, Rhoton AL Jr, Cruz OR, Peace DA. Suboccipital burr holes and craniectomies: an anatomical study of surgical landmarks. Neurosurg Focus. 2005;19(2):E1.
3. Bucy PC. Exposure of the posterior or cerebellar fossa. J Neurosurg. 1966;24:820–32.
4. Prell J, Rachinger J, Scheitzach J, et al. Midline-craniotomy of the posterior fossa with attached bone flap: experiences in pediatric and adult patients. Acta Neurochir. 2011;153:541–5.
5. Deshmukh VR, Figueiredo EG, Spetzler RF. Quantification and comparison of telovelar and transvermian approaches to the fourth ventricle. Neurosurgery. 2006;58(ONS Suppl 2):ONS-202–7.
6. Legnani FG, Saladino A, Casali C, et al. Craniotomy vs. craniectomy for posterior fossa tumors: a prospective study to evaluate complications after surgery. Acta Neurochir. 2013;155(12):2281–6.
7. Hadanny A, Rozovski U, Nossek E, et al. Craniectomy versus craniotomy for posterior fossa metastases: complication profile. World Neurosurg. 2016;95:3680.
8. Ganslandt O, Merkel A, Schmitt H, et al. The sitting position in neurosurgery: indications, complications, and results. Acta Neurochir. 2013;155(10):1887–93.
9. Jadik S, Wissing H, Friedrich K, et al. A standardized protocol for the prevention of clinically relevant venous air embolism during neurosurgical interventions in the semi-sitting position. Neurosurgery. 2009;64(3):533–9.
10. Porter JM, Pidgeon C, Cunningham AJ. The sitting position in neurosurgery: a critical appraisal. Br J Anaesth. 1999;82(1):117–28.

14 The Retrosigmoid Approach

14.1 Introduction

The retrosigmoid approach is a well-established surgical corridor to the posterior cranial fossa, and it is primarily used for accessing lesions in the cerebellopontine angle (CPA), such as acoustic neuromas, meningiomas, and vascular compression syndromes [1–3]. This approach involves a curvilinear incision behind the ear, followed by craniotomy that provides direct access to the CPA while minimizing cerebellar retraction [4]. The key anatomical landmarks include the transverse and sigmoid sinuses, which dictate the craniotomy boundaries to prevent iatrogenic vascular injury [5]. Studies have refined the optimal burr hole placement to reduce complications, such as excessive sinus bleeding, and to ensure a safe surgical corridor [5]. Advancements in microsurgical techniques and neuronavigation have further enhanced the efficacy and safety of this approach, making it a preferred option for posterior fossa tumor resection and neurovascular decompression [3].

The choice between craniectomy and craniotomy for the retrosigmoid approach is clinically relevant and depends on surgical goals, pathology, and patient factors. Craniotomy is associated with a lower risk of cerebrospinal fluid (CSF) leakage, pseudomeningocele formation, and wound infections, which can contribute to shorter hospital stays. Craniectomy provides a faster and broader surgical exposure but may leave the posterior fossa less protected, increasing the risk of brainstem compression, CSF-related complications, and postoperative headaches. Craniotomy is preferred when preserving normal anatomy, such as in reoperations and cases requiring precise reconstruction to reduce CSF leakage. While both approaches provide access to the cerebellopontine angle, the decision is guided by tumor size, expected complications, and the need for future interventions [6].

Supplementary Information The online version contains supplementary material available at https://doi.org/10.1007/978-3-032-04664-2_14. The videos can be accessed individually by clicking the DOI link in the accompanying figure caption or by scanning this link with the SN More Media App.

H. de Oliveira Manduca Palmiero, E. G. Figueiredo, *Neurosurgical Approaches Video Atlas*, https://doi.org/10.1007/978-3-032-04664-2_14

The asterion is a critical surgical landmark in the suboccipital approach, marking the junction of the lambdoid, occipitomastoid, and parietomastoid sutures. Correlations with the inferior half of the transverse sinus serve as a reliable reference point for burr hole placement and craniectomy planning [4]. The transition between the transverse and sigmoid sinuses occurs anteriorly to the asterion. It is a key strategy for preventing venous injury during posterior fossa and cerebellopontine angle surgery [3]. Proper identification of the asterion allows for systematic bone removal, optimizing access while minimizing complications in retrosigmoid and lateral suboccipital craniectomies [4].

Superior Petrosal Vein The superior petrosal vein, also known as Dandy's, is a crucial venous structure in the posterior cranial fossa that drains the anterior cerebellum and brainstem into the superior petrosal sinus. It is often encountered during the retrosigmoid approach, where its preservation or sacrifice poses a neurosurgical dilemma. While sacrificing the SPV can enhance surgical exposure, it carries risks, such as cerebellar venous infarction, brainstem edema, and hydrocephalus, with complication rates ranging from negligible to 30% across various studies. Therefore, SPV preservation is recommended whenever possible to minimize postoperative complications [7].

14.2 Indications for the Approach

The retrosigmoid approach is a standard technique for accessing the cerebellopontine angle (CPA) and posterior fossa. The procedure is widely used resection resections, vascular decompression, and aneurysm surgery. The main indications include *vestibular schwannomas, meningiomas*, epidermoid cysts, and other CPA lesions that require a posterolateral surgical corridor [1, 7]. It is also the preferred approach for microvascular decompression procedures, such as *Jannetta's procedure*, which treats trigeminal neuralgia [8], hemifacial spasm, and glossopharyngeal neuralgia by relieving neurovascular compression. The retrosigmoid approach also allows access to brainstem cavernomas and vertebrobasilar aneurysms [7]. The advantages of this approach include minimized cerebellar retraction and direct visualization of CPA structures, making it a versatile and practical choice for posterior fossa surgery.

14.3 Operative Set-Up [1, 9, 10]

Patient Positioning To perform the suboccipital approach, the patient can be positioned in three main ways: supine with head rotation, lateral decubitus (park-bench position), or semisitting. The supine position with head rotation is widely used, especially in retrosigmoid approaches for vestibular schwannoma and microvascular decompression. It is preferred due to its ease of setup, better cardiovascular stability, and reduced risk of air embolism. However, some surgeons favor the lateral or park-bench position for improved gravity-assisted cerebellar relaxation and

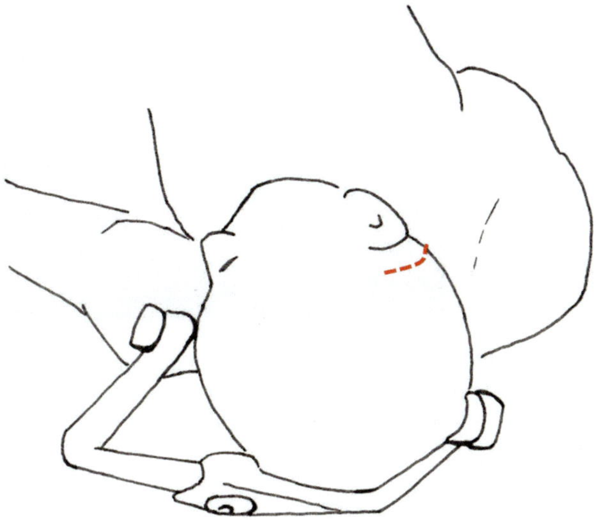

Fig. 14.1 In this illustration, the patient is in a supine position with the head rotated contralaterally to the craniotomy. This positioning is specific to the retrosigmoid and presigmoid approaches. In addition, note the retroauricular linear or arc-shaped incision (red dashed line)

better venous drainage. Proper padding is essential to prevent brachial plexus injury and pressure sores, with the dependent arm placed on a padded support (Fig. 14.1).

Head Positioning The head is secured in a three-pin Mayfield or Surgita head holder. For the supine position with head-rotation positioning, the following steps were followed to optimize surgical exposure:

(a) Elevation. The head is elevated slightly above the heart to reduce venousRetrosigmoid approachoperative set-up congestion. We recommend elevating the head of the table using the inverted Trendelenburg maneuver.
(b) Rotation. The head is rotated 30°–45° away from the side of the lesion to align the surgical corridor.
(c) Flexion. Mild flexion increases the suboccipital working angle, whereas excessive flexion is avoided to prevent jugular venous compression.

Skin Preparation The surgical field is shaved in a limited manner, preserving hair when possible. The area was prepared with shampoo and antiseptic solution (chlorhexidine or povidone-iodine).

14.4 Surgical Technique [1, 9, 10] (Video 14.1)

Skin Incision A C-shaped or curvilinear retroauricular incision is made, starting 2 cm above the pinna and extending 2 cm below the mastoid tip, ensuring sufficient exposure while preserving vascular supply. The distance from the incision to the auricle was approximately two finger widths. We recommend using a cold scalpel

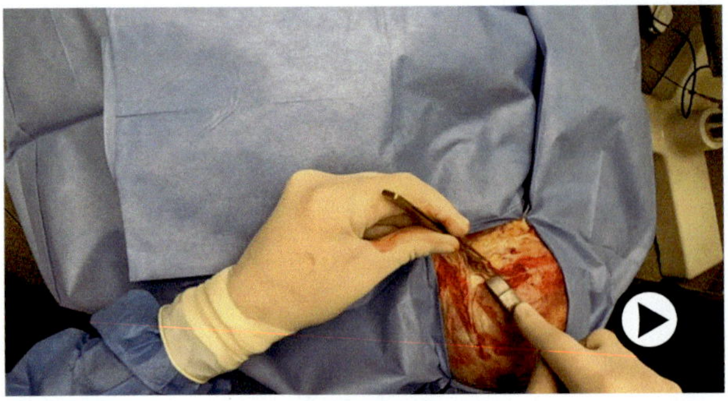

Video 14.1 This video demonstrates the retrosigmoid approach step-by-step, emphasizing key anatomical landmarks, bone work, dural opening, and cerebellar relaxation techniques for safe and effective access to the cerebellopontine angle and posterior fossa pathologies (▶ https://doi.org/10.1007/000-ht5)

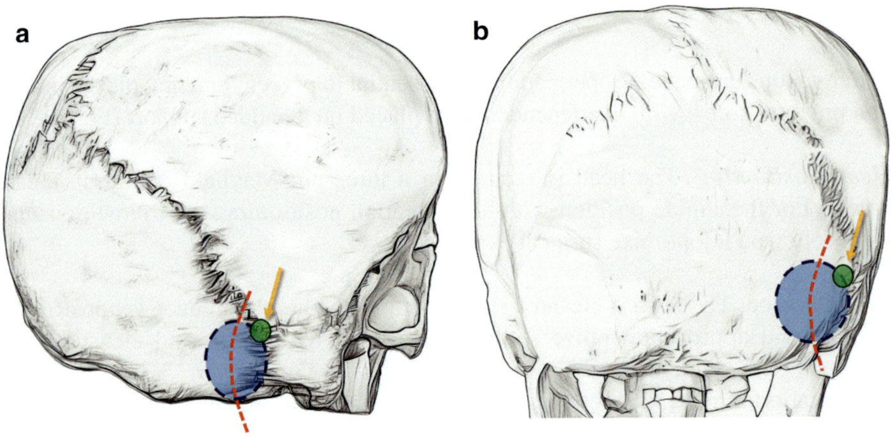

Fig. 14.2 Anatomical illustration of the retrosigmoid craniotomy is presented in two views: in (**a**), a more lateral view; and in (**b**), posteroanterior view. The first burr hole is highlighted by the green circle over the asterion (yellow arrow). The red-dashed line corresponds to the retroauricular arc-shaped incision

for the skin and monopolar cautery for deeper structures. The greater auricular and lesser occipital nerves are identified and preserved when possible (Fig. 14.2).

Muscle A myocutaneous flap is created by incising the suboccipital musculature in a layered fashion to allow adequate retraction. The sternocleidomastoid, splenius capitis, and semispinalis capitis muscles are dissected using a monopolar cautery and periosteal elevator. The suboccipital triangle is exposed, and the mastoid emissary vein is coagulated, or sealed with bone wax to control bleeding.

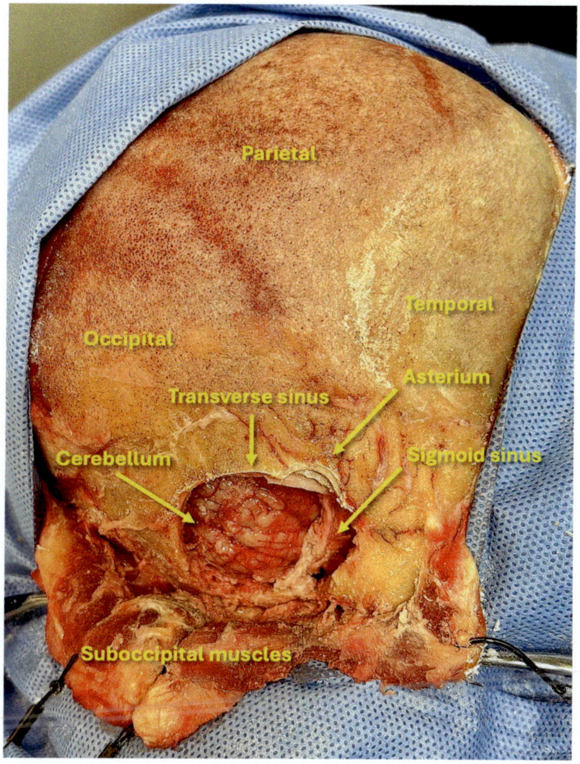

Fig. 14.3 Photograph showing the retrosigmoid craniotomy; the asterion region, the initial burr hole, and the anatomical landmarks for identifying the transverse and sigmoid venous sinus; the musculature was reflected inferiorly, although in surgical procedures, we reflect it laterally with a retractor

Craniotomy A burr hole is placed at the asterion or slightly below it to target the transverse-sigmoid sinus junction. Using a high-speed drill, a 3–4-cm craniotomy is performed to expose the sigmoid and transverse sinuses while avoiding excessive cerebellar compression. The bone flap is either replaced (craniotomy) or excluded (craniectomy) based on the surgical goals. Any exposed mastoid air cells were sealed with bone wax or fibrin glue to prevent postoperative CSF leakage (Figs. 14.2, 14.3, 14.4, 14.5, and 14.6).

Dural Opening The dura is opened in a C-shaped fashion, with the base medial to preserve the venous sinuses, approximately 3–5 mm from the transverse and sigmoid sinuses. Initial CSF drainage from the lateral cerebellomedullary cistern helps to relax the cerebellum, minimizing the need for retraction.

Once the microsurgery has been completed, identification of the internal auditory canal is challenging. *The Tübingen line* is a reliable dural landmark for identifying the inferior limit of the internal auditory canal (IAC) during the retrosigmoid approach, particularly in cases of large and giant vestibular schwannomas in which direct visualization is challenging. This anatomical line was formed by the termination of dural foldings near the vestibular aqueduct, creating a consistent reference for safe drilling of the posterior wall of the IAC. Once identified, the removal of

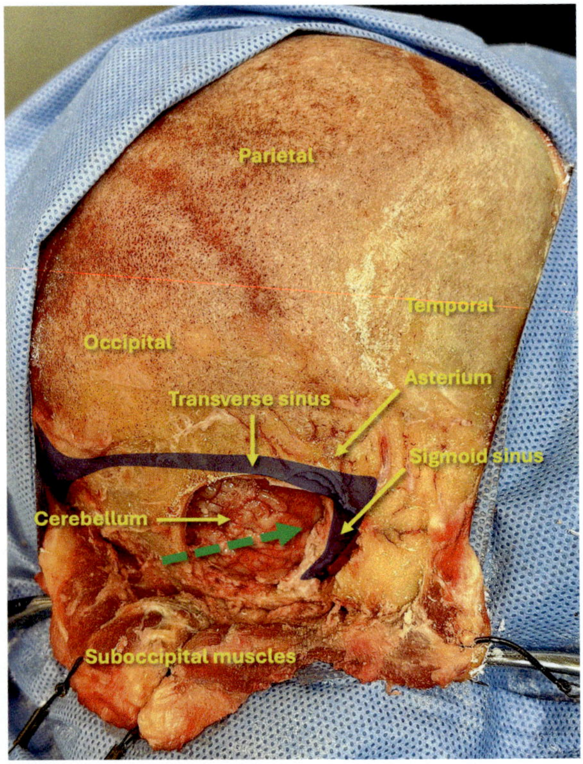

Fig. 14.4 Surface anatomy and key landmarks for the retrosigmoid approach to the cerebellopontine angle (CPA). The transverse and sigmoid sinuses are illustrated over the photograph to emphasize their important role in guiding the craniotomy and dural opening. Note the anatomical relationship of the asterion to these venous sinuses, which serves as a crucial external reference point. The green arrow indicates the surgical corridor toward the CPA

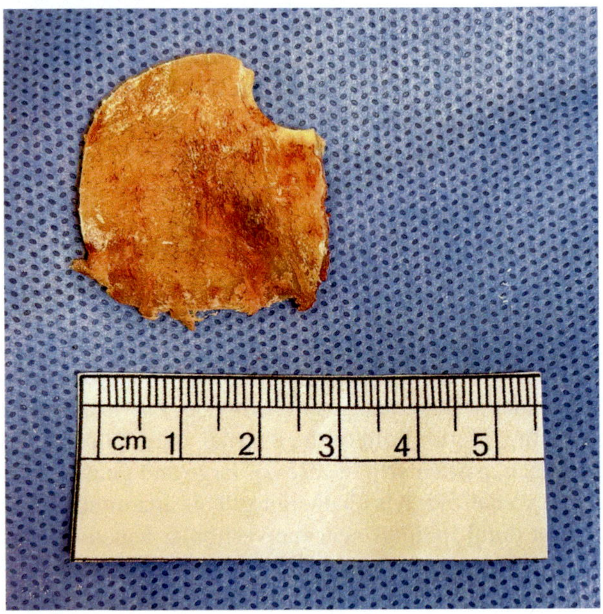

Fig. 14.5 Photograph of the bone flap, which has a diameter of 3 cm

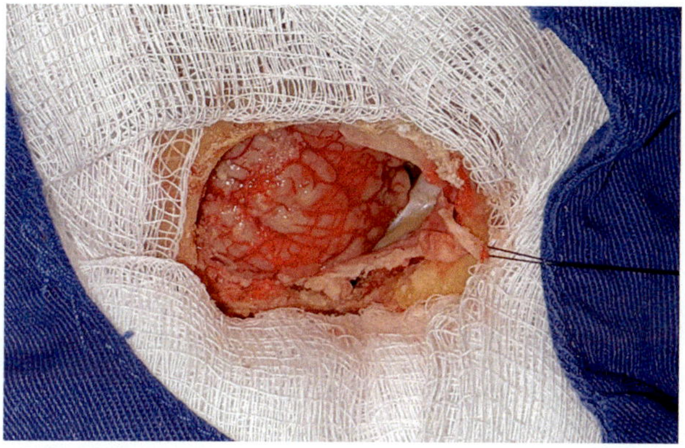

Fig. 14.6 In this image, the area of the retrosigmoid craniotomy was covered with gauze and a blue fenestrated drape, which were prepared for microsurgery

bone just above the Tübingen line consistently exposes the IAC, making it a valuable surgical guide to prevent facial and cochlear nerves [11].

Closure After tumor resection or neurovascular decompression, hemostasis is ensured, and the dura is closed in a watertight fashion using primary sutures or a dural graft. The bone flap is secured with titanium plates. The muscle and skin were meticulously reexpanded in anatomical layers to reduce dead space and minimize the risk of CSF leakage.

14.5 Pearls and Pitfalls

- Burr HoleRetrosigmoid approachpearls and pitfalls Placement: Positioning the burr hole at or slightly below the asterion optimizes access to the transverse-sigmoid sinus junction, reducing venous injury; use a diamond burr and gently dissect the dura.
- Dural Opening: A C-shaped dural opening with a medial base preserves the sigmoid and transverse sinuses, facilitating better dural reapproximation.
- CSF Drainage: Opening the cerebellum medullary cistern early allows gradual CSF release, thereby preventing sudden decompression and reducing cerebellar retraction injuries.
- Cerebellar Relaxation: Overretraction may cause cerebellar contusion or cranial nerve injury. Progressive CSF drainage minimizes the need for cerebellar retraction, thereby reducing the risk of venous congestion and infarction.
- Superior Petrosal Vein: Sacrificing the superior petrosal vein increases the risk of cerebellar infarction and brainstem edema; preserve it when possible.
- Facial and Cochlear Nerves: Excessive bipolar coagulation near the internal auditory canal can damage the cochlear and facial nerves; prioritize sharp dissection and nerve monitoring.
- Dural Closure: A watertight dural repairRetrosigmoid approachpearls and pitfalls using primary sutures or a dural substitute can prevent CSF leakage and pseudomeningocele formation.

References

1. Bambakidis NC, Megerian CA, Spetzler RF. Chapter 5 - Surgical Approaches to the Cerebellopontine Angle. In: Surgery of the cerebellopontine angles. Shelton: BC Decker; 2009. p. 80–5.
2. Fossett DT, Caputy AJ. Chapter 13 - Retrosigmoid Craniotomy. In: Operative neurosurgical anatomy. New York: Thieme; 2001. p. 81–5.
3. Rhoton AL Jr. The cerebellopontine angle and posterior fossa cranial nerves by the retrosigmoid approach. Neurosurgery. 2000;47(3):S93–129.
4. Ribas GC, Rhoton AL Jr, Cruz OR, Peace D. Suboccipital burr holes and craniectomies. Neurosurg Focus. 2005;19(2):E1.
5. Lang J Jr, Samii A. Retrosigmoidal approach to the posterior cranial fossa: an anatomical study. Acta Neurochir. 1991;111:147–53.
6. Gnanalingham KK, Lafuente J, Thompson D, Harkness W, Hayward R. Surgical procedures for posterior fossa tumors in children: does craniotomy lead to fewer complications than craniectomy? J Neurosurg. 2002;97(4):821–6.
7. Narayan V, Savardekar AR, Patra DP, et al. Safety profile of superior petrosal vein (the vein of Dandy) sacrifice in neurosurgical procedures: a systematic review. Neurosurg Focus. 2018;45(1):E3.
8. Kaufmann AM, Price AV. A history of the Jannetta procedure. J Neurosurg. 2020;132(2):639–46.
9. Elhammady MS, Telischi FF, Morcos JJ. Retrosigmoid approach: indications, techniques, and results. Otolaryngol Clin N Am. 2012;45(2):375–97.
10. Rodriguez Rubio R, Xie W, Vigo V, et al. Immersive surgical anatomy of the retrosigmoid approach. Cureus. 2021;13(6):e16068.
11. Campero A, Martins C, Rhoton AL Jr, Tatagiba M. Dural landmark to locate the internal auditory canal in large and giant vestibular schwannomas: the Tübingen line. Neurosurgery. 2011;69(ONS Suppl 1):ONS99–ONS102.

The Presigmoid Approach

15

15.1 Introduction

The presigmoid approach is a surgical technique used to access lesions in the cerebellopontine angle, petroclival region, and adjacent areas of the skull base. This approach involves creating a corridor anterior to the sigmoid sinus and posterior to the petrous part of the temporal bone, allowing surgeons to reach both the middle and posterior cranial fossae, facilitating the resection of complex lesions, such as petroclival meningiomas of cerebellopontine angle tumors [1, 2].

Initially described as a temporal-translabyrinthine approach for the treatment of vestibular schwannomas [3, 4] and later as an anatomical route to the clivus [4, 5], this approach has evolved through the work of leading surgeons, with Ossama Al-Mefty playing a crucial role in its clinical application, particularly for petroclival tumors [6, 7]. The presigmoid approach combines elements of the retrosigmoid and subtemporal routes, allowing for optimal visualization while minimizing brain retraction and neurovascular manipulation. It is highly effective in improving tumor resectability and increasing operability in cases in which lesions extend medially to the brainstem and neurovascular structures [3, 4].

Variations and Combinations [1, 6, 8] The presigmoid approach can be combined with other surgical corridors to increase exposure as follows:

(a) *Retrosigmoid Approach*: Combining retrosigmoid and retrosigmoid craniotomies provides a broader view of the cerebellopontine angle, which is beneficial for large acoustic schwannomas.

Supplementary Information The online version contains supplementary material available at https://doi.org/10.1007/978-3-032-04664-2_15. The videos can be accessed individually by clicking the DOI link in the accompanying figure caption or by scanning this link with the SN More Media App.

H. de Oliveira Manduca Palmiero, E. G. Figueiredo, *Neurosurgical Approaches Video Atlas*, https://doi.org/10.1007/978-3-032-04664-2_15

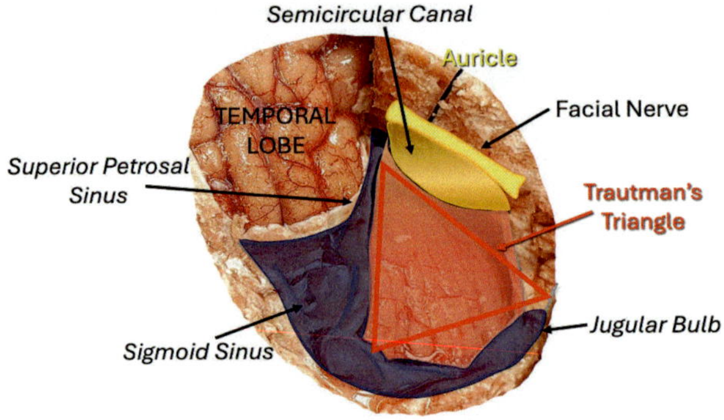

Fig. 15.1 Trautman's triangle is represented in this illustration over photograph (red triangle), corresponding to the dural region in the presigmoid approach that can be opened. Its boundaries are as follows: superior, toward the temporal lobe—*the superior petrosal sinus* (which can be ligated during the approach); anteriorly—*the semicircular canal and otic capsule*; and postero-inferiorly—*the sigmoid sinus and jugular bulb*. In this figure, we can also see the course of the facial nerve (highlighted), its relationship with this approach, and the rationale for electrophysiological monitoring during mastoidectomy

(b) *Supratentorial Approach*: Incorporating temporal craniotomy improves the visualization of lesions that involves the tentorium.
(c) *Anterior Petrosal (Kawase's) Approach*: Combining anterior petrosectomy with the presigmoid route provides access to lesions extending into the middle cranial fossa.

Neuronavigation and Electrophysiological Monitoring Understanding the anatomy of the temporal bone, its relationship with the transverse and sigmoid sinuses, the jugular bulb, and the superior petrosal sinus, as well as the course of the facial nerve through the temporal bone, is fundamental for performing the retrosigmoid approach. Neuronavigation is a crucial tool in this approach, providing an additional layer of guidance during surgery and assisting the surgeon in reaching key areas, such as the petroclival region. Furthermore, given the close anatomical relationship of this surgical corridor with the brainstem, cerebellopontine angle (CPA), and cranial nerves IV, V, VI, VII, and VIII, neurophysiological monitoring plays a vital role in protecting the functionality of these neural structures during the procedure (Fig. 15.1) [3].

15.2 Indications for the Approach

The presigmoid approach is primarily indicated for lesions in the cerebellopontine angle (CPA), brainstem, and petroclival region, particularly when traditional retrosigmoid or subtemporal approaches do not provide adequate exposure. Often used for petroclival meningiomas, vestibular schwannomas, epidermoid cysts, chordoma, brainstem cavernoma, and basilar artery aneurysms. This approach is especially advantageous for lesions that extend both supra- and infratentorially, necessitating a combined view of the middle and posterior cranial fossae. In addition, it offers a broad surgical field while minimizing brain retraction and reducing the risk of injury to vital neurovascular structures. However, its application must be considered carefully in cases where hearing preservation is a priority, as some variations, such as translabyrinthine or transcochlear modifications, may lead to permanent hearing loss [1–3].

15.3 Operative Set-Up [1, 2, 4, 9, 10]

Patient Positioning The patient is then placed in the supine position on the operating table. The head is fixed with Mayfield or Sugita head holders, ensuring rigid fixation. Electrophysiological monitoring is mostly set up to prevent facial nerve injury during drilling near the facial nerve canal because of the localization of the brainstem and cranial nerves localized in the corridor (Fig. 15.2).

Head Positioning

(a) *Elevation.* The head is elevated 10°–15° to reduce venous congestion. The inverted Trendelenburg maneuver is helpful at this point.

(b) *Rotation.* The head is rotated approximately 90° to the contralateral side to optimize the surgical corridor. We recommend placing a padded support under the ipsilateral shoulder to facilitate rotation because relying solely on cervical rotation may cause brachial plexus injuries and jugular compression. The sagittal suture should remain parallel to the ground [4].

(c) *Flexion.* Mild neck flexion is recommended to align the posterior fossa with the surgical approach. Excessive flexion should be avoided to prevent jugular vein compression and intracranial hypertension.

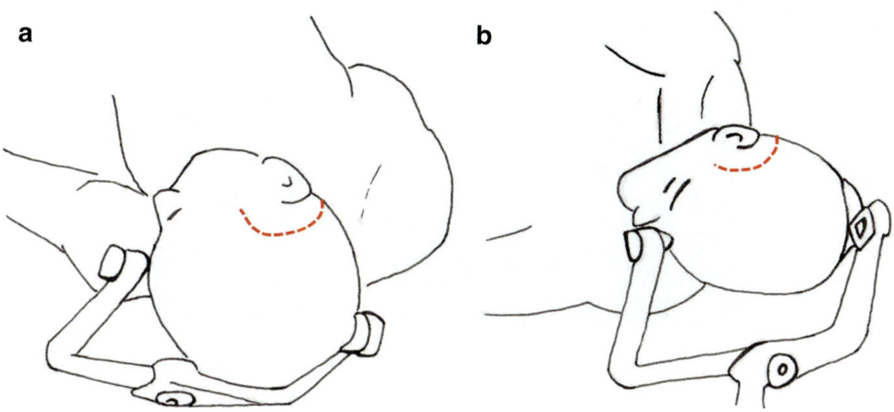

Fig. 15.2 For the presigmoid approach, the positioning can be the same as for the retrosigmoid approach (**a**) or lateral (**b**). The arc-shaped incision is marked in red

Skin Preparation Standard antiseptic preparation with shampoo, chlorhexidine, or povidone-iodine is performed, covering the auricle, mastoid region, and upper cervical area. Draping includes isolating the ear and covering the operative field from the temporal region to the upper cervical spine, thereby allowing access to both the presigmoid and retrosigmoid regions.

15.4 Surgical Technique [1, 2, 4, 9, 10] (Video 15.1)

Skin Incision A C-shaped retroauricular incision is made with two fingers behind the ear, starting at the pinna, extending posteriorly around the auricle, and curving down 3 cm below the mastoid tip. The greater auricular nerve was preserved to minimize postoperative numbness. The incision was extended to the temporalis fascia and mastoid periosteum to provide adequate exposure.

Muscle Flap The sternocleidomastoid and splenius capitis muscles are retracted inferiorly, while the temporalis muscle is dissected with a monopolar cautery and the periosteal elevator is reflected anteriorly. The periosteum and soft tissue are dissected to expose the mastoid process, supramastoid crest, and asterism, which serve as landmarks for the sigmoid sinus. The digastric groove and spine of Henle were identified to assist in locating the mastoid antrum and sinodural angle (Citelli's angle).

Craniotomy (Figs. 15.3, 15.4, 15.5, 15.6, and 15.7)
Mastoidectomy. A mastoidectomy is performed using a high-speed drill with continuous irrigation to expose the sigmoid sinus posteriorly, superior petrosal sinus superiorly, and presigmoid dura medially. The bone covering the venous sinuses has a more cortical consistency, serving as an anatomical landmark near the sinuses

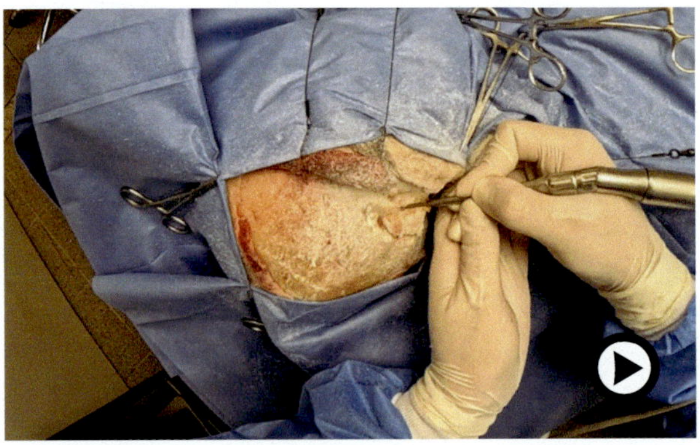

Video 15.1 This video demonstrates the presigmoid approach, highlighting the step-by-step execution of mastoidectomy and temporal craniotomy to access the cerebellopontine angle and petroclival region through Trautman's triangle and anterior to the sigmoid sinus, with emphasis on key anatomical landmarks, surgical technique, and neurovascular preservation (▶ https://doi.org/10.1007/000-ht6)

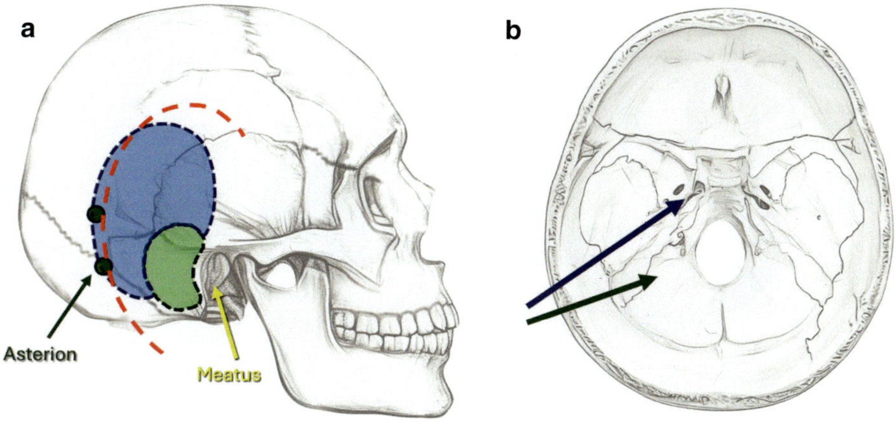

Fig. 15.3 In (**a**), the illustration shows the presigmoid approach where is designed the skin incision (red dashed C-shaped) and craniotomy area formed by the mastoidectomy (light green area) and the temporal craniotomy (blue area); also see the burr holes (green circles), the Asterion, and the meatus. In (**b**), we can observe the intracranial reach of the retrosigmoid approach: the cerebellopontine angle region through the mastoidectomy (green arrow) and the petroclival region through the temporal craniotomy combined with the mastoidectomy (navy blue arrow)

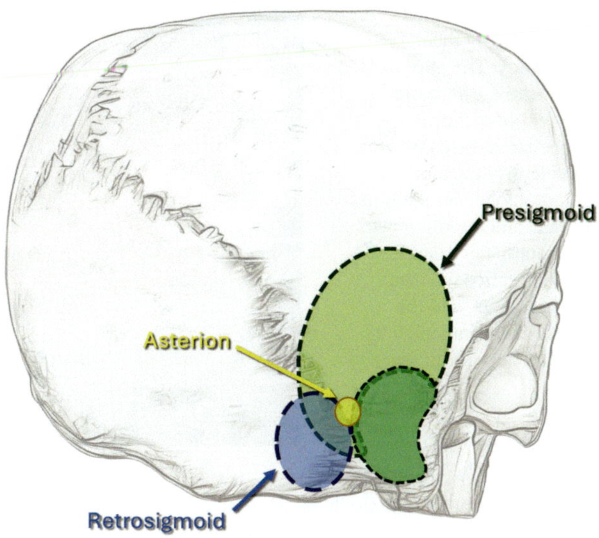

Fig. 15.4 In this illustration, we see the retrosigmoid (blue area) and presigmoid (green area) approaches compared, along with their relationship to the Asterion, a craniometric reference point for identifying the sigmoid sinus

(Figs. 15.4, 15.5, 15.6, and 15.7). The tegmen mastoideum was carefully thinned to prevent CSF leakage. The presigmoid dura was exposed by drilling as follows:

(a) Laterally, to reveal the sinodural angle.
(b) Medially to expose the *Trautman* triangle identified by the a. jugular bulb and the sigmoid sinus postero-inferiorly; b. superior petrosal sinus superiorly; c. otic capsule anteriorly.

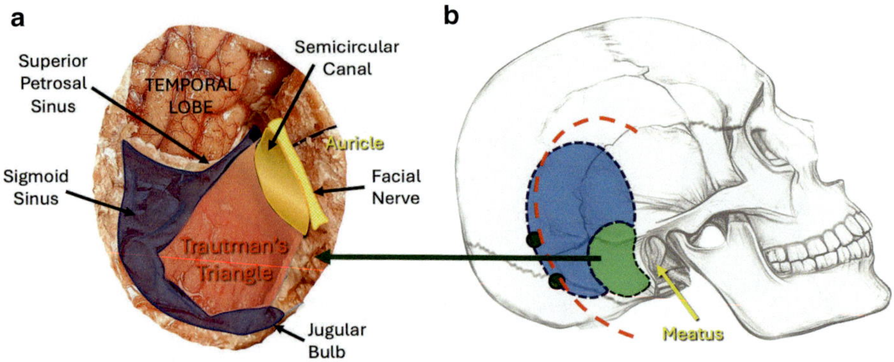

Fig. 15.5 This illustration shows the microscopic view (on the left, **a**) of the mastoidectomy region, corresponding to the light green area on the right (**b**). Observe Trautman's triangle in (**a**) and its relationships with surrounding structures

Fig. 15.6 Operative photograph showing the combined presigmoid approach with temporal craniotomy, with gauze and a blue fenestrated drape covering the craniotomy. The approach anterior to the sigmoid sinus exposes the cerebellar surface. We can also identify the auricle, temporal lobe, cerebellum surface, and the references for Trautman's triangle: superior petrosal sinus, sigmoid sinus, and the jugular bulb (indicated by the direction of the arrow)

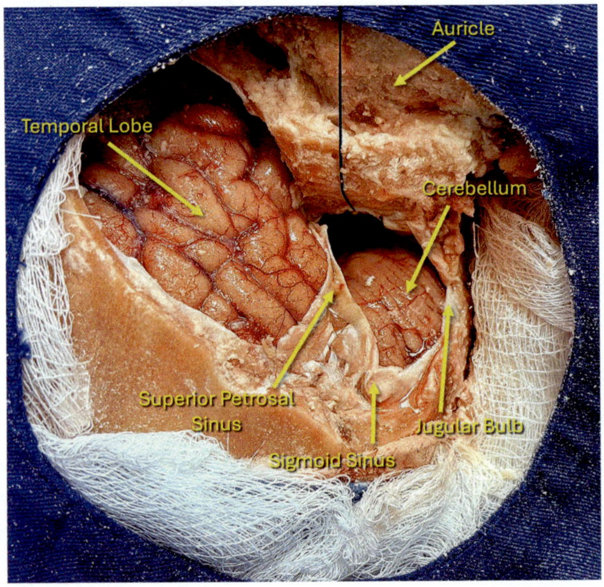

The posterior fossa dura is identified, and the approach is extended anteriorly if needed by removing part of the petrous apex. If more exposure is necessary, the labyrinth can be drilled (translabyrinthine approach) or the cochlea (transcochlear approach), sacrificing hearing.

Temporal Craniotomy Some authors have suggested [4], and we also recommend performing temporal craniotomy after completing mastoidectomy to facilitate sigmoid sinus retraction, improve posterior fossa exposure, and expand the surgical corridor to the middle fossa. For this procedure, one or two burr holes are made at

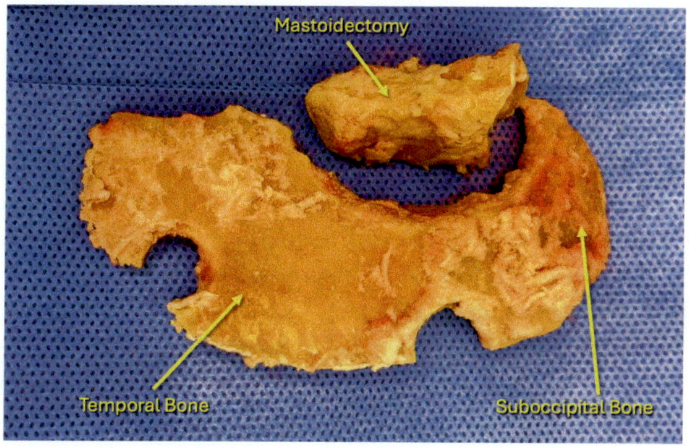

Fig. 15.7 Photograph showing the bone flaps associated with the mastoidectomy and the temporal-suboccipital bone flap

the posterior limit of the temporal craniotomy, followed by dural detachment and finally bone cutting.

In anatomical terms and for comparison purposes, see in Fig. 15.4 the retrosigmoid and presigmoid approaches and their relationship with the Asterion, the landmark for identifying the sigmoid sinus.

Dural Opening The dura is incised parallel to the superior petrosal sinus in a T- or C-shaped manner, with one limb along the presigmoid dura and the other extending into the posterior fossa. The superior petrosal sinus may be ligated and divided if additional exposure is required. Microsurgical dissection continues to expose the cerebellopontine angle, petroclival region, and brainstem (Fig. 15.6).

Closure Dural closure is performed using a watertight primary closure or patch graft to prevent CSF leakage. A fat graft or muscle plug is placed in the mastoid defect to prevent further CSF fistula. The temporal bone flap is fixed with mini plates and screws, and the mastoid bone defect is covered with a titanium mesh or hydroxyapatite cement, particularly if extensive petrosectomy is performed. The muscle flap is repositioned, and the skin is closed in layers. A pressure dressing is applied to minimize postoperative swelling and hematoma formation.

15.5 Pearls and Pitfalls

- *Patient Positioning*: The supine position with 90° head rotation and mild neck flexion optimizes surgical exposure while avoiding jugular compression and brachial plexus injury.
- *Mastoidectomy* must be carefully performed to expose the sigmoid sinus, superior petrosal sinus, and presigmoid dura while using the cortical bone consistency near the venous sinuses for guidance.

- *Temporal craniotomy after mastectomy* facilitates sigmoid sinus retraction, improves posterior fossa exposure, and expands the surgical corridor to the middle fossa.
- *Identifying the Trautman* triangle enhances access to the posterior fossa and CPA.
- *Dural Opening* should follow a T- or C-shaped incision, with ligation of the superior petrosal sinus if needed for greater exposure.
- *Neuronavigation and Neurophysiological Monitoring* are essential for avoiding facial nerve, cranial nerves IV–VIII, and brainstem structures.
- *Closure* requires watertight dural repair with a fat graft or muscle plug in the mastoid defect to prevent CSF leakage. A titanium mesh or hydroxyapatite cement may be used to reconstruct extensive petrosectomy defects.

References

1. Alejandra J, Mariana R, Andrea D, Fernando M. Edgardo south anatomy of surgical presigmoid approach. Indian J Anat Surg Head Neck Brain. 2017;3(4):110–4.
2. Bambakidis NC, Megerian CA, Spetzler RF. Chapter 5 - Surgical Approaches to the Cerebellopontine Angle. In: Surgery of the cerebellopontine angles. Shelton: BC Decker; 2009. p. 80–5.
3. Morrison AW, King TT. Experiences with a translabyrinthine-transtentorial approach to the cerebellopontine angle. J Neurosurg. 1973;38(3):382–90.
4. Siqueira MG. Chapter 10 - Acesso pré-sigmoide. In: Tratado de Neurocirurgia: volume I. Barueri: Manole; 2016. p. 84–90.
5. Hakuba A, Nishimura S, Tanaka K, Kishi H, Nakamura T. Clivus meningioma: six cases of total removal. Neurol Med Chir (Tokyo). 1977;17(2):127–39.
6. Al-Mefty O, Aum D, Rassi MS. Petroclival meningiomas and the petrosal approach. In: McDermott MW, editor. Handbook of clinical neurology, Meningiomas, Part II, vol. 170. Amsterdam: Elsevier; 2020.
7. Al-Mefty O, Dunn IF, Pravdenkova S, Abolfotoh M. True petroclival meningiomas: results of surgical management. J Neurosurg. 2014;120(1):40–51.
8. Albairmani SS, Muthana A, Mohammed TF, Al-Zaidy MF, Atallah O, Aljuboori A, et al. Combined presigmoid approach: a literature review. Surg Neurol Int. 2024;15:342.
9. Troude L, Baucher G, Lavieille J-P, Roche P-H. The presigmoid-retrolabyrinthine approach: technical note. Neurochirurgie. 2021;67(6):503–7.
10. Moreira LB, Meybodi AT, Zhao X, Almefty KK, Lawton MT, Preul MC. Dissection of the petrosal presigmoid-retrolabyrinthine approach for the petroclival region on a cadaver: 2-dimensional operative video. Oper Neurosurg (Hagerstown). 2020;19:1–2.

The Far Lateral Approach

16

16.1 Introduction

The far lateral approach is a skull base surgical technique that provides access to the craniocervical junction, including the lower clivus, anterior foramen magnum, and upper cervical spine. Originally described by Roberto Heros in 1986 [1, 2], this approach has since evolved into a versatile method for treating various pathologies, such as vertebrobasilar aneurysms, foramen magnum meningiomas, and schwannomas of the lower cranial nerves [2, 3]. By extending the lateral suboccipital route and incorporating bony resection techniques, including transcondylar, supracondylar, and paracondylar modifications, the far lateral approach enhances surgical exposure while minimizing brainstem retraction [3, 4]. A thorough understanding of the surgical anatomy, including the vertebral artery's extradural course, the cranial nerve pathways, and the bony landmarks of the occipital condyle, is essential to perform the approach, optimize patient outcomes, and reduce complications [3, 4].

As initially described by Heros [1], the far lateral approach is a modification of the lateral suboccipital approach, in which accessing the proximal basilar trunk, vertebrobasilar junction, vertebral artery, inferolateral cerebellum, and the anterior and lateral portions of the foramen magnum requires additional bone removal from the rim of the foramen magnum toward the occipital condyle, as well as removal of the posterolateral arch of the atlas to expose the vertebral artery. This approach allows exposure of the lateral suboccipital-cervical region with minimal retraction of the brainstem [1], mainly the medulla.

Supplementary Information The online version contains supplementary material available at https://doi.org/10.1007/978-3-032-04664-2_16. The videos can be accessed individually by clicking the DOI link in the accompanying figure caption or by scanning this link with the SN More Media App.

H. de Oliveira Manduca Palmiero, E. G. Figueiredo, *Neurosurgical Approaches Video Atlas*, https://doi.org/10.1007/978-3-032-04664-2_16

Anatomical Landmarks The far lateral approach relies on key anatomical landmarks to provide safe and effective access to the craniocervical junction and anterior foramen magnum. The superior nuchal line and external occipital protuberance mark the upper limit of the approach, whereas the inferior nuchal line provides an attachment for muscles that must be dissected. The occipital condyle, which articulates with the atlas, is a crucial bone structure that can be partially resected to improve exposure. The vertebral artery, especially its V3 segment, courses through the sulcus arteriosus of the C1 posterior arch and may be carefully mobilized. The hypoglossal canal housing the cranial nerve XII serves as the medial boundary, while the jugular foramen marks the lateral extent. Safe execution of the approach requires preserving vital neurovascular structures, including the occipital artery, sigmoid sinus, and lower cranial nerves (IX, X, XI, XII), ensuring adequate exposure while minimizing complications [1, 3, 5].

Muscle Layers The far lateral approach requires sequential dissection of multiple muscle layers, progressing from superficial to deep [3].

(a) The superficial layer includes the *sternocleidomastoid* and *trapezius muscles*, which expose the deeper muscles.
(b) The second layer comprises the *splenius capitis* and *semispinalis capitis*, which must be carefully detached to reveal the suboccipital triangle.
(c) The third layer includes the *longissimus capitis* and *posterior belly of the digastric muscle*, which overlay the deeper suboccipital muscles.
(d) The fourth layer, crucial for exposing the vertebral artery and bony landmarks, comprises the *posterior major and minor*, *obliquus capitis superior*, and *obliquus capitis inferior*, forming the suboccipital triangle. Proper identification and reflection of these layers allow access to the vertebral artery, occipital condyle, and foramen magnum, ensuring a safe surgical corridor [3, 5].

Occipital Condyle and the Arch of C1 The necessity of removing the C1 arch during the far lateral approach depends on the location of the lesion and the surgical exposure requirements. Studies have shown that C1 laminectomy is not always required, especially when the lesion is positioned above the lower margin of the foramen magnum, as adequate exposure can be achieved without it, thereby reducing surgical morbidity [6]. However, in cases where extensive exposure is needed, such as for lesions extending inferiorly or involving the vertebral artery's course, C1 laminectomy may be necessary [7]. Regarding occipital condyle resection, partial drilling is generally safe and improves the surgical corridor, particularly for lesions located below the hypoglossal canal. Cadaveric studies have indicated that up to 40% of the condyle can be removed without compromising the atlanto-occipital joint's stability, provided the hypoglossal canal remains intact [8]. The balance between maximizing exposure and preserving structural integrity is crucial for optimizing surgical outcomes.

16.2 Indications for the Approach

The far lateral approach is indicated for lesions in the ventrolateral and anterior regions of the foramen magnum, craniocervical junction, and lower clivus. It is commonly used for resecting anterior foramen magnum meningiomas, chordoma, epidermoid lesions, and schwannomas, as well as for vascular lesions, such as posterior inferior cerebellar artery aneurysms. This approach is advantageous when lesions are obstructed by the brainstem, lower cranial nerves, or vertebral artery, making traditional posterior approaches inadequate. Additionally, the far lateral approach is preferred for decompressing brainstem compression caused by vascular loops and microvascular decompression. The ability to provide direct access while minimizing brainstem and cerebellar retraction is essential for safely and effectively treating complex skull base pathologies [2, 3].

16.3 Operative Set-Up [1, 4, 9]

Patient Positioning The patient is typically positioned in either the lateral or park-bench position, ensuring optimal access to the craniocervical junction while minimizing brainstem and cerebellar retraction. In the lateral position, the patient lies with the operative side facing upward, and the body is stabilized with adequate padding, including an axillary roll to prevent brachial plexus compression. The park-bench position provides additional exposure by allowing the head to be rotated downward while maintaining a neutral spinal alignment (Fig. 16.1).

Head Positioning

(a) *Elevation.* The head is positioned slightly above the level of the heart to promote venous drainage and reduce the risk of air embolism by using the inverted Trendelenburg position.

(b) *Rotation.* A 30° tilt toward the ipsilateral shoulder improved access to the foramen magnum and lateral skull base.

(c) *Flexion.* The head is flexed so that the chin is approximately one finger width (3 cm) from the sternum, optimizing the surgical angle while avoiding jugular vein compression. Care should be taken to prevent excessive flexion, which could compromise vertebral artery flow and brainstem perfusion.

The ipsilateral shoulder is gently pulled down and secured with tape to improve access to the craniocervical junction and to reduce obstruction by the shoulder. This maneuver enhances the surgical corridor while ensuring that the head remains in a stable and optimized position. Adequate padding should be used to prevent brachial plexus compression.

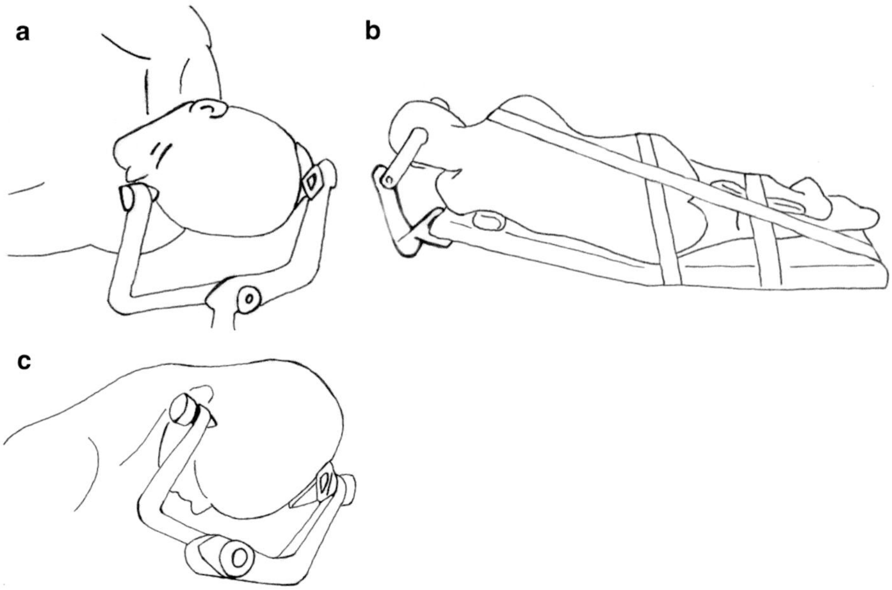

Fig. 16.1 Illustration showing the park bench positioning (**a**): front view of the patient and (**b**): back view of the patient, noting the use of adhesive tapes over the shoulder, applying traction toward the foot of the table, pelvis, and lower limbs) and the lateral positioning (**c**). (Source: Personal Archive)

Skin Preparation The scalp was shaved approximately 2 cm beyond the planned incision to facilitate drape adhesion and reduce infection risk. Antisepsis is performed using shampoo and povidone-iodine or chlorhexidine, ensuring coverage of the occipital and mastoid regions, extending to the upper cervical spine.

16.4 Surgical Technique [1, 4, 5, 9] (Video 16.1)

Skin Incision A hockey-stick or inverted "L" incision is made, beginning 3 cm above the mastoid tip, extending superiorly, curving medially just below the superior nuchal line, and then extending inferiorly to C2–3. The incision follows natural anatomical landmarks, ensuring adequate exposure while preserving vascular integrity for proper healing. The skin flaps are reflected laterally with meticulous hemostasis using bipolar cautery.

Muscle Dissection According to Heros' original description [1], the muscle mass is dissected with monopolar cautery, but first, the sternocleidomastoid, splenius capitis, and semispinalis capitis muscles are dissected and retracted laterally to expose the deeper suboccipital muscles. Subsequently, and more carefully, the

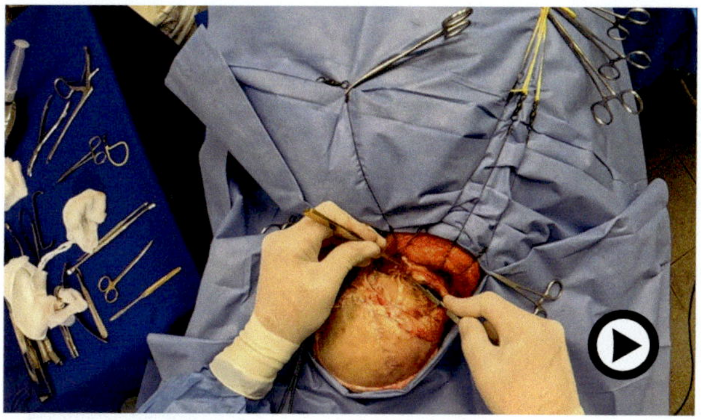

Video 16.1 This video demonstrates the far lateral approach, outlining the step-by-step process of suboccipital exposure, removal of the C1 arch, and partial drilling of the occipital condyle to access the craniocervical junction and anterior foramen magnum. It emphasizes anatomical landmarks, safe dissection and preservation of the vertebral artery, and dural opening (▶ https://doi.org/10.1007/000-ht7)

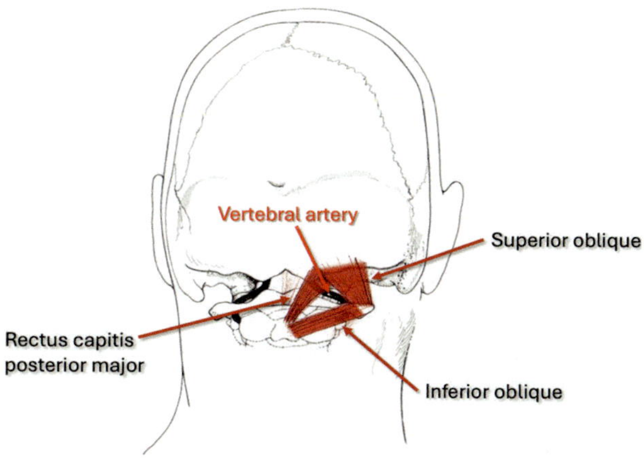

Fig. 16.2 Illustration showing the deepest muscle layer forming the suboccipital triangle: rectus capitis posterior major, obliquus capitis superior, and obliquus capitis inferior. At the center of the triangle, we can identify the vertebral artery. (Source: Personal Archive)

longissimus capitis, rectus capitis posterior major, obliquus capitis superior, and obliquus capitis inferior are reflected to preserve the vertebral artery and the surrounding venous plexus. The suboccipital triangle is exposed, providing access to the C1 posterior arch and vertebral artery (Fig. 16.2).

Craniotomy *Suboccipital Craniotomy*: At least two burr holes are placed, one near the asterion and another medially at the inferior occipital bone. A lateral suboccipital craniotomy is performed, exposing the sigmoid sinus, transverse sinus, and foramen magnum. The bony exposure extends laterally to improve surgical access without excessive cerebellar retraction (Figs. 16.3, 16.4, 16.5, 16.6, and 16.7).

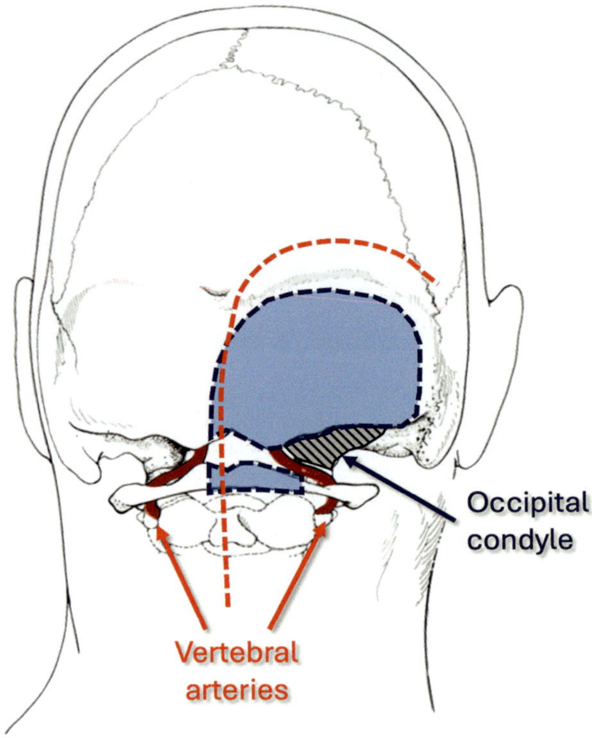

Fig. 16.3 Illustration showing the craniotomy (blue area), the arch of C1, the occipital condyle (striped area), and the vertebral arteries. See the L-shaped incision (red dashed line). (Source: Personal Archive)

Removal of the C1 Arch: The posterior arch of C1 is removed using a high-speed drill and Kerrison rongeurs, extending from the midline to the sulcus arteriosus of the vertebral artery. Care should be taken to avoid excessive venous bleeding from the vertebral venous plexus. A safer way to dissect the C1 arch while identifying the vertebral artery follows two principles: a. the vertebral artery is related to the superior surface of the C1 arch from 1 cm lateral to the midline; b. the use of a blunt dissector is more prudent than monopolar cautery when working near the C1 arch.

Partial Condyle Resection: when required, the posterior third of the occipital condyle is drilled, ensuring that the hypoglossal canal remains intact to prevent cranial nerve XII injury. Drilling is performed stepwise, removing the bone incrementally while preserving the atlanto-occipital joint's stability.

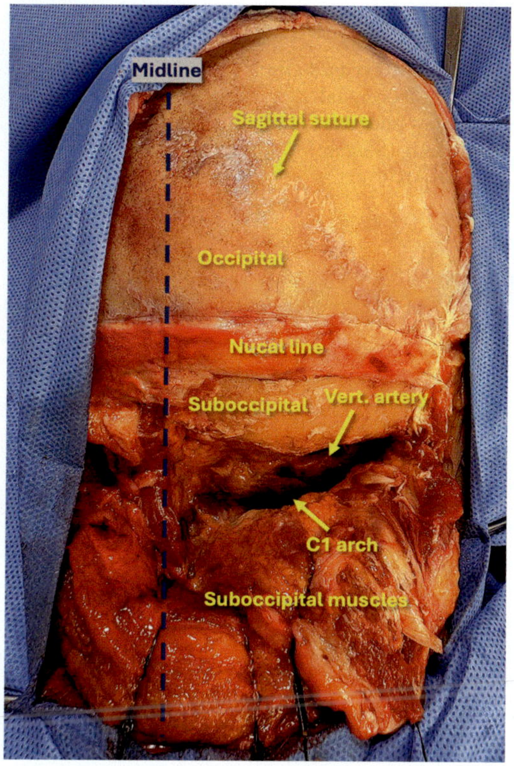

Fig. 16.4 Surgical photograph demonstrating the occipital-suboccipital region on the right side, the nuchal line, the suboccipital muscles dissected and reflected inferiorly, and the right vertebral artery resting on the C1 arch. (Source: Personal Archive)

Dural Opening The dura is opened using a C- or Y-shaped incision starting from the transverse-sigmoid junction down to the foramen magnum and C1. The dura is tented laterally toward the mastoid to optimize surgical exposure and minimize brainstem retraction. After the start of microscopy, cerebrospinal fluid is drained from the cisterna magna to relax the cerebellum and improve visualization.

Closure The dura is closed and watertight using a 4-0 absorbable suture, with fascia lata or dural substitute grafts used for reinforcement. The occipital bone flap is repositioned and secured with a miniplate and screws. The muscles are reapproximated layer by layer, and the skin is closed using subcutaneous and skin sutures. A compressive sterile dressing is applied to minimize postoperative hematoma formation.

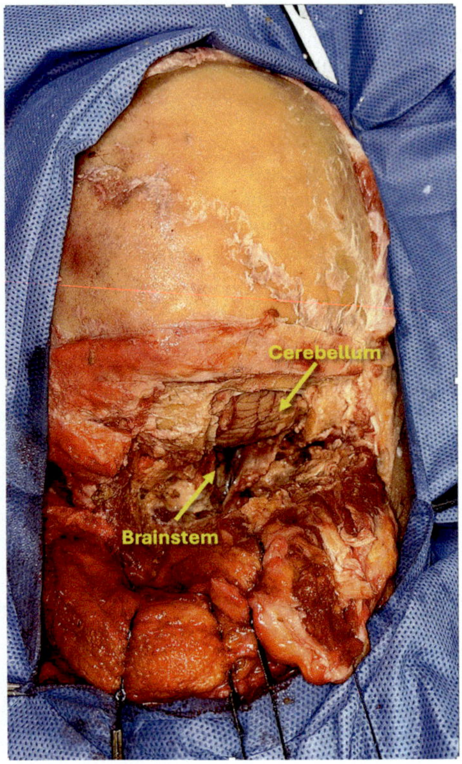

Fig. 16.5 In this image, the cerebellum and brainstem are exposed after the right suboccipital craniotomy and removal of the C1 arch. (Source: Personal Archive)

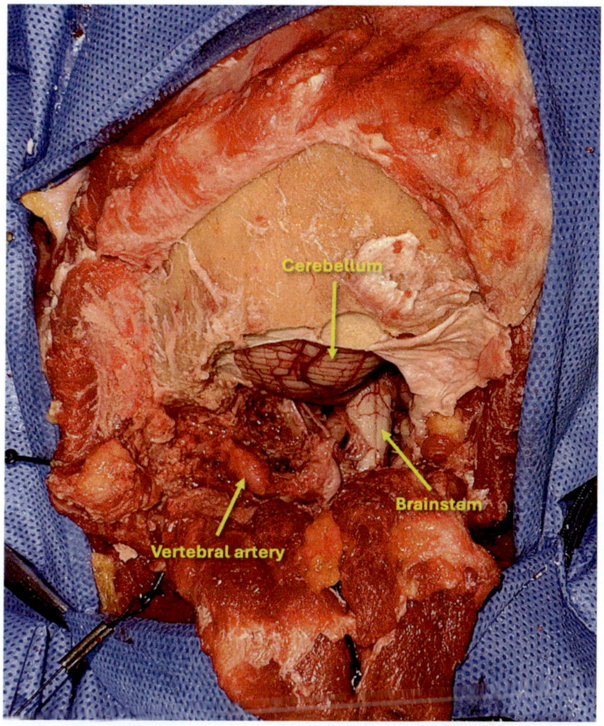

Fig. 16.6 Photograph of the far lateral approach in another specimen, exposing the cerebellum and brainstem. (Source: Personal Archive)

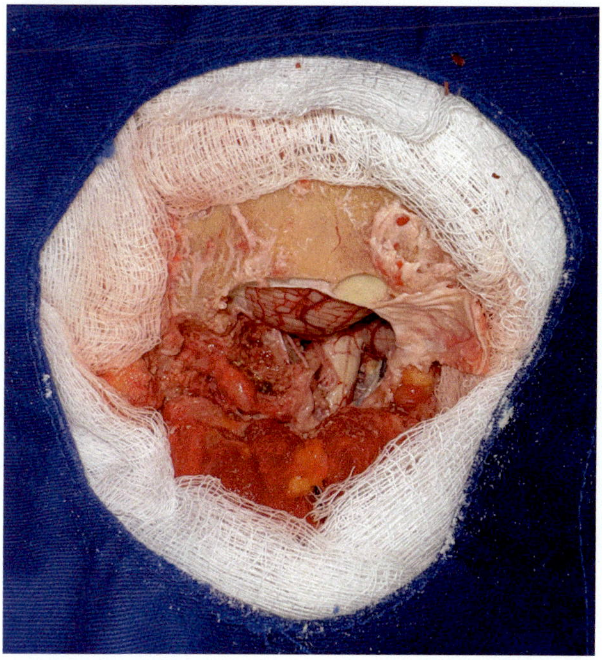

Fig. 16.7 In this picture, the far lateral approach was performed on the right side, with gauze and a blue fenestrated drape prepared for microsurgery. (Source: Personal Archive)

16.5 Pearls and Pitfalls

- *Head Positioning*: Avoid excessive flexion to prevent jugular vein compression and impaired venous drainage.
- *Muscle dissection*: *The* sternocleidomastoid and suboccipital muscles *are* carefully *retracted* to minimize venous bleeding.
- *Vertebral Artery*: Identify the artery lateral to the midline on the superior surface of the C1 arch; use a blunt dissector instead of a monopolar cautery near C1.
- *C1 Arch*: Only remove when necessary to improve access; excessive resection increases craniocervical instability.
- *Occipital Condyle*: Up to 40% of the occiput is possible if the hypoglossal canal remains intact.
- *Dural opening*: *A* C- or Y-shaped incision reflects the dura laterally toward the mastoid to optimize exposure while minimizing brainstem retraction.
- *Cerebrospinal fluid drainage*: *The* cerebellum medullary cistern *is opened* early to relax the cerebellum and reduce retraction.
- *Closure*: Ensure watertight dural repair using 4-0 absorbable sutures with fascia lata or dural substitutes. Reapproximate muscle layer by layer to ensure proper healing and reduce dead space. The occipital bone flap was secured with a miniplate and screws for structural stability.

References

1. Heros RC. Lateral suboccipital approach for vertebral and vertebrobasilar artery lesions. J Neurosurg. 1986;64(4):559–62.
2. Luzzi S, Giotta Lucifero A, Brambilla I, et al. Far lateral approach. Acta Biomed. 2021;92(Suppl 4):e2021352.
3. Payman A, Shoakazemi A, Safdarian R, et al. Immersive surgical anatomy of the far-lateral approach. Cureus. 2022;14:e31257.
4. El Ahmadieh TY, Figueroa SA, Cavallo C, et al. The far-lateral suboccipital approach to the lesions of the craniovertebral junction. World Neurosurg. 2021;155:218–28.
5. Fossett DT, Caputy AJ. Chapter 15 - Extreme Lateral Approach. In: Operative neurosurgical anatomy. New York: Thieme; 2001. p. 90–9.
6. Sriamornrattanakul K, Akharathammachote N, Chonhenchob A, et al. Far-lateral approach without C1 laminectomy for microsurgical treatment of vertebral artery and proximal posterior inferior cerebellar artery aneurysms: experience from 48 patients. World Neurosurg X. 2023;19:100216.
7. Pai SB, Raghuram G, Keshav GC, Rodrigues E. Far-lateral transcondylar approach to anterior foramen magnum lesions – our experience. Asian J Neurosurg. 2018;13(3):651–5.
8. Wen HT, Rhoton AL Jr, Katsuta T, Oliveira E. Microsurgical anatomy of the transcondylar, supracondylar, and paracondylar extensions of the far-lateral approach. J Neurosurg. 1997;87(4):555–85.
9. Chaddad-Neto F, Doria-Netto HL, Campos-Filho JM, Reghin-Neto M, Rhoton AL Jr, Oliveira E. The far-lateral craniotomy: tips and tricks. Arq Neuropsiquiatr. 2014;72(9):699–705.

The Endoscopic Transsphenoidal Approach

17

17.1 Introduction

The transsphenoidal approach has become the preferred surgical route for accessing the sellar and parasellar regions, particularly for pituitary tumors. The adoption of this approach has been driven by advancements in microsurgical and endoscopic techniques, allowing for improved visualization and precision while minimizing trauma to the brain and surrounding structures [1]. Pituitary surgery evolved from transcranial approaches, prompting Schloffer's first successful transsphenoidal tumor removal in 1906. Cushing initially adopted and refined the transsphenoidal technique, using it selectively between 1910 and 1925 before favoring transcranial surgery for better optic decompression, while Dott preserved the transsphenoidal approach, later revitalized by Guiot and Hardy with microsurgical advancements. The endoscopic transsphenoidal approach evolved from Hardy's microsurgical refinements, and it gained popularity in the 1990s with improved visualization, minimally invasive techniques, and reduced morbidity [2].

A comprehensive understanding of sellar and parasellar anatomy is important for successful transsphenoidal surgery. The sellar region is bordered superiorly by the diaphragm sellae and optic chiasm, laterally by the cavernous sinuses, and posteriorly by the clivus [3]. The pituitary gland resides within the sellar turcica, and its blood supply is primarily derived from the superior and inferior hypophyseal arteries [4]. The sphenoid sinus, which provides the natural corridor for transsphenoidal access, exhibits significant anatomical variations that must be considered preoperatively [5]. The intercarotid distance at the sellar floor averages approximately 18 mm, with variations that may impact surgical planning [6]. Additionally, the sphenoid sinus may be classified as sellar, presellar, or conchal, influencing the ease of surgical access [7].

Supplementary Information The online version contains supplementary material available at https://doi.org/10.1007/978-3-032-04664-2_17. The videos can be accessed individually by clicking the DOI link in the accompanying figure caption or by scanning this link with the SN More Media App.

H. de Oliveira Manduca Palmiero, E. G. Figueiredo, *Neurosurgical Approaches Video Atlas*, https://doi.org/10.1007/978-3-032-04664-2_17

The transsphenoidal approach can be performed using either a microscopic or endoscopic technique. The microscopic approach, which is traditionally favored by neurosurgeons, provides stereoscopic visualization and remains the gold standard in many institutions [8]. On the other hand, endoscopic transsphenoidal surgery offers a broader field of view and greater maneuverability, especially in cases with complex anatomical variations or extended approaches to the skull base [9]. The choice of technique often depends on surgeon preference, institutional resources, and patient-specific anatomical factors; however, in recent years, the endoscopic transsphenoidal approach has become the gold standard for pituitary surgery.

Transsphenoidal surgery is the primary treatment modality for pituitary adenomas, craniopharyngiomas, and skull base tumors [10]. The minimally invasive nature of transcranial approaches reduces morbidity and length of hospital stay and improves postoperative recovery compared to transcranial approaches [11]. However, challenges such as cerebrospinal fluid leaks, vascular injury, and incomplete tumor resection necessitate ongoing refinements in technique and adjunctive technologies [11]. Preoperative anatomical studies using CT of the paranasal sinuses and their sellar relationship, combined with MRI for analyzing brain structures adjacent to the sellar lesion, as well as intraoperative neuronavigation, will optimize the transsphenoidal approach for treating sellar and parasellar lesions, enhancing procedural safety. Thus, the transsphenoidal approach remains a cornerstone of neurosurgical treatment for sellar region pathologies.

17.1.1 Anatomical Landmarks

Nasal Approach The nasal phase of the transsphenoidal approach begins by identifying the *middle turbinate*, which serves as an initial landmark for navigating toward the sphenoid sinus. The *superior turbinate* helps locate the *sphenoid ostium*, which is typically positioned in the sphenoethmoidal recess approximately 1.5 cm above the choana. Access to the sphenoid sinus requires widening of the natural sphenoid ostium and removal of the interspinous septa to expose the sellar floor. A crucial anatomical consideration is the *major septum*, which provides a midline reference point but can be variable, with deviations or multiple septations that may attach to the internal carotid artery, increasing the risk of injury during the procedure [12, 13].

Sellar Region from Sphenoidal View From within the sphenoid sinus, the *sellar bulge* is the primary landmark, flanked laterally by the carotid prominences, which indicate the position of the *cavernous internal carotid arteries*. Specifically, the *opticocarotid recess* separates the optic nerves from the carotid arteries and serves as a key corridor for extended skull base approaches. The optic chiasm is located superior to the sellar region, and there are potential anatomical variations, such as a prefixed or postfixed chiasm, that can influence surgical exposure. The *clivus* is located inferior to the sella and provides access to the posterior skull base. The *planum sphenoidale,* which forms the roof of the sphenoid sinus, is an important reference for extended transsphenoidal approaches targeting the suprasellar region [4, 13].

17.2 Indications for the Approach

The transsphenoidal approach is primarily indicated for sellar and parasellar lesions, particularly pituitary adenomas, due to its minimally invasive nature and direct access to the sella turcica. It is the preferred route for microadenomas, nonfunctioning macroadenomas, hormonally active tumors unresponsive to medical therapy, recurrent adenomas, Rathke's cleft cysts, and some craniopharyngiomas, as well as select cases of skull base tumors with limited lateral extension [8, 11, 12].

17.3 Operative Set-Up [12, 14]

Patient Positioning The patient is supine on the operating table, with the trunk elevated by approximately 10°–30° to promote venous drainage and reduce intracranial pressure. The arms are tucked at the sides, and a slight reverse Trendelenburg position may be used to optimize the anatomical alignment for the endonasal approach.

Head Positioning Depending on the surgeon's preference, the head is stabilized either in a horseshoe headrest or by a Mayfield head holder (Figs. 17.1 and 17.2).

Elevation: The head and trunk are elevated 10° in the neutral position to promote venous drainage, reduce intracranial pressure, and minimize cerebrospinal fluid leaks. This maneuver optimizes the surgical corridor by aligning the endoscopic trajectory with the nasal cavity, sphenoid sinus, and sella turcica [12, 15].

Extension: The head is slightly *extended* (10°–20°) to align the nasal cavity and sphenoid sinus with the surgical trajectory, facilitating direct endoscopic visualization.

Rotation is generally maintained in a neutral position or with a slight turn (5°–15°) toward the surgeon when a unilateral nostril approach is planned.

Skin Preparation A standard sterile preparation uses chlorhexidine or povidone-iodine solution to cover the entire face, anterior neck, and upper chest. The nasal cavity is decongested preoperatively using phenylephrine-soaked pledgets to minimize intraoperative bleeding. The oral cavity is covered with a sterile drape or throat pack to prevent fluid aspiration. If neuronavigation is used, fiducial markers or a stereotactic frame may be placed preoperatively for image guidance.

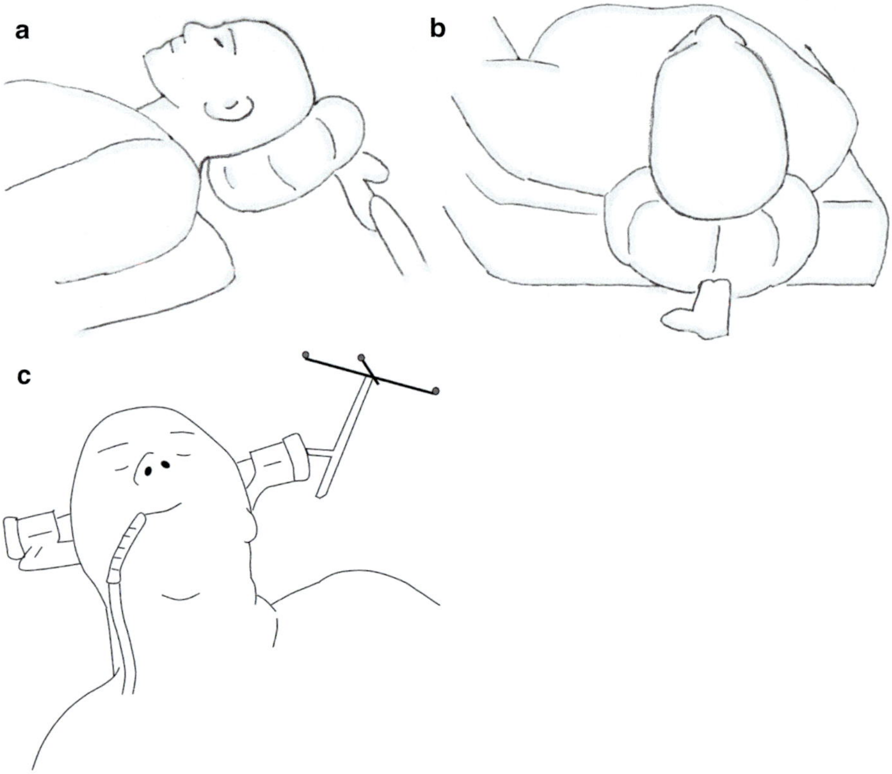

Fig. 17.1 Illustration showing the patient supine in a horseshoe headrest (**a** in lateral view and **b** from vertex). In (**c**), we can see a patient in the supine position with the head fixed in Mayfield and the neuronavigation system positioned

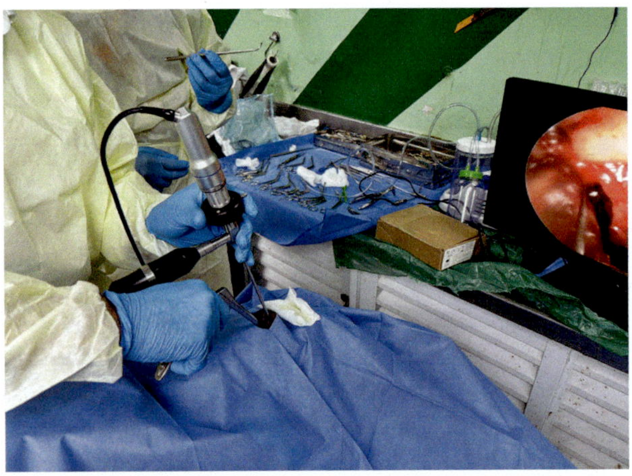

Fig. 17.2 Observe the surgeon's positioning in front of the patient (in an anatomy laboratory setting), looking at the monitor while performing the transnasal endoscopic approach

The anterolateral thigh region is prepared, ensuring coverage from the inguinal crease to just above the knee. Sterile drapes are applied. A wide area is prepared if a fat graft or fascial lata is necessary for closure.

17.4 Surgical Technique [4, 12, 13] (Video 17.1)

Endoscopic Transnasal Approach The procedure begins by introducing a 0-degree rigid endoscope (4 mm in diameter, 18–30 cm long) through one nostril (Fig. 17.3a). The *middle turbinate* is gently lateralized to increase the exposure while preserving nasal function (Fig. 17.3b). The *superior turbinate* is a key landmark for locating the *sphenoid ostium* (Figs. 17.3b and 17.4). A contralateral speculum or suction instrument is introduced to facilitate bimanual dissection when using the binostril approach. The endoscope is advanced along the *sphenoethmoidal recess*, and the *sphenoid ostium* is identified approximately 1.5 cm above the choana.

Mucosal Flap A vascularized nasoseptal flap is elevated from the posterior nasal septum to the posterior septal branch of the *sphenopalatine artery* for later reconstruction (Fig. 17.3c). The mucosal incision extends from the choana to the rostrum of the sphenoid sinus. If no flap is required, the mucosa is carefully removed while preserving the key anatomical structures. The flap is stored in the nasopharynx until closure.

Sphenoid Approach A wide sphenoidotomy is performed by removing the rostrum and intersinus septations to expose the sellar floor in full. Attention should be paid to prevent injury to the *internal carotid artery*, especially in patients in whom the *major septum* is asymmetrically attached to the carotid prominence. The sellar bulge was identified along with key landmarks such as the *opticocarotid recess*,

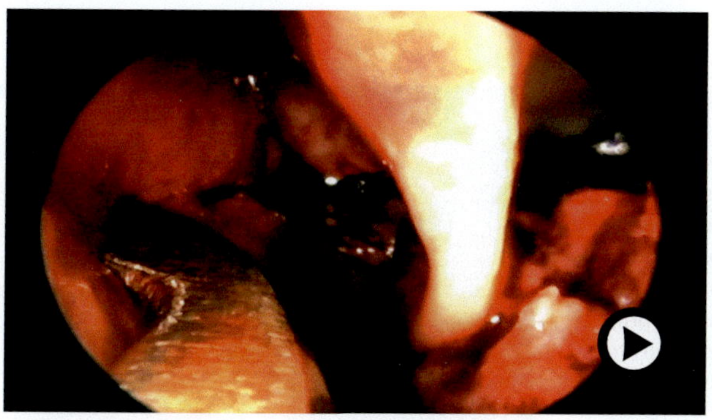

Video 17.1 This video presents the step-by-step execution of the endoscopic transsphenoidal approach to the sellar region, highlighting nasal corridor preparation, sphenoid sinus entry, sellar floor drilling, dural opening, and key anatomical landmarks essential for safe and effective access to sellar and parasellar lesions via the transsphenoidal approach (▶ https://doi.org/10.1007/000-ht8)

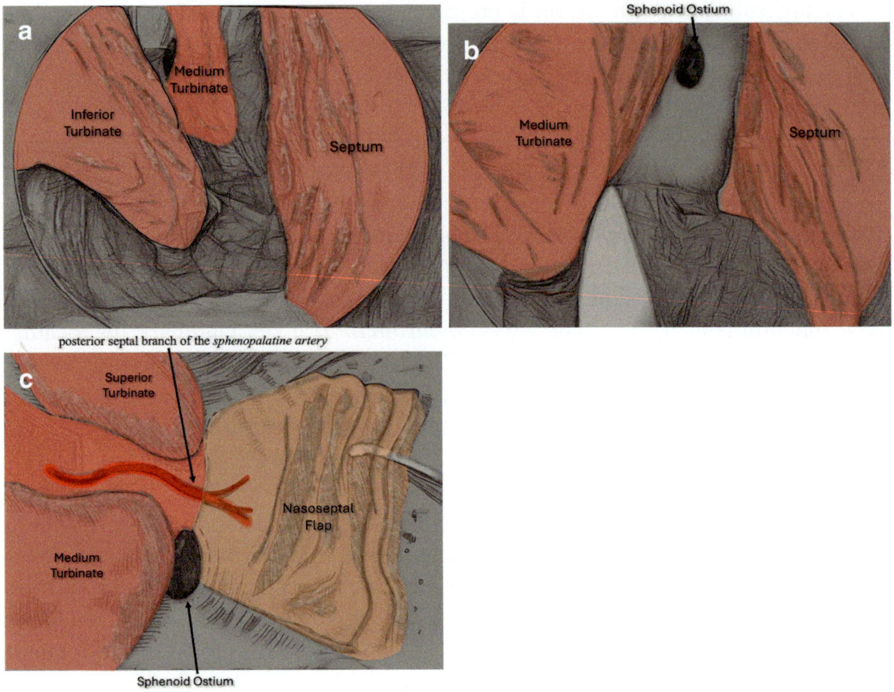

Fig. 17.3 Illustration showing the steps for transnasal access to the sphenoid sinus. In (**a**), as we enter the nasal cavity with the endoscope through the right nostril, we identify the inferior and middle turbinates and, laterally, the nasal septum. In (**b**), by laterally retracting the middle turbinate, we more clearly identify the sphenoidal ostium, which is located near the superior turbinate. In (**c**), using a dissector, we elevate the nasoseptal flap toward the sphenoidal ostium while preserving the posterior septal branch of the sphenopalatine artery, which is situated above the sphenoidal ostium. Once the flap is created, it is positioned toward the nasopharynx. (Source: Personal Archive and based on literature [4, 12, 13])

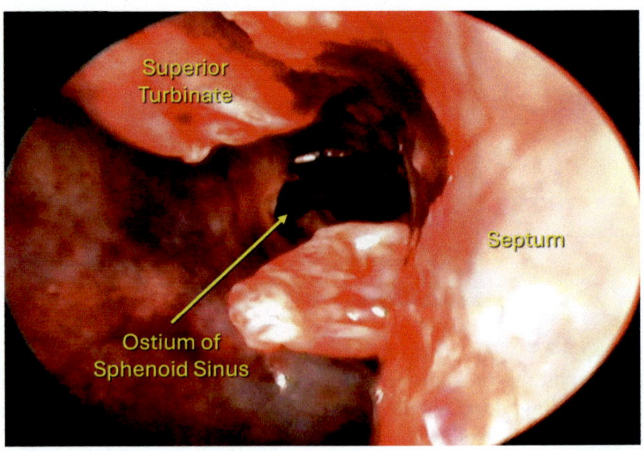

Fig. 17.4 Intraoperative cadaveric endoscopic view showing the right nasal cavity. The sphenoid sinus ostium is seen medial to the superior turbinate and lateral to the nasal septum, marking a reference point for sphenoidotomy during transnasal transsphenoidal approaches

planum sphenoidale, and *clivus* (Figs. 17.5, 17.6, and 17.7). The neurosurgeon opens the sellar region using a high-speed drill until eggshell consistency is achieved and, with the aid of Kerrison rongeurs, carefully removes the sellar floor to achieve wide exposure of the underlying dura while preserving the adjacent structures, including the carotid arteries.

Dural Opening The dura is incised using a U-shaped or cruciate technique, depending on tumor consistency and extent. If a cerebrospinal fluid (CSF) leak is anticipated, gasket-sealing may be planned for closure. The tumor is removed in a piecemeal fashion using suction, curettes, and angled instruments. If the residual tumor remains within the cavernous sinus or suprasellar compartment, angled endoscopes (30°–45°) may be used to improve visualization.

Closure The sellar defect is reconstructed using a multilayer technique, often involving autologous fat grafts, fascial lata, or synthetic dural substitutes. If a significant intraoperative CSF leak occurs, the nasoseptal flap is rotated into place and reinforced with fibrin glue. After identifying the intraoperative fistula, it should be

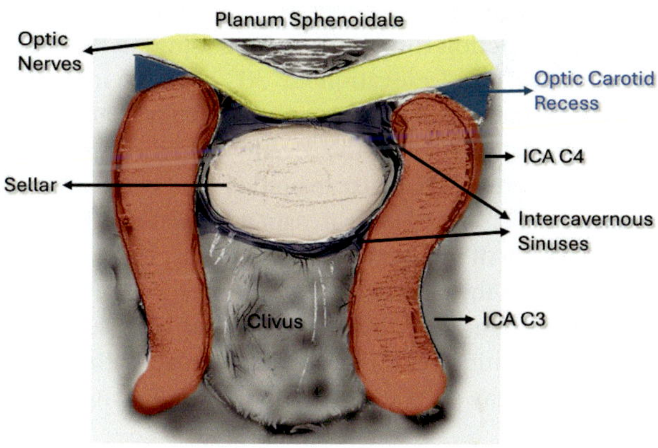

Fig. 17.5 Illustration or picture showing the sphenoid structures once complete the access (Sellar, Internal Carotids, Intercavernous Sinuses, Optic Nerves, Opticocarotid Recess, Planum Sphenoidale, Clivus). See the Optic Carotid Recess (blue triangles)

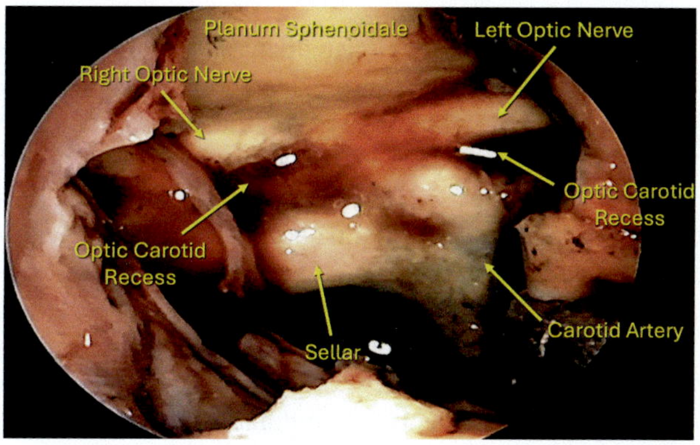

Fig. 17.6 Intraoperative photograph showing the sellar region before opening. We can identify the surrounding structures: planum sphenoidale, optic nerves, optic carotid recesses, and carotid arteries

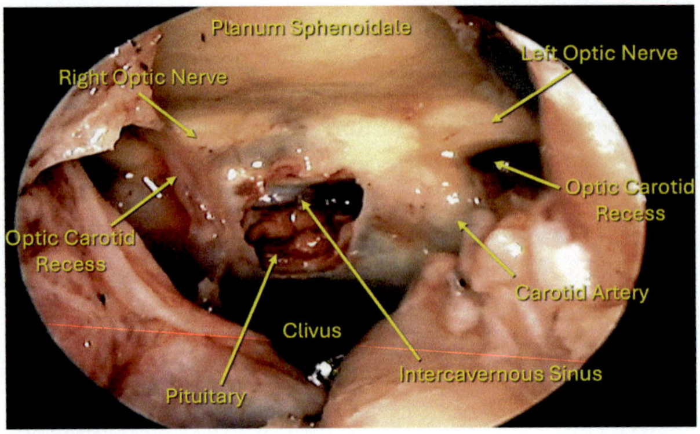

Fig. 17.7 This anatomical dissection photograph shows the sella after bone and dural opening. We can identify the planum sphenoidale, optic nerves, opticocarotid recesses, carotid arteries, intercavernous sinus, pituitary, and clivus

immediately treated. A lumbar drain may be placed in high-risk patients to reduce postoperative CSF leakage. The nasal cavity is packed with absorbable materials, and the patient is monitored for postoperative complications, particularly diabetes insipidus and CSF rhinorrhea.

Postoperative Care Postoperative care following transsphenoidal surgery includes bed rest restriction for 24–48 h, depending on the presence of a cerebrospinal fluid (CSF) leak. Head elevation to 30° reduces intracranial pressure by facilitating venous drainage and prevents CSF leakage. Patients are monitored for CSF leaks, with early detection vital to prevent meningitis; if a leak is suspected, a lumbar drain may be inserted. Diabetes insipidus was evaluated using urine output and serum sodium levels, with desmopressin administered if persistent polyuria occurred. The typical length of inpatient stay after transsphenoidal surgery ranges from 2 to 5 days, depending on the patient's recovery, presence of CSF leaks, and endocrine stability. Patients without complications, such as CSF leaks or diabetes insipidus, may be discharged within 48–72 h, whereas those with persistent CSF leaks or hormonal imbalances may need extended monitoring or lumbar drainage [16].

17.5 Endoscope Versus Microscope

In neurosurgical practice, visualization techniques are tailored to specific anatomical regions to optimize surgical outcomes. Endoscopic approaches have become preferred for pituitary surgery due to their minimally invasive nature and enhanced visualization capabilities. The endoscope provides panoramic and angled views of the sellar and parasellar regions (Fig. 17.8a), facilitating more complete tumor resections and improved surrounding structure assessment. Studies have demonstrated that endoscopic transsphenoidal surgery is associated with higher rates of gross-total resection and better postoperative visual outcomes compared to microscopic approaches [17]. In contrast, microscopic techniques remain the standard for intracranial brain surgeries, offering high-resolution, three-dimensional visualization essential for precise manipulation within the brain's complex architecture.

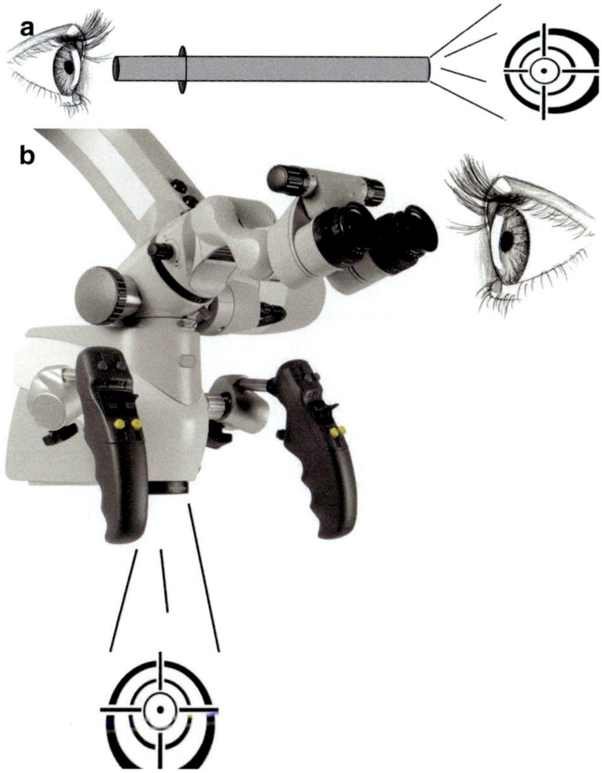

Fig. 17.8 Illustrations comparing the views offered to the neurosurgeon by the endoscope in (**a**) and the microscope in (**b**). Note how the endoscope reaches deeper, illuminating the target structures and projecting the image to the surgeon. The microscope illuminates more superficial structures, magnifies them, reconstructs them in three dimensions, and presents the image to the neurosurgeon while being less dynamic than the endoscope

The operating microscope's superior depth perception and magnification are crucial for navigating delicate neural structures and vascular networks, enhancing surgical accuracy and safety in brain tumor resections and other intracranial procedures (Fig. 17.8b). While both modalities have distinct advantages, the selection between endoscopic and microscopic visualization is contingent upon the specific surgical context and anatomical considerations.

17.6 Pearls and Pitfalls

- *Preoperative Planning*: *Computed tomography and magnetic resonance imaging* to assess sphenoid sinus pneumatization and carotid artery position. Neuronavigation improves accuracy in complex cases.
- *Surgical Technique*: The sphenoid ostium (~1.5 cm above choana) for correct sinus entry. Angled endoscopes (30°–45°) for suprasellar and cavernous sinus access.
- *Surgical Entry*: Misidentification of the sphenoid ostium leads to a misplaced approach. Carotid dehiscence increases the risk of vascular injury.
- *Tumor Resection*: Blind curettage can cause cavernous sinus damage. Inadequate resection of fibrous tumors may require staged surgery.

- *Reconstruction*: If CSF leakage is anticipated, a nasoseptal flap should be used. Multilayer closure with autologous grafts reduces CSF leakage.
- *Postoperative Care*: Unrecognized diabetes insipidus leads to delayed complications.

Acknowledgments We would like to thank the ENT doctors and Fellows in Endonasal Endoscopic and Skull Base Surgery who assisted us with the transnasal transsphenoidal approach: Carolina Arcoverde de Oliveira, Guilherme Rodrigues Marinho, Igor Almeida Nascimento, and Marcio Ribeiro Studart da Fonseca Filho.

References

1. Cappabianca P, Cavallo LM, de Divitiis E. Endoscopic endonasal transsphenoidal surgery. Neurosurgery. 2002;50(3):738–46.
2. Liu JK, Das K, Weiss MH, Laws ER Jr, Couldwell WT. The history and evolution of transsphenoidal surgery. J Neurosurg. 2001;95(6):1083–96.
3. Rhoton AL. The sellar region. Neurosurgery. 2002;51(4 Suppl):S335–74.
4. Renn WH, Rhoton AL Jr. Microsurgical anatomy of the sellar region. J Neurosurg. 1975;43(3):288–98.
5. Perondi GE, Solari D, Cavallo LM, et al. Endoscopic anatomy of the sellar region. Pituitary. 2013;16(2):251–9.
6. Fuji K, Chambers SM, Rhoton AL Jr. Neurovascular relationships of the sphenoid sinus. Neurosurgery. 1979;4(4):333–52.
7. Wang J, Yang G, Dong Y. Anatomical variations of the sphenoid sinus and their impact on transsphenoidal surgery. Surg Radiol Anat. 2011;33(2):147–54.
8. Jho HD, Carrau RL. Endoscopic endonasal transsphenoidal surgery: experience with 50 patients. J Neurosurg. 1997;87(1):44–51.
9. Fatemi N, Dusick JR, de Paiva Neto MA, Malkasian D, Kelly DF. Endonasal versus open craniotomy for clival chordomas. Neurosurg Focus. 2012;32(6):E7.
10. Laws ER Jr, Kanter AS. Pituitary surgery. Neurosurgery. 2007;61(3):881–90.
11. Gondim JA, Schops M, de Almeida JP, et al. Endoscopic endonasal approach for pituitary adenomas: surgical complications in 301 patients. Pituitary. 2011;14(2):174–83.
12. Cappabianca P, Cavallo LM, Colao A, et al. Endoscopic endonasal transsphenoidal surgery: procedure, endoscopic equipment, and instrumentation. Childs Nerv Syst. 2004;20(11–12):796–801.
13. García-Garrigós E, Gámez M, Venegas M, et al. Transsphenoidal approach in endoscopic endonasal surgery for skull base lesions: what radiologists and surgeons need to know. Radiographics. 2015;35(4):1019–42.
14. Fossett DT, Caputy AJ. Chapter 7 - Transphenoidal Approach. In: Operative neurosurgical anatomy. New York: Thieme; 2001. p. 32–6.
15. Cappabianca P, Cavallo LM, Solari D, Stagno V, Esposito F, de Angelis M. Endoscopic endonasal surgery for pituitary adenomas. World Neurosurg. 2014;82(6 Suppl):S3–S11.
16. Prete A, Corsello SM, Salvatori R. Current best practice in the management of patients after pituitary surgery. Ther Adv Endocrinol Metab. 2017;8(3):33–48.
17. Guo S, Wu J, Zhao Y, et al. A meta-analysis of endoscopic vs. microscopic transsphenoidal surgery for non-functioning and functioning pituitary adenomas: comparisons of efficacy and safety. Front Neurol. 2021;12:614382.

Decompressive Craniectomy 18

18.1 Introduction

Decompressive craniectomy is a life-saving neurosurgical procedure designed to alleviate the effects of uncontrolled intracranial hypertension due to conditions like severe traumatic brain injury (TBI) and malignant cerebral edema following an ischemic stroke [1–3]. Time is critical; medical decisions must be made as soon as indications arise, and the procedure should be conducted as quickly as possible. By removing a section of the skull and opening the dura, decompressive craniectomy reduces intracranial pressure (ICP), prevents brain herniation, and enhances cerebral perfusion [1, 3]. The strongest indication for decompressive craniectomy is failure of maximal medical management to control elevated ICP, as persistent intracranial hypertension considerably heightens the risk of mortality and severe disability [3]. Although it remains controversial due to the potential for long-term morbidity, decompressive craniectomy has shown survival benefits, particularly in patients with malignant middle cerebral artery infarction and refractory posttraumatic intracranial hypertension [2, 3]. Ongoing trials are further refining patient selection criteria, optimal surgical techniques, and long-term outcomes to maximize the benefits of this intervention [1].

The size of the craniotomy in decompressive hemicraniectomy is a critical factor in its effectiveness in reducing ICP and preventing secondary brain injury. Studies have shown that a minimum craniectomy diameter of 12 cm is necessary for sufficient decompression, with larger craniectomies offering further advantages in decreasing shear stress, avoiding venous compression, and lowering the risk of external cerebral herniation [4, 5]. Suboptimal hemicraniectomies, especially those

---

Supplementary Information The online version contains supplementary material available at https://doi.org/10.1007/978-3-032-04664-2_18. The videos can be accessed individually by clicking the DOI link in the accompanying figure caption or by scanning this link with the SN More Media App.

H. de Oliveira Manduca Palmiero, E. G. Figueiredo, *Neurosurgical Approaches Video Atlas*, https://doi.org/10.1007/978-3-032-04664-2_18

smaller than 12 cm, are associated with a higher incidence of infarcts, hemorrhages, and parenchymal shear stress because of limited brain expansion [5]. A more extensive decompression (≥18 cm anterior-posterior diameter) is often recommended for optimal ICP control, reducing the risk of postsurgical complications, and enhancing long-term neurological outcomes [6]. Additionally, bone removal extending to the temporal base is vital for preventing uncal herniation and ensuring complete hemispheric expansion [6]. Therefore, while a 12-cm craniectomy is the accepted minimum, a more extensive craniotomy improves the safety and efficacy of the procedure in patients with malignant cerebral edema and refractory intracranial hypertension [4].

Intracranial Pressure (ICP) Decompressive craniectomy effectively reduces ICP by increasing intracranial volume through skull removal and opening of the dura, thereby mitigating the risk of herniation and secondary brain injury [6, 7]. The immediate result of decompressive craniectomy is a significant decrease in ICP, with studies showing a 66% reduction after bone removal and an additional 50% drop following dural opening, highlighting the important role of dural decompression [7]. The effectiveness of the procedure hinges on the degree of bony removal, with a minimum diameter of 12 cm being crucial to prevent shear stress, venous compression, and ischemic injury [6]. Furthermore, sufficient decompression to the temporal base ensures further reduction of ICP, decreasing the chance of uncal herniation and optimizing cerebral perfusion [7]. While variations in craniotomy size exist, the combination of extensive bony decompression and duraplasty is essential for achieving sustained ICP control and enhancing neurological outcomes [6] (Fig. 18.1).

Complications Decompressive craniectomy is associated with various complications, including hydrocephalus, external cerebral herniation, subdural hygromas, and hemorrhagic progression of contusions [4, 8, 9]. Post-traumatic hydrocephalus occurs in up to 31.6% of patients following decompressive craniectomy, with approximately 10% requiring ventriculoperitoneal shunting [8, 9]. External cerebral

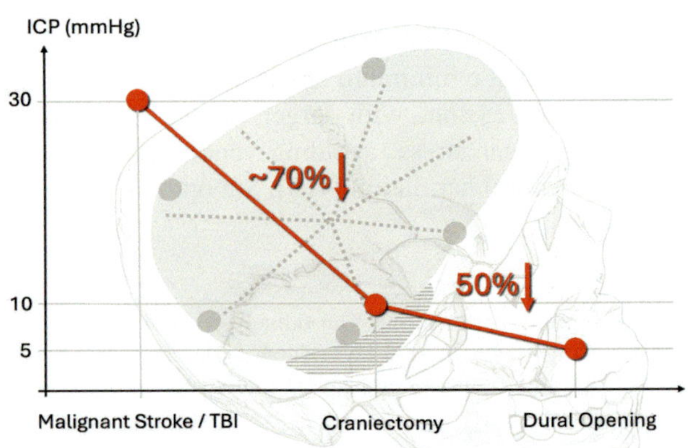

Fig. 18.1 In this figure, we see the relationship between the decrease in ICP with craniectomy (by 70%) and dural opening (an additional 50%) [7]

herniation, often due to a small craniectomy defect, can lead to infarction and cortical damage; ensuring a craniectomy diameter of at least 12 cm helps minimize this risk [4]. Subdural hygromas, which occur in nearly 50% of cases, typically resolve spontaneously but require monitoring to differentiate them from hydrocephalus [4]. Hemorrhagic complications, particularly at the craniectomy edges, are associated with inadequate hemicraniectomy size and improper dural handling [10]. Solutions include early detection of hydrocephalus through imaging, performing duraplasty to prevent excessive brain expansion, ensuring appropriate timing for cranioplasty, and using larger craniectomies to avoid shear stress and ischemia [4, 8, 9].

18.2 Indications for the Approach

Decompressive craniectomy is indicated for refractory intracranial hypertension in conditions such as severe traumatic brain injury and malignant middle cerebral artery infarction, in which medical management fails to control elevated ICP [3, 11, 12]. In cases of traumatic brain injury (TBI), decompressive craniectomy is recommended for patients with sustained ICP greater than 25 mmHg despite maximal medical therapy, particularly those with diffuse brain swelling or contusions that result in significant midline shift [3]. For ischemic stroke, decompressive craniectomy is performed in cases of malignant middle cerebral artery infarction associated with severe cerebral edema, midline shift exceeding 5 mm, and impending herniation. Evidence suggests that early surgery (within 48 h) can lead to improved survival and functional outcomes [11, 12]. Furthermore, decompressive craniectomy may be considered for other conditions, including intracerebral hemorrhage, venous sinus thrombosis, and postoperative brain swelling, when elevated ICP threatens neurological integrity [13]. Patient selection, timing, and surgical technique are crucial factors for optimizing outcomes in candidates undergoing decompressive craniectomy [3, 12].

18.3 Operative Set-Up [2, 13]

Before positioning the patient for decompressive craniectomy, cervical spine clearance is crucial to prevent exacerbation of undiagnosed cervical spine injuries, which can lead to secondary neurological deficits; therefore, cervical spine imaging (CT in an emergency setting) should be performed in all trauma cases before head manipulation [14, 15].

Patient Positioning The patient is positioned supine with a slight elevation to 30° to improve cerebral venous drainage and reduce ICP. The Trendelenburg maneuver elevates the head compared with the heart. A shoulder roll may be placed to facilitate proper head positioning while ensuring adequate access to the surgical field. The arms are positioned at the sides or tucked to prevent excessive flexion or pressure points.

Head Positioning The head is positioned on a horseshoe support, although some surgeons prefer the *Mayfield* headholder to provide stability and prevent unintended movements during surgery. In trauma surgery, the horseshoe is preferred when there are fractures or suspicion of fractures, or even for ease of positioning. One advantage of the Mayfield headholder is that it keeps the head fixed when using a Gigli saw (Fig. 18.2).

Once again: Before positioning, check for cervical fractures and ensure that the collar can be removed. Keep the cervical collar on if a fracture is suspected and avoid rotation.

(a) *Elevation.* A 30-degree head elevation is maintained to reduce venous congestion; keep the head elevated above the level of the heart.
(b) *Rotation.* The degree of rotation depends on the side of the craniectomy: for *hemicraniectomy*, the head is turned approximately 30° to the contralateral side to expose the temporal and frontal regions; the *bifrontal craniectomy*, the head remains neutral to allow bilateral access.
(c) *Extension.* Minimal extension is preferred to prevent excessive neck and brainstem tension.

Skin Preparation The surgical field is shaved and prepared with chlorhexidine or povidone-iodine to minimize infection risk. The incision is infiltrated with a local anesthetic (epinephrine) to reduce bleeding. A sterile drape is applied to ensure optimal access to the entire hemicranium.

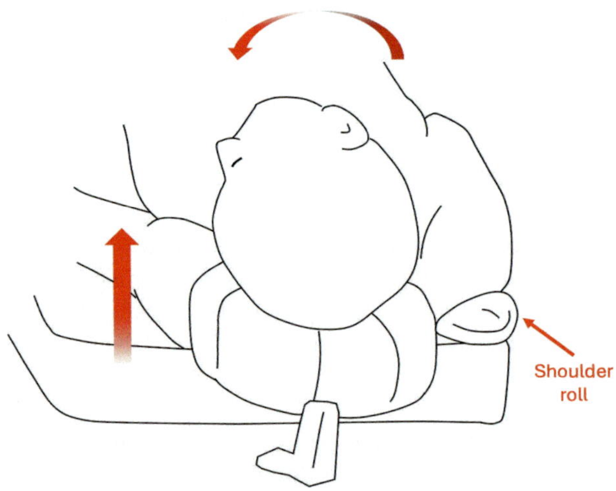

Fig. 18.2 In this image, we see the head positioning using a horseshoe. Note the elevation and for contralateral rotation by 30° assisted by shoulder roll placement

18.4 Surgical Technique [2, 13] (Video 18.1)

Skin Incision The incision choice depends on the extent of decompression required. The *reverse question mark* incision is the most common, but some authors advocate for the *T-incision described* by Kempe [16].

A reverse *question mark* incision starts from the midline near the forehead, extends laterally above the ear, and curves down toward the zygoma (Fig. 18.3a).

The *T-incision* described by Kempe is an alternative to the *question mark* that allows broader exposure while maintaining a robust blood supply to the scalp. This incision consists of: (1) a midline vertical incision extending from the widow's peak posteriorly to the inion, and (2) a transverse incision at the coronal level extending laterally toward the superior temporal line [16] (Fig. 18.3b).

Muscle Flap The temporalis muscle is incised in a myocutaneous flap and reflected anteriorly and inferiorly with monopolar electrocautery to expose the cranial surface. Some surgeons prefer myofascial dissection for later cranioplasty. Maintaining the vascular pedicles in the muscle reduces postoperative atrophy.

Craniotomy A flap (>12 cm in anterior-posterior diameter) is removed, extending from the frontal, temporal, parietal, and occipital bones, ensuring adequate opening. Avoid extending too far toward the occipital region, as this can complicate postoperative care and increase the difficulty of brain compression. A high-speed drill is used to place the burr holes. Burr holes are created at the temporal base and MacCarthy's point, but additional burr holes may be created along the planned craniotomy path to facilitate dural dissection. The Gigli saw can be used when needed or when a craniotome is unavailable (Figs. 18.4, 18.5, 18.6, 18.7, and 18.8). The bone flap is stored in a subcutaneous pocket or frozen for future cranioplasty.

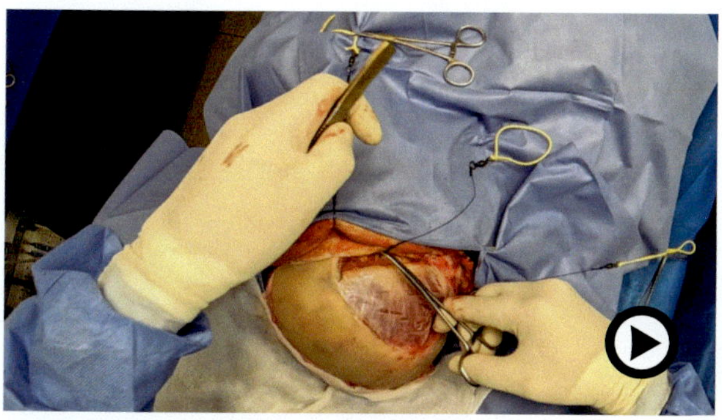

Video 18.1 This video provides a step-by-step demonstration of decompressive hemicraniectomy, highlighting key anatomical landmarks for the procedure, the bone flap removal technique, nuances of dural opening, and temporal fossa decompression to effectively reduce intracranial pressure in cases of malignant cerebral edema (▶ https://doi.org/10.1007/000-ht9)

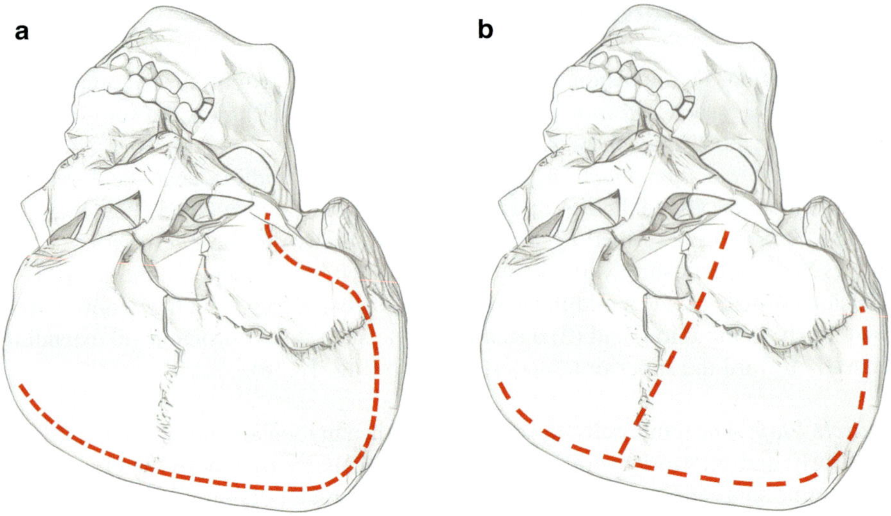

Fig. 18.3 Illustration showing the reverse question mark skin incision (**a**) and the alternative T-incision described by Kempe in (**b**)

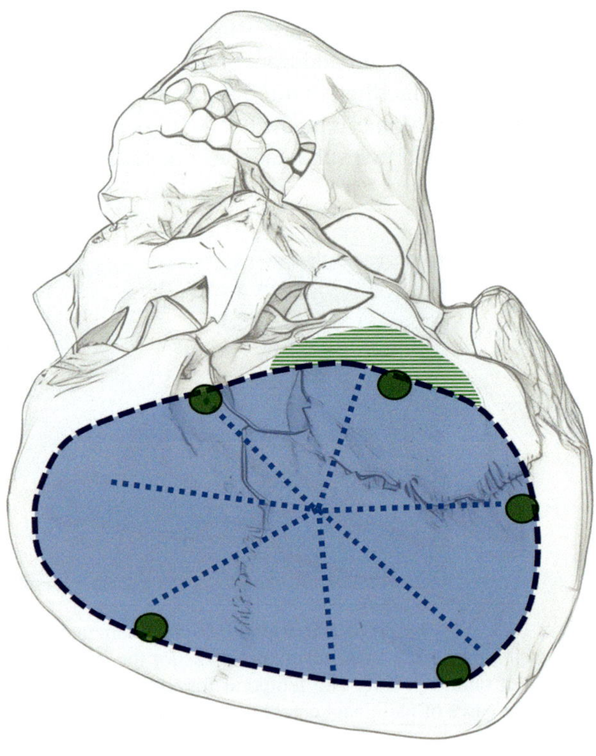

Fig. 18.4 Figure showing the craniotomy area (blue area) and burr holes (green circles). The green striped area corresponds to the extent of craniectomy using a rongeur toward the temporal base to avoid or treat uncal herniation. The star-shaped dural opening (light blue dashed lines) is also represented

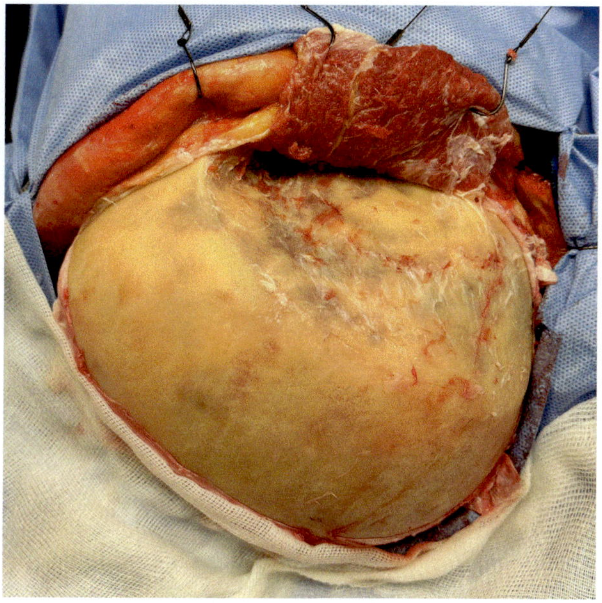

Fig. 18.5 Photograph of the skull with the temporal muscle dissected and reflected inferiorly, the sutures visible, and the entire craniectomy area ready

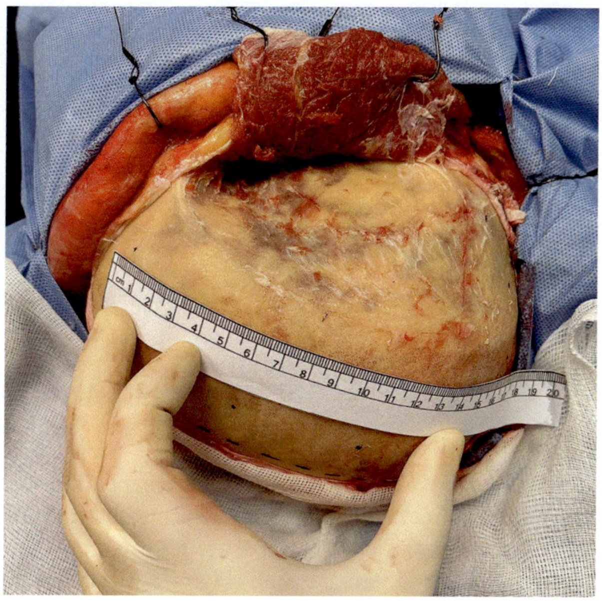

Fig. 18.6 In this photograph, we identify the craniectomy coverage area, and using a ruler, we can determine how much we need to expand the craniectomy to achieve a diameter greater than 12 cm

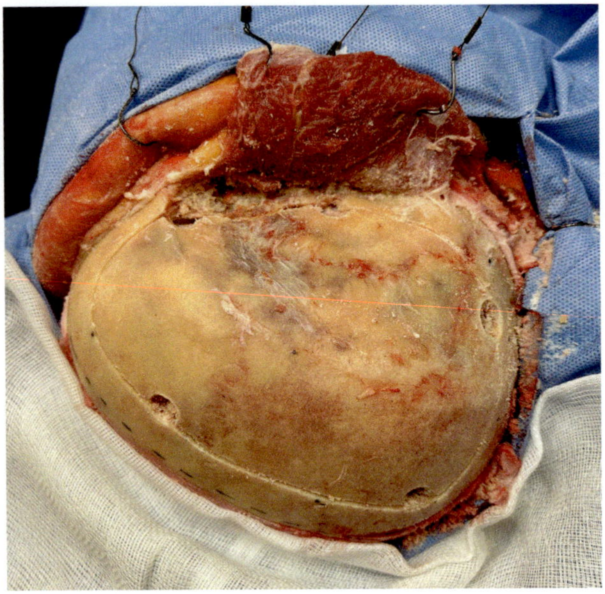

Fig. 18.7 Intraoperative photograph showing right-sided decompressive craniectomy with no bone flap still not removed. The craniectomy should be approximately wide, with an anatomical extent, involving the frontal, temporal, parietal, and occipital bones. Observe the star-shaped dural opening

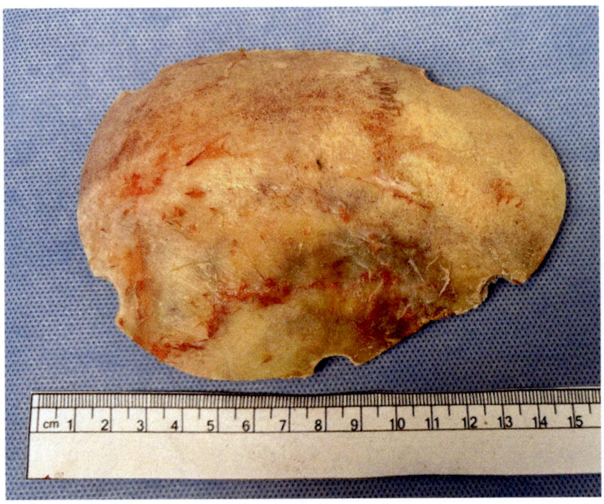

Fig. 18.8 Photograph of the bone flap with a ruler showing an anteroposterior diameter greater than 12 cm; in this example: 15 cm

Dural Opening We recommend a star-shaped durotomy to widely open the dura and relieve intracranial pressure, ensuring that the underlying brain is not under excessive tension. The dural flaps are reflected outward to the periphery to prevent constriction during re-expansion (Figs. 18.4 and 18.9).

Duroplasty Without Dural Closure Duroplasty is a crucial step in decompressive craniectomy aimed at accommodating brain expansion, lowering intracranial pressure, and preventing complications, such as external cerebral herniation [17].

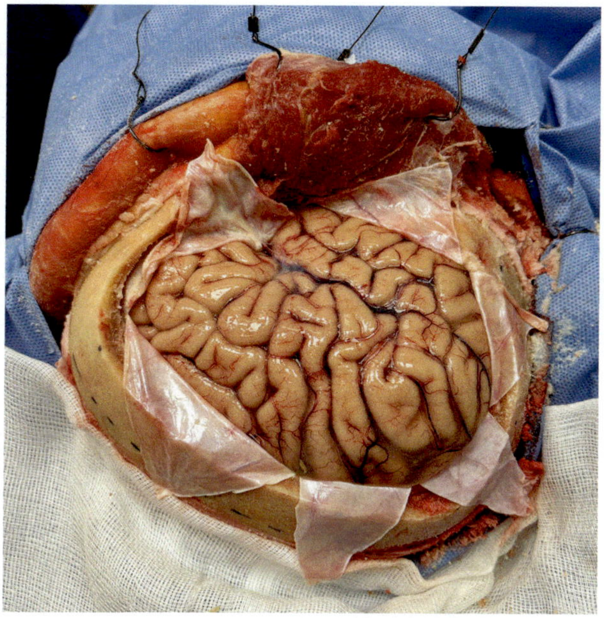

Fig. 18.9 The star-shaped dural opening. This dural opening allows the expansion of the entire brain, thus relieving intracranial pressure

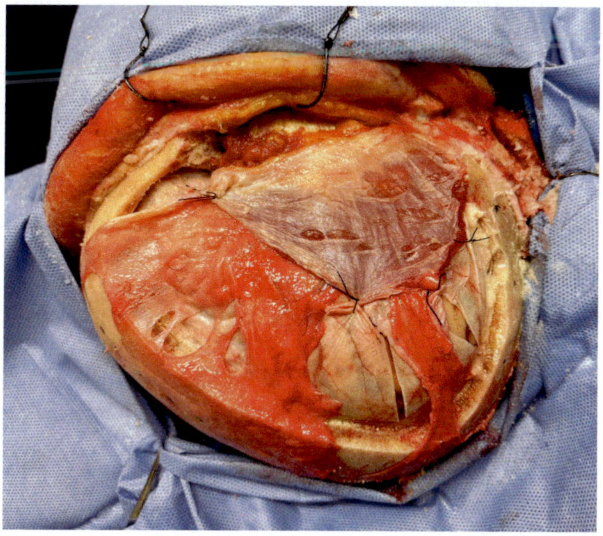

Fig. 18.10 The periosteal tissue positioned over the dura mater and the temporalis muscle were reflected and secured with anchoring sutures. With this technique, the brain has no restriction of expansion, and the drain can be placed in the subcutaneous space without moving the dura, periosteal, and muscular tissues. The dissection area is also preserved for future cranioplasty

Various techniques and materials have been suggested, including autologous pericranium, synthetic dural substitutes, and nonruptured duraplasty [18]. Studies comparing these approaches indicate that vascularized galea pericranium duraplasty results in better long-term outcomes with reduced rates of complications like CSF leaks and infections, compared with synthetic grafts [17]. Non-sutured duraplasty has been investigated as a time-saving alternative, decreasing operative duration and blood loss while maintaining similar safety profiles [18, 19] and without a statistically significant increase in CSF leaks and postoperative hydrocephalus [18] (Fig. 18.10).

Closure For closure, we recommend repositioning the temporalis muscle over the dura mater and periosteal tissue without suturing to avoid additional brain compression. The skin flap is repositioned, and subcutaneous sutures with absorbable thread ensure proper skin alignment and reduce tension during closure. Skin closure can be performed using continuous or simple interrupted Nylon or clear monocryl sutures or skin staples, but the sutures must be watertight. We also recommend using a subcutaneous drain to prevent and drain postoperative subcutaneous hematoma collection. Delayed cranioplasty is planned after the resolution of cerebral edema.

18.5 Pearls and Pitfalls

- *Time is brain, early decision-making*: Prompt recognition of refractory intracranial hypertension and early surgical intervention improves survival.
- *Adequate Craniectomy Size*: A minimum diameter of 12 cm is required; suboptimal craniectomy increases the risk of venous compression, shear stress, and infarction. Larger craniotomies (>18 cm AP diameter) improve decompression and reduce complications.
- *Temporal Base Decompression*: Extending craniectomy to the temporal base prevents uncal herniation and optimizes ICP control.
- *Dural Opening*: Failure to perform a wide durotomy leads to insufficient decompression and worsens brain swelling. A star-shaped durotomy prevents tension; duraplasty closure or closure without suturing does not affect CSF leakage and hydrocephalus.
- *Patient positioning*: The cervical spine must be cleared before positioning. Horseshoe head support is preferred in trauma cases; a *Mayfield* head holder provides better stability, especially when a *Gigli* saw is used.
- *Improper skin closure*: Watertight skin closure is critical. Avoid excessive muscle compression over the dura. Use of subcutaneous drains to prevent hematoma formation.
- *Cranioplasty Timing*: A premature cranioplasty for unresolved edema increases the risk of complications. Wait until the brain swelling resolves.
- *Hydrocephalus and CSF Leaks*: Monitor for posttraumatic hydrocephalus; early detection prevents ventriculoperitoneal shunting delays.

References

1. Kolias AG, Kirkpatrick PJ, Hutchinson PJ. Decompressive craniectomy: past, present and future. Nat Rev Neurol. 2013;9(7):405–15.
2. Cannarsa GJ, Simard JM. Decompressive craniectomy for stroke: who, when, and how. Neurol Clin. 2022;40(2):321–36.
3. Hawryluk GWJ, Rubiano AM, Totten AM, et al. Guidelines for the management of severe traumatic brain injury: 2020 update of the decompressive craniectomy recommendations. Neurosurgery. 2020;87(3):427–34.

4. Stiver SI. Complications of decompressive craniectomy for traumatic brain injury. Neurosurg Focus. 2009;26(6):E7.
5. Wagner S, Schnippering H, Aschoff A, Koziol JA, Schwab S, Steiner T. Suboptimum hemicraniectomy as a cause of additional cerebral lesions in patients with malignant infarction of the middle cerebral artery. J Neurosurg. 2001;94(5):693–6.
6. Tanrikulu L, Oez-Tanrikulu A, Weiss C, et al. The bigger, the better? About the size of decompressive hemicraniectomies. Clin Neurol Neurosurg. 2015;135:15–21.
7. Beez T, Munoz-Bendix C, Steiger HJ, Beseoglu K. Decompressive craniectomy for acute ischemic stroke. Crit Care. 2019;23:209.
8. Ovenden CD, Barot DD, Gupta A, et al. Incidence of hydrocephalus following decompressive craniectomy for ischemic stroke: a systematic review and meta-analysis. Clin Neurol Neurosurg. 2023;234:107989.
9. Rufus P, Moorthy RK, Joseph M, Rajshekhar V. Post-traumatic hydrocephalus: incidence, pathophysiology, and outcomes. Neurol India. 2021;69(Suppl 2):S420–8.
10. Wagner S, Schnippering H, Aschoff A, et al. Suboptimum hemicraniectomy as a cause of additional cerebral lesions in malignant infarction. J Neurosurg. 2001;94(5):693–6.
11. Elsawaf A, Galhom A. Decompressive craniotomy for malignant middle cerebral artery infarction: optimal timing and literature review. World Neurosurg. 2018;116:e71–8.
12. Lin J, Frontera JA. Decompressive hemicraniectomy for large hemispheric strokes. Stroke. 2021;52(4):1500–10.
13. Holland M, Nakaji P. Craniectomy: indications and technique. Oper Tech Neurosurg. 2004;7(1):10–5.
14. Como JJ, Diaz JJ, Dunham CM, et al. Practice management guidelines for identifying cervical spine injuries following trauma: update from the Eastern Association for the Surgery of Trauma. J Trauma Acute Care Surg. 2009;67(3):651–9.
15. Holly LT, Kelly DF, Counelis GJ, Blinman TA, McArthur DL, Cryer HG. Cervical spine clearance in unconscious trauma patients: a prospective study. J Neurosurg. 2002;96(1 Suppl):3–8.
16. Abecassis IJ, Young CC, Caldwell DJ, et al. The Kempe incision for decompressive craniectomy, craniotomy, and cranioplasty in traumatic brain injury and stroke. J Neurosurg. 2021;135(6):1807–16.
17. Ramola M, Singh J, Khurana L, et al. Comparative analysis of duroplasty techniques in decompressive craniectomy: the CANDID study. Oper Neurosurg. 2025;28(3):357–67.
18. Jeong TS, Yee GT, Lim TG, Kim WK, Yoo CJ. Efficacy and safety of decompressive craniectomy with non-suture duraplasty in patients with traumatic brain injury. PLoS One. 2020;15(10):e0232561.
19. Kumar P, Srivastava C, Bajaj A, Yadav A, Ojha BK. Dural opening without closure in decompressive craniectomy: a prospective, randomized, controlled study. J Clin Neurosci. 2023;108:30–6.

Microsurgical Approaches to the Ventricles

19

19.1 Introduction

Microsurgical access to the ventricles remains the gold standard for treating intraventricular lesions, offering superior precision and safety when navigating deep brain structures. Although endoscopic techniques have revolutionized ventricular surgery by providing minimally invasive options for procedures such as endoscopic third ventriculostomy and colloid cyst resection, their application is limited by constraints in bimanual manipulation and visualization [1]. Neuronavigation has significantly enhanced ventricular surgery by permitting precise intraoperative localization of lesions, reducing cortical transgression, and optimizing surgical trajectories, particularly in cases requiring stereotactic accuracy [2]. However, microsurgical techniques using specialized craniotomies, such as the transcallosal interhemispheric and transcortical approaches, remain the most reliable methods for accessing ventricular structures while preserving surrounding neurovascular integrity [3, 4]. These approaches integrate microsurgical instruments, intraoperative imaging, neuronavigation, and neuroanatomical knowledge to ensure maximal lesion resection while minimizing morbidity, maintaining their role as the cornerstone of ventricular surgery.

19.2 Ventricular Drainage

During specific neurosurgical procedures, it is necessary to access the lateral ventricles or the third ventricle for CSF drainage, promoting brain relaxation or serving as a landmark for accessing lesions [3]. *Kocher's point* is a commonly utilized entry

Supplementary Information The online version contains supplementary material available at https://doi.org/10.1007/978-3-032-04664-2_19. The videos can be accessed individually by clicking the DOI link in the accompanying figure caption or by scanning this link with the SN More Media App.

H. de Oliveira Manduca Palmiero, E. G. Figueiredo, *Neurosurgical Approaches Video Atlas*, https://doi.org/10.1007/978-3-032-04664-2_19

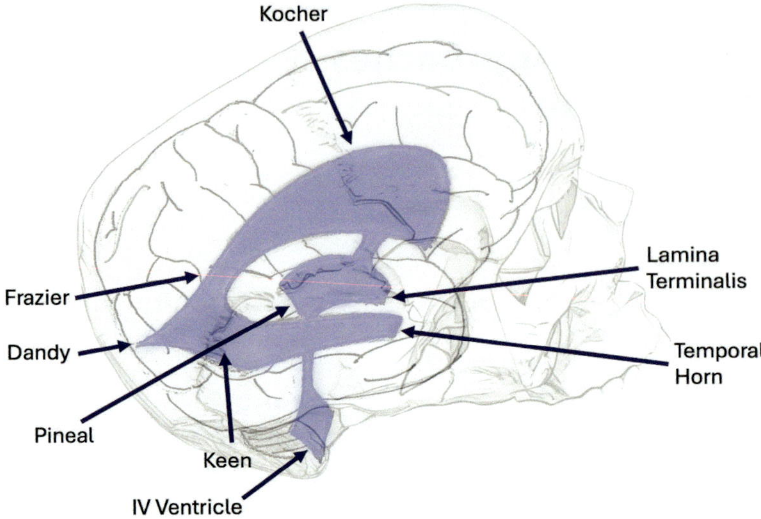

Fig. 19.1 Illustration showing access to the frontal horn of the lateral ventricles through Kocher's point (11–13 cm along the nasion-to-inion line and 3 cm lateral to the midline for EVD; or 1 cm anterior to the coronal suture and 3 cm lateral to the midline for endoscopic access), access to the lateral ventricles via the parietal and occipital approaches through Frazier's point (3–4 cm from the midline and 6–7 cm above the inion), Dandy's point (3 cm above the inion and 2 cm lateral to the midline), and Keen's point (2.5–3 cm posterior and 2.5–3 cm superior to the top of the pinna); as well as access to the fourth ventricle via the telovelar or endoscopic approach. The lateral ventricle's temporal horn is also identified [5, 6]

site for accessing the lateral ventricle through the frontal lobe, positioned 2–3 cm lateral to the midline at the level of the coronal suture through the cranium [5]. *Kocher's point* is also anatomically referenced using the sulci and gyri on the surface of the frontal lobe [5]. At the junction of the superior frontal and precentral gyri, the gyri are typically aligned with the superior frontal sulcus. This positioning ensures a direct and safe trajectory into the frontal horn of the lateral ventricle, minimizing damage to the eloquent cortex and subcortical structures [6] (Fig. 19.1).

To access the lateral ventricles from the parietal and occipital lobes, whether for ventriculoperitoneal shunt (VPS) placement or during neurosurgical approaches to these lobes, two ventricular access points are commonly used: *Keen's point* and *Frazier's point* [5].

19.3 Frontal Horn and Monro Foramen

The frontal horn of the lateral ventricle is a vital anatomical landmark for intraventricular surgeries, particularly for accessing the foramen of Monro. It is bordered medially by the septum pellucidum and laterally by the head of the caudate nucleus, with the corpus callosum forming its roof. The foramen of Monro, an essential pathway between the lateral and third ventricles, is anatomically defined by the fornix and thalamostriate vein, structures crucial for maintaining cognitive and motor functions. Surgical approaches to this region require precise anatomical knowledge to minimize disruption of the surrounding periventricular structures, particularly the fornices, to prevent memory impairment. The transcallosal interhemispheric approach is often used for accessing lesions within this area, offering a direct route while avoiding cortical transgression, thus preserving eloquent brain regions [7].

The surgical approach for the frontal horn and foramen of Monro depends on the lesion and its spatial relationship with critical neurovascular structures. Tumors in this area, such as central neurocytomas and colloid cysts, are often accessed through the anterior interhemispheric transcallosal corridor, allowing for safe dissection with minimal retraction of the cingulate gyrus and superior sagittal sinus bridging veins [8]. Preoperative imaging, including magnetic resonance imaging (MRI) and magnetic resonance venography, is essential for defining the foramen's patency and planning the best surgical trajectory. In patients with hydrocephalus, intraoperative cerebrospinal fluid drainage can facilitate ventricular decompression and enhance exposure. Furthermore, microsurgical techniques, including neuronavigation and intraoperative monitoring, are crucial for minimizing morbidity and maximizing tumor resection [9].

19.3.1 Lamina Terminalis and Temporal Horn

Accessing the third ventricle through the *lamina terminalis* provides a direct and safe route, which is often used in endoscopic third ventriculostomy (ETV) or tumor resection [3]. We can also access the *lamina terminalis* through the Sylvian fissure following the optic nerve toward the chiasma and the l*amina terminals* [4] (Fig. 19.1).

The *temporal horn* of the lateral ventricle is accessed following the incisura line, which is an imaginary trajectory along the tentorial incisura that helps avoid critical neurovascular structures [5] (Fig. 19.1). This access is useful during amygdalo-hippocampectomy through an anterior approach to the Sylvian fissure via supraorbital, supraorbital-zygomatic, and pterional craniotomies [4].

19.3.2 Atrium

The lateral ventricle atrium, or trigone, is a complex anatomical region where the body, temporal horn, and occipital horn converge. This deep-seated structure is bordered superiorly by the corpus callosum, medially by the calcar avis, and laterally by the tapetum of the corpus callosum, making surgical access particularly challenging [3]. The atrium frequently harbors lesions such as meningiomas, gliomas, and choroid plexus tumors, which, due to their ventricular location and slow-growing nature, can reach substantial sizes before symptomatic presentation. Primary clinical manifestations of homonymous hemianopia and intracranial hypertension resulting from optic radiation compression and cerebrospinal fluid obstruction [10]. The transparietal transcortical approach is commonly used to access tumors in the atrium, offering a direct path while minimizing injury to surrounding eloquent areas. However, interhemispheric transcallosal and parieto-occipital interhemispheric approaches remain viable alternatives, particularly in cases requiring preservation of the optic pathways [4]. Given the rich vascular supply from the anterior and posterior choroidal arteries, meticulous microsurgical dissection is essential to prevent excessive blood loss and preserve adjacent neural structures, ensuring optimal postoperative functional outcomes.

19.3.3 Telovelar

Suboccipital approach is the standard route, involving a midline incision and opening the cerebellomedullary fissure by dissecting the uvulotonsillar cleft and mobilizing the tonsils without splitting the vermis. It provides a broad exposure of the ventricular floor while preserving cerebellar function [3]. The *far-lateral approach*, which is used for lateral recess lesions, extends access through the *foramen of Luschka* by opening the cerebellomedullary cistern and mobilizing the tonsils [4].

The telovelar approach has been increasingly favored over the traditional transversion approach because it avoids direct injury to the vermis, thereby reducing the risk of cerebellar mutism and ataxic syndromes [11]. This approach provides extensive exposure from the calamus scriptorius to the Sylvian aqueduct, allowing resection of lesions located along the entire fourth ventricle while preserving the dentate nuclei and related cerebellar structures [4]. Additionally, modifications such as C1 laminectomy and unilateral or bilateral tonsillar retraction have been shown to enhance further access to the lateral recesses and superior fourth ventricular regions, optimizing surgical control and minimizing neurological morbidity [11].

19.3.4 Pineal

Surgical access to the pineal region is among the most challenging neurosurgical procedures due to its deep midline location and proximity to vital neurovascular structures, including the vein of Galen, internal cerebral veins, and the quadrigeminal cistern [12]. The supracerebellar infratentorial approach, first described by Krause and later refined with microsurgical techniques, remains the preferred method for pineal region lesions because it provides a direct midline trajectory with minimal brain retraction [13]. This approach can be midline or paramedian, with the latter offering better visualization of the collicular plate and cerebellomesencephalic fissure while reducing the need for venous sacrifice [14]. In cases in which superior exposure is required, occipital transtentorial and posterior interhemispheric transcallosal approaches serve as viable alternatives, particularly for tumors extending into the third ventricle or corpus callosum [15]. The surgical route is dictated by lesion size, extension, and venous anatomy to preserve the deep venous system and to avoid postoperative complications, such as Parinaud syndrome and cerebellar ataxia.

The posterior wall of the third ventricle, which is closely related to the pineal region, extends from the suprapineal recess to the cerebral aqueduct and includes the habenular and posterior commissures, pineal recess, and collicular plate [15]. The third ventricle is a critical corridor for surgical access to tumors and cystic lesions extending into the third ventricle, necessitating precise microsurgical dissection to avoid injury to the tectal plate and periaqueductal gray matter. The posterior interhemispheric transcallosal approach is instrumental in accessing lesions that extend superiorly into the third ventricle [15]. At the same time, the supracerebellar infratentorial route is more suitable for tumors confined to the pineal recess and quadrigeminal cistern [15]. Neuronavigation and intraoperative neuromonitoring are essential adjuncts in these procedures, ensuring accurate targeting while minimizing collateral damage to eloquent structures.

19.4 Surgical Set-Up and Surgical Technique

19.4.1 Frontal Horn and Foramen of Monro

Access to the frontal horn of the lateral ventricle and foramen of Monro is primarily achieved through two well-established microsurgical approaches: frontal craniotomy with transcortical access and the interhemispheric transcallosal approach. The frontal transcortical route, often performed via a tailored frontal craniotomy, provides direct entry into the lateral ventricle, especially for lesions such as colloid cysts, intraventricular tumors, and hydrocephalus-related obstructions. This approach offers a shorter surgical pathway, but it risks cortical injury and potential seizures if not meticulously planned. In contrast, the interhemispheric transcallosal approach enables access to the foramen of Monro via the interhemispheric fissure, avoiding cortical incisions and minimizing damage to eloquent brain areas. This route is particularly useful for midline lesions, tumors extending into the third ventricle, and bilateral pathology, providing a wider exposure while preserving periventricular structures [16].

Operative Set-Up Proper patient positioning is critical for optimizing surgical exposure and reducing the risk of complications. The patient is placed in the supine position, with a pad under the shoulders to facilitate a slight extension of the neck, thereby preventing excessive venous congestion (Fig. 19.2a). The head is secured

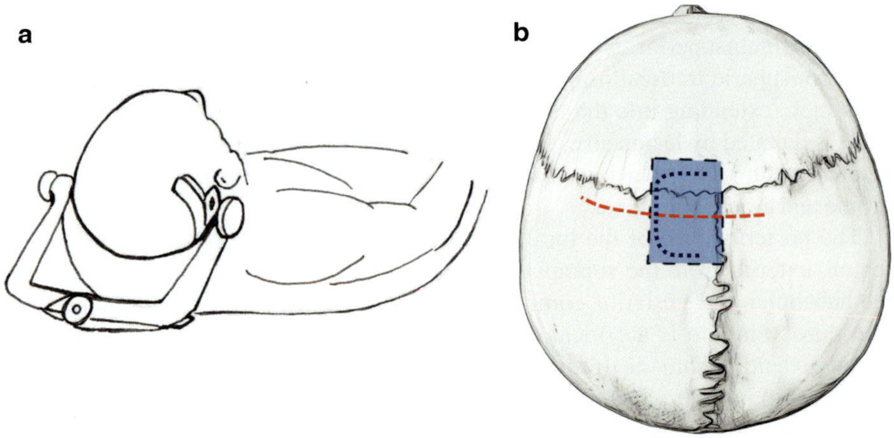

Fig. 19.2 Illustrations showing the supine positioning (**a**) and the interhemispheric craniotomy area (**b**)

using a Mayfield or Sugita head holder to ensure precise immobilization. For the interhemispheric transcallosal approach, the head is elevated approximately 15° to enhance venous drainage and brain relaxation, with minimal or no rotation to maintain a direct midline trajectory. Slight head flexion aligns the interhemispheric fissure with the surgeon's line of vision while avoiding excessive bridging vein tension [17]. For the transcortical approach, a neutral or slightly rotated head position may be used, depending on the lesion's lateralization and surgical target. Neuronavigation is highly recommended for refining trajectory and craniotomy placement.

Surgical Technique A curvilinear incision is made anterior to the coronal suture, based on the planned craniotomy. A frontal craniotomy is tailored for the selected approach, ensuring adequate exposure while preserving the superior sagittal sinus and bridging veins (Fig. 19.2b). In the interhemispheric transcallosal approach, burr holes are placed along the midline, and a U-shaped dural incision is created, reflecting the dura toward the sagittal sinus to expose the interhemispheric fissure (Fig. 19.3). The transcortical route requires a careful cortical incision over the superior frontal gyrus using cortical mapping and ultrasound guidance to minimize functional impairment. The interhemispheric fissure is gently dissected using microsurgical techniques, and a 2 cm callosotomy is performed over the pericallosal arteries to access the foramen of Monro. Controlled cerebrospinal fluid drainage via ventricular tap is often used to relax the brain and facilitate a retraction-free approach [18]. The surgical corridor was then expanded to ensure optimal visualization of the ventricular system while preserving delicate neural and vascular structures (Fig. 19.4).

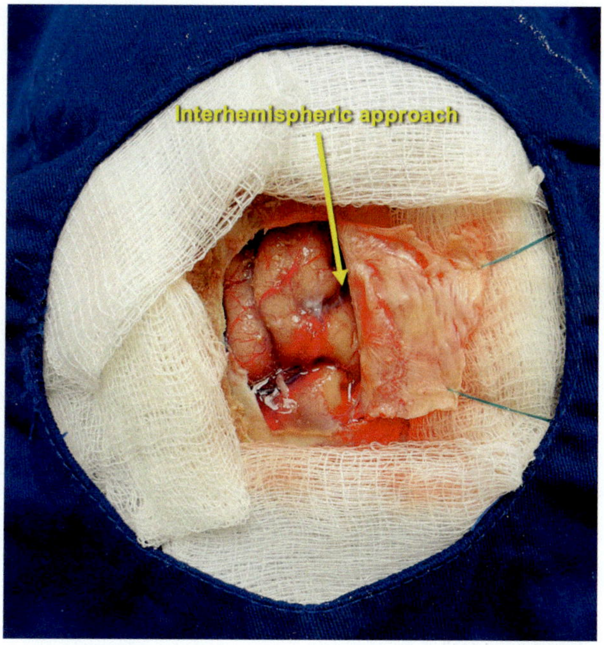

Fig. 19.3 Anatomical dissection showing the interhemispheric craniotomy with blue and white drapes for microsurgery. The yellow arrow indicates the direction from which the microscope view can be used to perform the interhemispheric approach

19.4.2 Lamina Terminalis and Temporal Horn

The lamina terminalis and temporal horn of the lateral ventricle can be accessed through various surgical approaches, including the pterional, mini-pterional, supra-orbitozygomatic, frontotemporal-orbitozygomatic, and pretemporal approaches. The pterional approach remains the most widely used because of its versatility in providing access to both the anterior and middle cranial fossae. This approach involves exposing the Sylvian fissure, thereby enabling safe entry into the basal cisterns, including the opticocarotid and lamina terminalis cisterns. By opening the lamina terminalis, direct access to the third ventricle is achieved, facilitating the management of tumors, hydrocephalus, and vascular lesions [19]. Additionally, the pterional approach offers an efficient route to the temporal horn, allowing for resection of mesial temporal tumors, amygdalo-hippocampectomy, and surgical treatment of temporal horn entrapment.

Operative Set-Up The patient is positioned in a supine position with a rolled sheet cushion under the ipsilateral shoulder to optimize cranial exposure while minimizing strain on the cervicobrachial plexus (Fig. 19.5a). A *Mayfield* or *Sugita* head holder is used to secure the head, thereby ensuring stability during the procedure. The head is elevated approximately 15° above the thoracic level to enhance venous

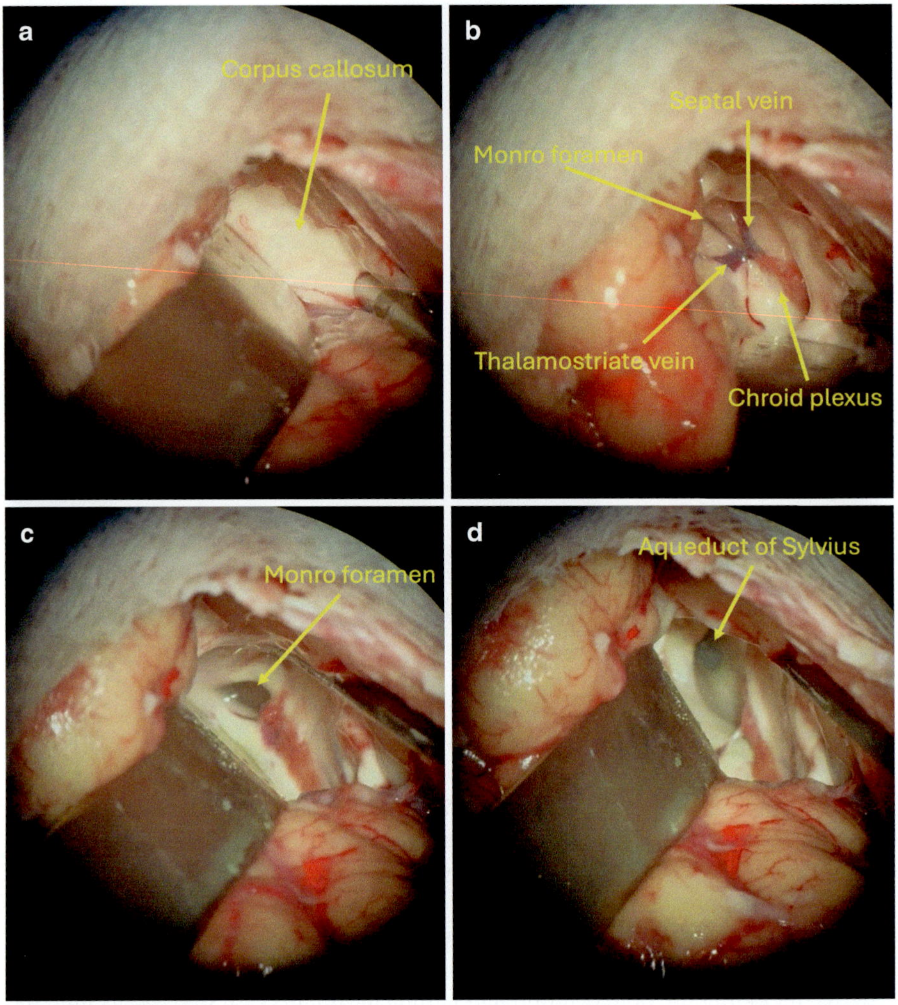

Fig. 19.4 Microsurgical photographs showing the interhemispheric approach. In (**a**), we present the initial step with the identification of the corpus callosum, which emits an intense white glow under microscopy. The septal vein, thalamostriate vein, and choroid plexus (**b**) are anatomical landmarks for identifying the foramen of Monro (**b**, **c**). After entering the third ventricle, we can locate the aqueduct of Sylvius (**d**) anteriorly

return and intracranial decompression. The degree of contralateral head rotation varies depending on the target structure (45°–60°) of the lamina terminalis [20]. Head extension is performed to align the malar eminence as the highest point in the field, which enhanced the visualization of the Sylvian fissure and basal cisterns.

Surgical Technique A standard arcuate skin incision is made, starting 1 cm anterior to the tragus and extending toward the midline, ensuring optimal exposure of the pterion while preserving the superficial temporal artery (Fig. 19.5b; Video 19.1).

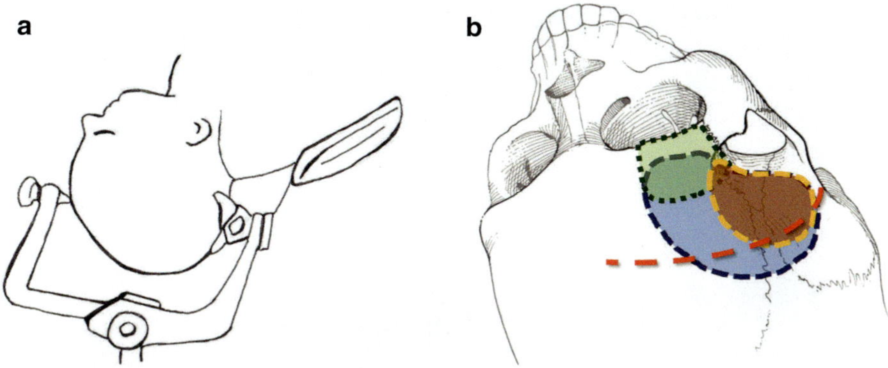

Fig. 19.5 Illustrations showing the supine positioning in (**a**) and the possible craniotomy areas for access to the lamina terminalis and temporal horn in (**b**) (supraorbital craniotomy in green, mini-pterional in orange, and pterional in blue)

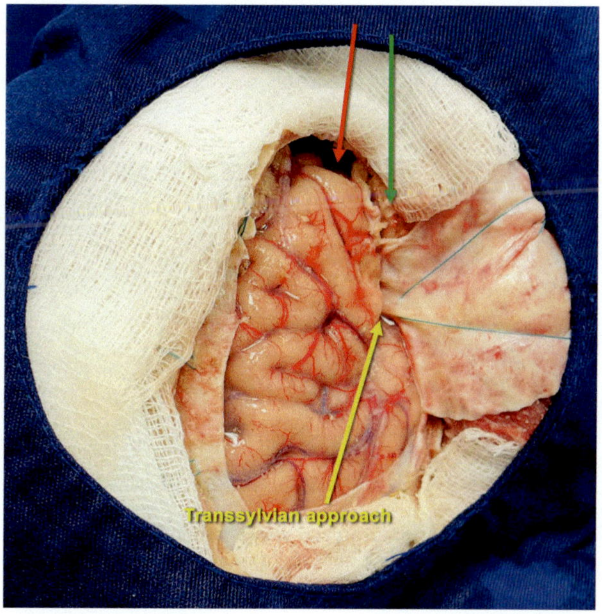

Fig. 19.6 Intraoperative photographs of the classic pterional approach prepared for microsurgery. The yellow arrow indicates the direction for the microscope view to perform the transsylvian approach, followed by changing the angle of view toward the lamina terminalis (red arrow) and the temporal horn (green arrow)

A muscle-sparing dissection technique is preferred to protect the temporal branch of the facial nerve. The pterional craniotomy is performed by placing a keyhole burr hole at the frontosphenoidal suture, with additional burr holes along the superior temporal line, if needed (Fig. 19.6). The bone flap is elevated, and the sphenoid ridge is placed to improve access to the Sylvian fissure and basal cisterns [21]. The dur is then opened in a curvilinear fashion, with the flap reflected anteriorly to maintain exposure and to avoid tension. Further dissection of the Sylvian fissure facilitates entry into the lamina terminalis cistern (Fig. 19.7), while anteroinferior

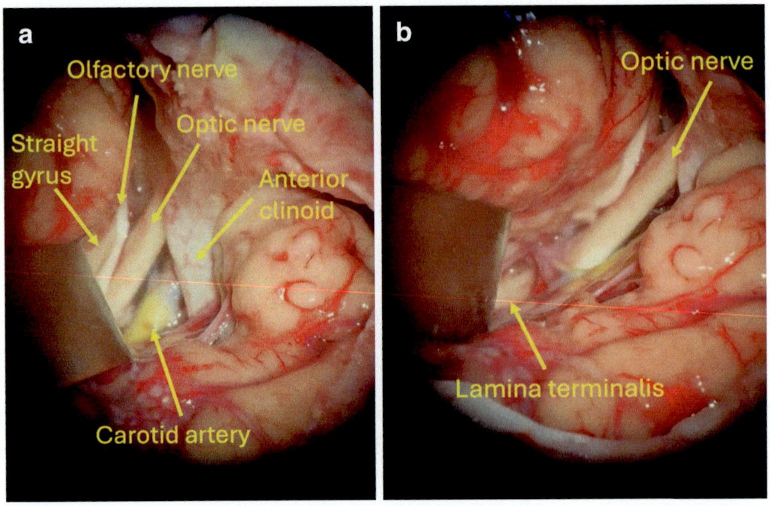

Fig. 19.7 Microsurgical photograph showing access to the lamina terminalis in (**a**), where we can see the olfactory nerve with the straight gyrus, the optic nerve, the anterior clinoid process, and the carotid artery. During the dissection, we follow the path of the optic nerve to identify the lamina terminalis (**b**)

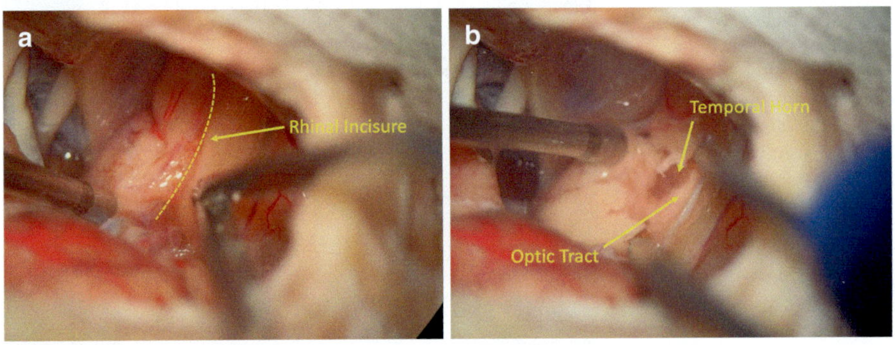

Fig. 19.8 During microsurgical access through the Sylvian fissure to the temporal horn of the lateral ventricle, the rhinal incisure (**a**) serves as the anatomical landmark for opening the temporal horn; observe the relationship between the optic tract and the temporal horn (**b**)

dissection allows access to the temporal horn, ensuring minimal brain retraction (Fig. 19.8).

19.4.3 Atrium

Access to the atrium (trigone) of the lateral ventricle can be achieved via the parietal, parieto-occipital, or interhemispheric approaches. The choice depends on the lesion's location, relationship with adjacent structures, and the need to preserve the

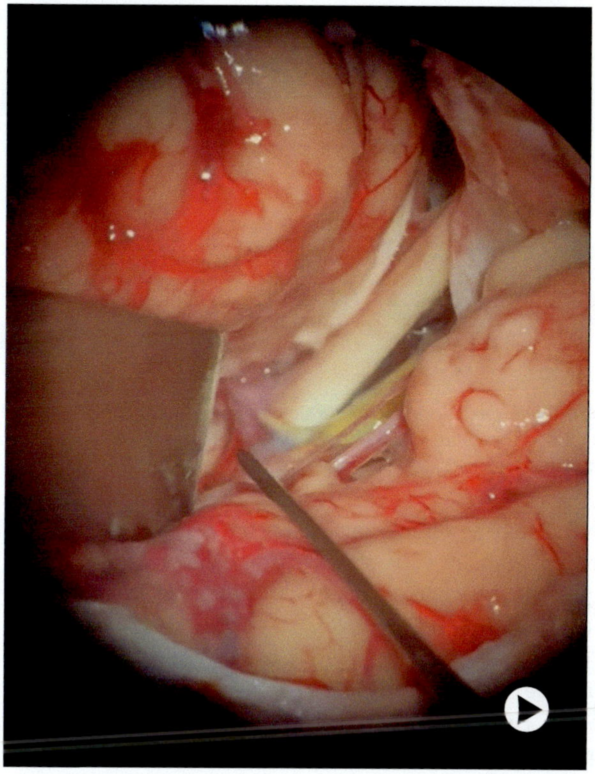

Video 19.1 This video demonstrates microsurgical access to the lateral ventricles through the lamina terminalis, frontal horn, temporal horn, and atrium, as well as to the third and fourth ventricles using tailored craniotomies. It highlights anatomical landmarks, approach trajectories, and technical nuances essential for safe and effective ventricular access (▶ https://doi.org/10.1007/000-hta)

eloquent cortex. Among these, the transparietal approach is commonly used due to its direct trajectory into the atrium, offering a relatively short path while minimizing retraction in deep neurovascular structures. This method involves transcortical or transsulcal entry through the superior parietal lobule, which allows a straightforward route to the ventricular cavity while avoiding excessive manipulation of the optic radiation, thereby reducing the risk of postoperative visual field deficits [3]. Neuronavigation and intraoperative ultrasound aid in optimizing trajectory and minimizing cortical disruption.

Operative Set-Up The patient is typically positioned in the supine or lateral position, depending on the surgical corridor and surgeon preference (Fig. 19.9a). In the supine position, a rolled sheet or gel pad is placed under the contralateral shoulder to facilitate mild head tilt while maintaining the surgical side elevated. The head is elevated from approximately 10° to 15° to enhance venous drainage and reduce intracranial pressure. Minimal to moderate rotation (20°–30° contralateral) is applied, depending on the target's lateralization, ensuring an optimal trajectory into

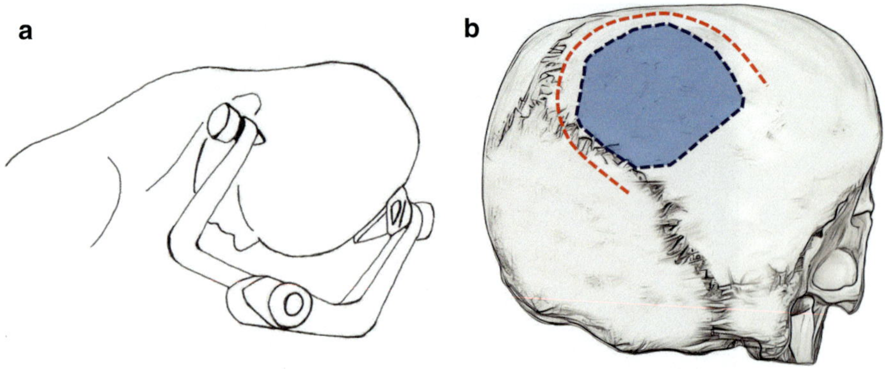

Fig. 19.9 In these illustrations, see (**a**) lateral positioning para a realização da craniotomia parietal (**b**). The red dashed line represents the horseshoe skin incision, and the parietal craniotomy is represented by the blue area

the atrium while avoiding undue tension on the bridging veins. Neck flexion was avoided to prevent jugular vein compression, and neuronavigation was used to refine the surgical corridor and enhance precision during cortical entry [22].

Surgical Technique A linear or horseshoe-shaped incision is made over the superior parietal lobule, centered along the planned craniotomy. The parietal craniotomy, measuring approximately 4–5 cm in diameter, is designed to expose the dura while avoiding injury to the superior sagittal sinus. Burr holes are placed strategically, one along the superior parietal region and another posterolaterally, facilitating gentle fural elevation (Fig. 19.9b). The dura is then opened in a C-shaped fashion, allowing for careful retraction while preserving major venous drainage (Fig. 19.10). Neuronavigation is employed to guide transcortical entry as well as ultrasound, ensuring precise localization of the atrial region while minimizing the risk of optic radiation injury. Cerebrospinal fluid drainage is controlled to aid brain relaxation, facilitating safe entry into the ventricle with minimal cortical disturbance [5] (Fig. 19.11).

19.4.4 Telovelar

Access to the telovelar region, particularly the fourth ventricle, is achieved primarily through suboccipital and far-lateral approaches. Among these, the suboccipital approach is the most widely used due to its midline access to the cerebellomedullary fissure, allowing for a natural dissection plane between the cerebellar tonsils without the need to split the vermis. This approach provides wide exposure of the fourth ventricle, making it particularly useful for the resection of intrinsic brainstem tumors, medulloblastomas, ependymoma, and fourth ventricle cystic lesions. Compared with the transversion approach, the telovelar route minimizes disruption

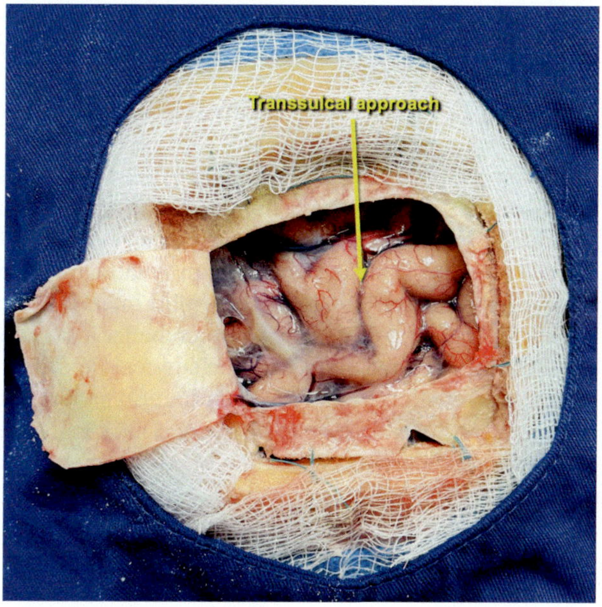

Fig. 19.10 In this anatomical dissection photograph, the parietal craniotomy is visible, and the patient is prepared for microsurgery. The yellow arrow indicates a microscope view of the transsulcal (transparietal) approach

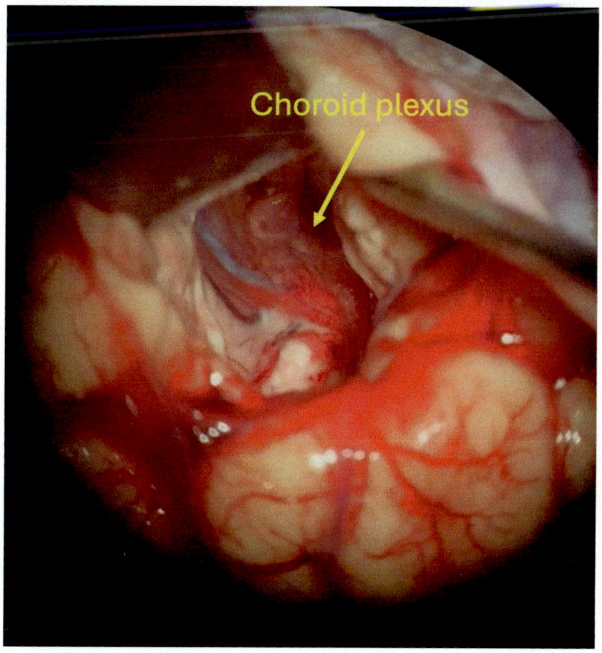

Fig. 19.11 Microsurgical photograph showing the ventricular atrium through the transparietal approach; the choroid plexus

of the cerebellar vermis, thereby reducing the risk of postoperative mutism and cerebellar dysfunction [23]. Suboccipital craniotomy, when performed with proper dural opening techniques, preserves venous structures while providing sufficient working space for microsurgical dissection.

Operative Set-Up The patient is placed in the prone, lateral park-bench, or semisitting position, with prone positioning being the most common for midline fourth ventricular lesions (Fig. 19.12a). The head is elevated (10°–15°) is employed to facilitate venous drainage and minimize intracranial pressure. The head remains neutral for midline lesions, while a mild lateral tilt may be used for paramedian targets. In cases requiring extensive cerebellar exposure, slight flexion is applied to align the foramen magnum with the surgical field to optimize access to the brainstem and cerebellomedullary fissure. Careful padding of pressure points is essential to prevent postoperative neuropathy, and intraoperative neuronavigation is recommended for the precise localization of deep-seated pathology [24].

Surgical Technique A midline straight skin incision is made that extends from the external occipital protuberance (inion) to the C2 level, depending on the extent of exposure required. The suboccipital craniotomy is initiated with burr holes placed bilaterally above the asterium to expose the transverse sinus and facilitate controlled elevation of the bone flap (Fig. 19.12b). If additional exposure is necessary, the posterior arch of C1 is removed using a Kerrison rongeur, ensuring careful dissection to avoid vertebral artery injury. The dura is opened in a Y- or U-shaped direction, reflecting flaps upward but avoiding excessive retraction on the venous sinuses [25] (Fig. 19.13). To achieve brain relaxation, an external ventricular drain is placed preoperatively at Dandy's or Frazier's point, allowing controlled cerebrospinal fluid drainage before dural opening. This step minimizes cerebellar retraction, thereby reducing the risk of venous infarction and brainstem distortion (Fig. 19.14).

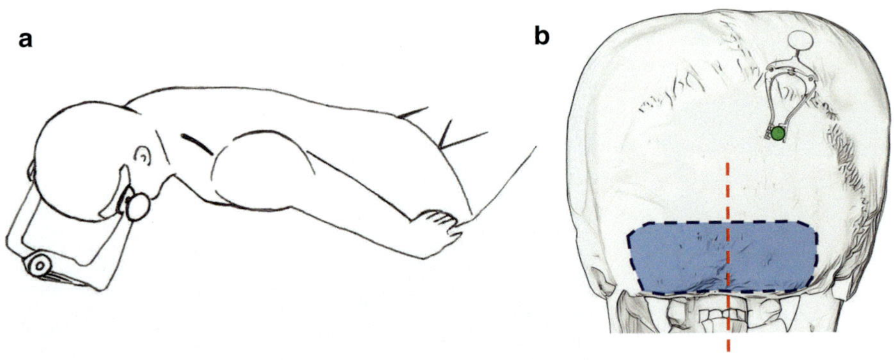

Fig. 19.12 For the suboccipital approach, the patient can be positioned in prone (**a**). The incision extends from the inion to C2 (red dashed line in **b**), and the blue area represents the suboccipital craniotomy in (**b**); Frazier's point is represented by the green circle with a Jansen retractor

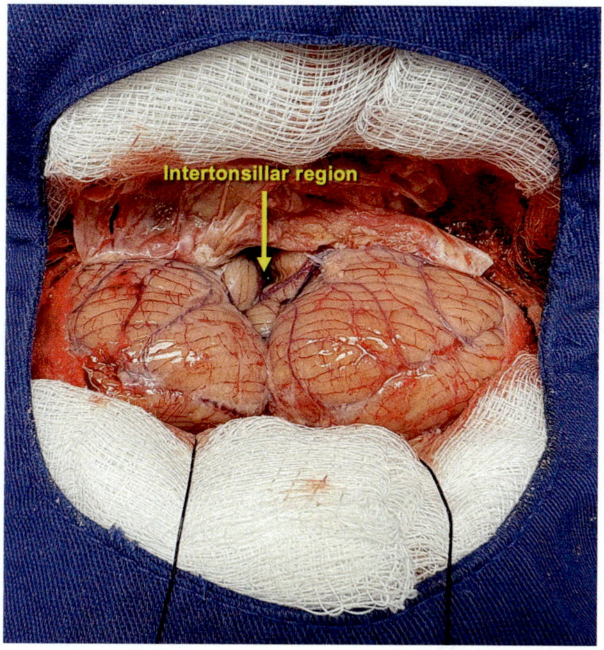

Fig. 19.13 Surgical approach: the suboccipital craniotomy is completed, and the intertonsillar region is identified for the telovelar approach. The yellow arrow indicates the microscope view

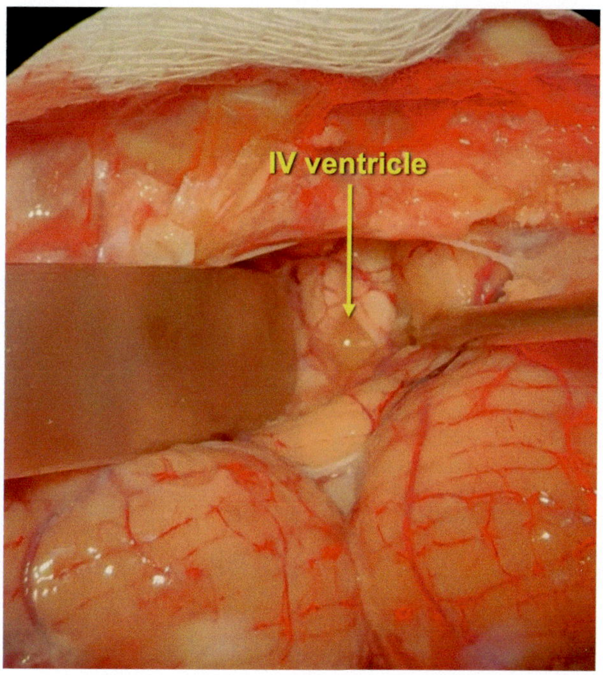

Fig. 19.14 Microsurgical image showing the fourth ventricle through the telovelar approach

19.4.5 Pineal

The pineal region can be accessed using the suboccipital supracerebellar, posterior interhemispheric, or occipital transtentorial approaches (Fig. 19.12a). The choice of approach depends on the lesion's size, extension, and relationship with critical neurovascular structures. The suboccipital supracerebellar approach is one of the most commonly used techniques for pineal region tumors, providing a direct midline route through the natural plane between the superior cerebellar surface and the tentorium. This method allows for excellent exposure while avoiding unnecessary cortical disruption, making it suitable for lesions below the tentorial plane or extending into the third ventricle [26]. Compared with the occipital transtentorial approach, which requires tentorial division and carries the risk of venous infarction, the supracerebellar infratentorial route is often preferred due to its preservation of supratentorial structures and reduced risk of visual field deficits.

Operative Set-Up and Surgical Technique The prone, park-bench, or semisitting positions can be used, with the prone position being the most frequently adopted to facilitate a natural downward displacement of the cerebellum while reducing venous congestion. The head is elevated from 10° to 15° with minimal rotation or flexion to maintain an optimal angle for accessing the quadrigeminal cistern and posterior third ventricle. The skin incision extends from the external occipital protuberance (inion) to C2 [24, 25]. A midline suboccipital craniotomy is performed, exposing the torcular Herophili, transverse sinuses, and superior cerebellar surface (Fig. 19.12b). The dura is opened in the Y- or U-s direction and appears upward but without retraction in the venous sinuses. Microsurgical dissection proceeds through the supracerebellar corridor using cerebrospinal fluid drainage to facilitate cerebellar relaxation and prevent excessive retraction [26] (Fig. 19.15). This technique allows for precise tumor resection while preserving the deep venous system and minimizing neurological morbidity (Fig. 19.16).

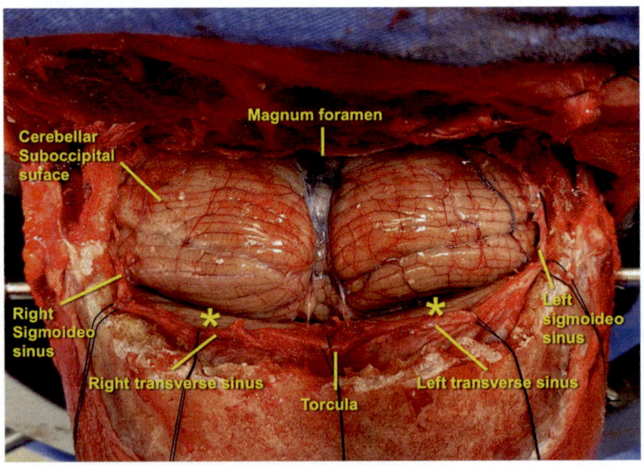

Fig. 19.15 Photograph of the suboccipital approach, showing a centered view of the supracerebellar infratentorial corridor (yellow stars). This image also identifies the foramen magnum, cerebellar surface, sigmoid sinuses, transverse sinuses, and torcula of Herophili

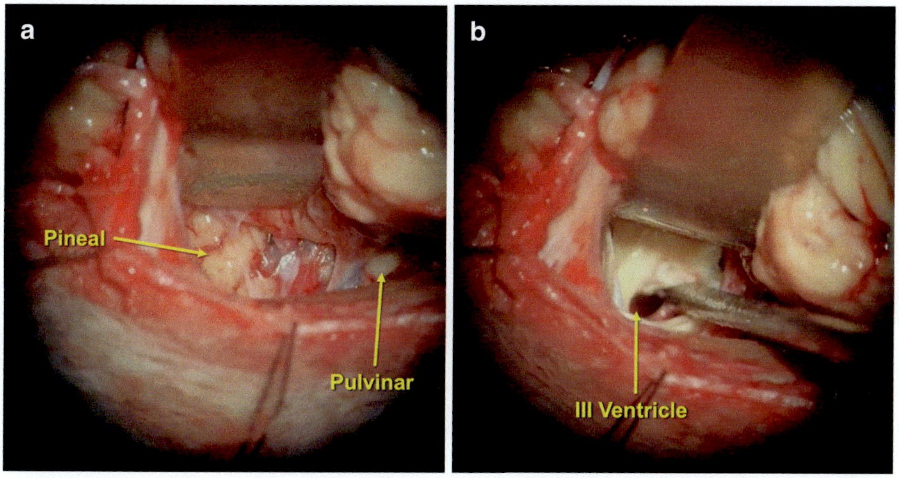

Fig. 19.16 Microsurgical photograph showing access to the pineal region. Note the surrounding venous structures and entry into the third ventricle. In (**a**), the pineal gland is observed in the midline and laterally in the pulvinar region. The third ventricle in (**b**) is accessible via the pineal gland

19.5 Pearls and Pitfalls

- *Preoperative imaging*: *MRI, magnetic resonance imaging*, and computed tomography angiography to assess the anatomy and avoid vascular injury.
- *Neuronavigation and intraoperative ultrasound* enhance tumor localization *accuracy*, ventricular access, and depth control while minimizing cortical damage and improving targeting.
- *CSF Drainage*: The EVD or lumbar drain aids brain relaxation, minimizing retraction.
- *Safe Surgical Corridor*: Transcallosal avoids cortical damage, whereas transcortical surgery requires careful trajectory planning.
- *Preserve Deep Veins*: Gentle dissection around the foramen of the Monro and pineal regions prevents venous infarction.
- *Cortical Injury*: Poor trajectory in transcortical approaches can result in optic radiation or injury to the motor cortex.
- *Venous Infarction*: Excessive traction on bridging veins in transcallosal access can cause ischemia; also, for the suboccipital approach, excessive traction while reflecting the dural flap can damage the venous sinuses.
- *Hemorrhage Risk*: Overaggressive tumor resection in the foramen of Monro or the atrium may disrupt the choroidal vessels.
- *Cerebellar Mutism*: Vermian splitting in fourth ventricle surgery increases risk; favor the telovelar approach.

- *Visual Deficits*: Poor atrial tumor trajectory can cause optic radiation injury, leading to homonymous hemianopia.
- *Meticulous planning, microsurgical precision, and neuronavigation* optimize safety and outcomes.

References

1. Schroeder HWS. General principles and intraventricular neuroendoscopy: endoscopic techniques. World Neurosurg. 2013;79(2S):S14.e23–8.
2. Ganslandt O, Behari S, Gralla J, Fahlbusch R, Nimsky C. Neuronavigation: concept, techniques, and applications. Neurol India. 2002;50:244–55.
3. Rhoton AL Jr. The lateral and third ventricles. Neurosurgery. 2002;51(4 Suppl):S207–71.
4. Winn HR, Youmans JR. Youmans and Winn neurological surgery. 8th ed. Philadelphia: Elsevier; 2023.
5. Greenberg MS. Handbook of neurosurgery. 9th ed. New York: Thieme; 2020.
6. Lozier AP, Cohen-Gadol AA. Operative techniques in neurosurgery: neurosurgical operative atlas, vol. 2. New York: Thieme; 2019.
7. Anderson RCE, Ghatan S, Feldstein NA. Surgical approaches to tumors of the lateral ventricle. Neurosurg Clin N Am. 2003;14(4):509–25.
8. Kasowski H, Piepmeier JM. Transcallosal approach for tumors of the lateral and third ventricles. Neurosurg Focus. 2001;10(6):Article 3.
9. Aftahy AK, Barz M, Wagner A, Liesche-Starnecker F, Negwer C, Meyer B, Gempt J. The interhemispheric fissure—surgical outcome of interhemispheric approaches. Neurosurg Rev. 2021;44:2099–111.
10. Zanini MA, Faleiros ATS, Almeida CR, Clara CA, Gabarra RC. Trigone ventricular meningiomas: surgical approaches. Arq Neuropsiquiatr. 2011;69(4):670–5.
11. Ghali MGZ. Telovelar surgical approach. Neurosurg Rev. 2019;42(4):865–78.
12. Simon E, Afif A, M'Baye M, Mertens P. Anatomy of the pineal region applied to its surgical approach. Neurochirurgie. 2015;61(2):70–6.
13. Matsuo S, Baydin S, Güngör A, et al. Midline and off-midline infratentorial supracerebellar approaches to the pineal gland. J Neurosurg. 2016;125(1):1–9.
14. Mottolese C, Szathmari A, Ricci-Franchi AC, et al. Supracerebellar infratentorial approach for pineal region tumors: surgical and technical considerations. Neurochirurgie. 2014;60(6):1–8.
15. Yamamoto I. Pineal region tumor: surgical anatomy and approach. J Neuro-Oncol. 2001;54(3):263–75.
16. Anetsberger SA, Marbacher S, Fandino J, et al. Interhemispheric approach. Acta Biomed. 2021;92(Suppl 4):e2021351.
17. Meyer FB. Atlas de Neurocirurgia: Acessos Básicos ao Crânio e Procedimentos Vascular. Rio de Janeiro: DiLivros; 2005.
18. Fossett DT, Caputy AJ. Operative neurosurgical anatomy. New York and Stuttgart: Thieme; 2001.
19. Rubio RR, Martinez E, Carceller F, et al. Immersive surgical anatomy of the pterional approach. Cureus. 2019;11(7):e5216.
20. Vishteh AG, Spetzler RF, Lawton MT, et al. The pterional approach. Oper Tech Neurosurg. 1998;1(1):39–49.
21. Yasargil MG. Microneurosurgery: volume 1. Stuttgart: Georg Thieme Verlag; 1984.
22. Yasargil MG. Microneurosurgery: Vol. IVB. Clinical considerations, surgery of the intracranial aneurysms and results. Stuttgart: Thieme; 1996.

23. Deshmukh VR, Figueiredo EG, Spetzler RF. Quantification and comparison of telovelar and transvermian approaches to the fourth ventricle. Neurosurgery. 2006;58(ONS Suppl 2):ONS-202–7.
24. Legnani FG, Saladino A, Casali C, et al. Craniotomy vs. craniectomy for posterior fossa tumors: a prospective study to evaluate complications after surgery. Acta Neurochir. 2013;155(12):2281–6.
25. Prell J, Rachinger J, Scheitzach J, et al. Midline-craniotomy of the posterior fossa with attached bone flap: experiences in pediatric and adult patients. Acta Neurochir. 2011;153:541–5.
26. Mottolese C, Szathmari A, Ricci-Franchi AC, et al. Supracerebellar infratentorial approach for pineal region tumors: our surgical and technical considerations. Neurochirurgie. 2014;60(6):1–8.

Summary of Cranial Approaches 20

Chapter #	Approach	Region	Key notes	Video #
3	Frontal and transbasal	Frontal/base	Accesses anterior cranial base, frontal lesions	3.1
4	The pterional	Frontal/temporal	Versatile; accesses sylvian fissure and parasellar region	4.1
5	Mini-pterional (minimally invasive)	Frontal/temporal	Smaller exposure; less invasive alternative to pterional	5.1
6	Supraorbital and supraorbital zygomatic (minimally invasive)	Frontal	Brow incision; less tissue disruption	6.1
7	Frontotemporo-orbitozygomatic	Frontal/temporal/orbital	Extended exposure for large or complex lesions	7.1
8	Clinoidectomy: Intradural and extradural	Sellar/parasellar	Used to access clinoidal and parasellar regions	8.1
9	Interhemispheric	Midline/interhemispheric	Good for falcine and corpus callosum lesions	9.1
10	Pretemporal and transcavernous (Dolenc's)	Temporal/cavernous sinus	Accesses cavernous sinus, upper basilar	10.1
11	Subtemporal and subtemporal-anterior-transpetrous (Kawase's)	Temporal/petrosal	Deep temporal and petroclival region	11.1
12	Parietal and occipital	Parietal/occipital	Accesses cortical and subcortical lesions	12.1
13	Suboccipital	Posterior fossa	Posterior fossa, midline or paramedian	13.1
14	Retrosigmoid	Cerebellopontine angle	For CPA tumors and retrosigmoid cerebellar access	14.1
15	Presigmoid	Cerebellopontine angle	Anterior CPA and petrosal lesions	15.1

(continued)

H. de Oliveira Manduca Palmiero, E. G. Figueiredo, *Neurosurgical Approaches Video Atlas*, https://doi.org/10.1007/978-3-032-04664-2_20

Chapter #	Approach	Region	Key notes	Video #
16	Far lateral	Posterior fossa/ craniovertebral junction	For lateral foramen magnum and lower brainstem	16.1
17	Endoscopic transsphenoidal	Sellar (endoscopic)	Endonasal approach to Sella and parasellar areas	17.1
18	Decompressive craniectomy	Frontal/temporal/ parietal/occipital	Used in trauma and malignant ICP cases such as malignant stroke	18.1
19	Microsurgical approaches to the ventricles	Intraventricular	Access lateral, third, or fourth ventricles	19.1

Future Directions in Cranial Approaches 21

21.1 Modern Neurosurgery: Origins and Legacy

Modern neurosurgery emerged from the intersection of precise anatomy, innovative operations, and groundbreaking technologies. In the early twentieth century, Harvey Cushing's (Fig. 21.1) meticulous approach and introduction of surgical hemostasis paved the way for cranial neurosurgery to advance beyond basic procedures like trephination and decompression. His pioneering work in brain tumor surgery and operative planning solidified neurosurgery as a distinct field and significantly improved the safety of intracranial operations [1].

The next leap occurred with the development of microneurosurgery. The advent of the operating microscope in the 1950s and 60s—particularly through the visionary work of Prof. Mahmut Gazi Yasargil (Fig. 21.2)—redefined surgical visibility

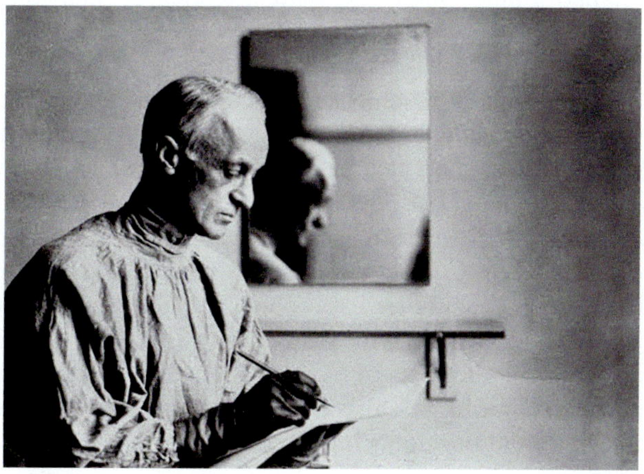

Fig. 21.1 Harvey Cushing, the father of modern neurosurgery, documenting operative notes. This iconic photograph captures Cushing's meticulous attention to detail, dressed in surgical attire, with his reflection in the background symbolizing both introspection and the duality of surgeon and scientist

H. de Oliveira Manduca Palmiero, E. G. Figueiredo, *Neurosurgical Approaches Video Atlas*, https://doi.org/10.1007/978-3-032-04664-2_21

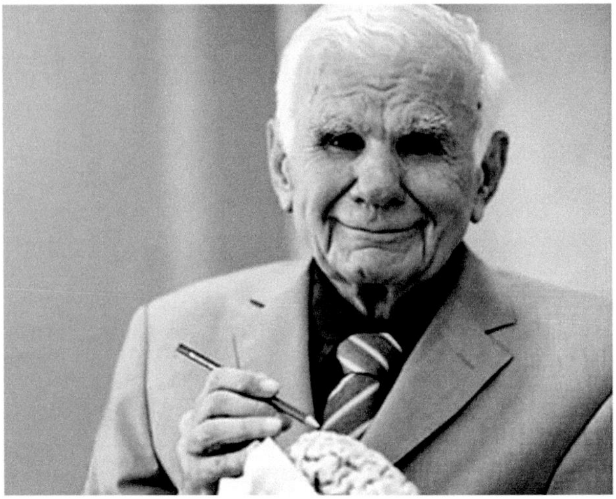

Fig. 21.2 Prof. Mahmut Gazi Yasargil, a legendary neurosurgeon, holds a model brain and a pencil, symbolizing a lifetime dedicated to the intricate art of neurosurgery. His gentle smile and steady hand reflect both wisdom and precision—hallmarks of a master who taught generations not only with his scalpel and microscope but also with his humility

and precision [2]. The introduction of bipolar coagulation, microsurgical instruments, and high-magnification visualization enabled previously unthinkable dissections along eloquent planes and neurovascular complexes [3]. Yasargil's systematic development of cranial approaches, particularly the pterional route, codified access to deep-seated lesions and neurovascular pathologies with minimal collateral damage [4].

Microsurgical approaches weren't just technical breakthroughs but also major anatomical advancements. They required a fresh look at skull base pathways, sulcal and cisternal navigation, and techniques for dissecting the subarachnoid space. This led to a deeper understanding of white matter tracts, vascular perforators, and key points of skull base attachment. Mastering anatomy became a crucial part of performing surgeries with excellence, and dissection became a nearly artistic skill.

This era also witnessed the proliferation of cadaveric dissection laboratories, training generations of neurosurgeons in the techniques that would become standard for aneurysm clipping, tumor resection, and complex skull base surgeries [5]. The culture of hands-on anatomical training, combined with technological mentorship, fostered a global diaspora of neurosurgeons steeped in the microsurgical ethic.

Today, modern neurosurgery stands at a crucial turning point. The principles established by Cushing and Yasargil remain, but they now intersect with groundbreaking technologies like robotics, tractography, virtual reality, and artificial intelligence, which will likely transform how we tackle brain-related issues. Recognizing the roots of modern neurosurgery is vital, not just to acknowledge its accomplishments but also to put them in perspective and inform the responsible integration of new tools into a field that has always strived for both innovation and precision.

21.2 Integration of Augmented Reality (AR) and Mixed Reality

Augmented reality (AR) and mixed reality (MR) technologies are rapidly transforming the visualization paradigm in cranial surgery. By superimposing segmented imaging data onto the surgical field, AR enables real-time intraoperative localization of lesions, vascular structures, and eloquent cortex without disrupting the operative flow. Platforms such as Surgical Theater and the Microsoft HoloLens provide immersive, stereoscopic environments in which preoperative planning and intraoperative navigation are seamlessly linked, allowing surgeons to "walk through" complex anatomy before making the first incision [6, 7].

These technologies augment—not replace—the meticulous anatomical planning that is foundational to neurosurgical approaches. However, their value lies in reducing cognitive load, improving spatial orientation, and enhancing team communication during high-stakes procedures. Early data suggest that AR-assisted procedures may shorten operative time and improve resection margins in tumor cases, although high-quality outcome studies remain limited [8]. As hardware improves in resolution, latency, and integration with neuronavigation platforms, AR is set to become a powerful adjunct in both open and endoscopic cranial procedures.

21.3 Advanced Tractography and Functional Imaging

The evolution of tractography and functional imaging has redefined surgical planning in cranial neurosurgery by enabling surgeons to move beyond purely anatomical constraints and incorporate patient-specific functional networks. High-resolution diffusion tensor imaging (DTI), constrained spherical deconvolution, and connectomic analyses now provide detailed visualization of white matter tracts such as the arcuate fasciculus, corticospinal tract, and optic radiation—structures often at risk during the resection of deep-seated or insular lesions [9]. When combined with resting-state fMRI, magnetoencephalography (MEG), and navigated transcranial magnetic stimulation (nTMS), these tools create a preoperative map of motor, language, and cognitive domains, empowering the surgeon to choose the least disruptive approach. This convergence of functional and anatomical imaging supports the modern ethos of "maximal safe resection," where the limits of surgery are defined not only by gross anatomical barriers but also by the connectomic integrity that underpins a patient's quality of life [10] (Fig. 21.3).

Intraoperative Ultrasound In parallel with preoperative tract-based planning, intraoperative ultrasound (iUS) has emerged as a dynamic, real-time modality for refining surgical navigation during cranial procedures. Unlike neuronavigation systems that rely on preoperative imaging, iUS provides continuous intraoperative feedback, overcoming challenges like brain shift and tissue deformation that reduce accuracy during resection. With advances in high-frequency probes, contrast enhancement, and fusion with tractography datasets, iUS has evolved from a basic

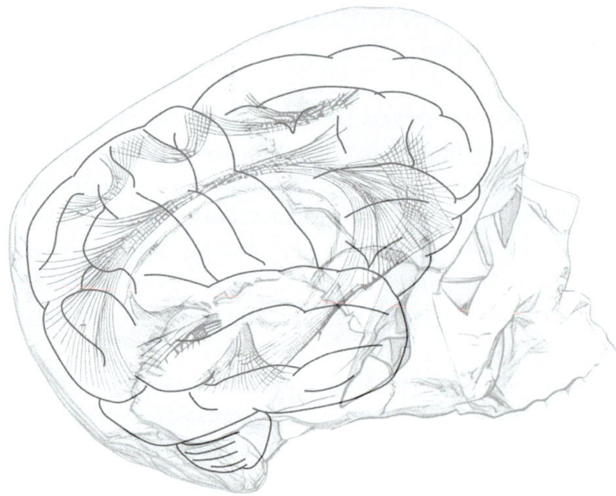

Fig. 21.3 Sagittal anatomical illustration demonstrating the major white matter tracts of the cerebral hemispheres superimposed on the skull base contour. This schematic emphasizes the spatial relationships between deep midline structures—such as the corpus callosum, cingulum, and internal capsule—and the overlying gyri and sulci. High-resolution tractography techniques aim to map these bundles preoperatively to preserve connectivity and function during cranial approaches

localization tool to a sophisticated adjunct that facilitates real-time tracking of lesion margins and vascular landmarks, particularly in deep-seated tumors or eloquent cortex regions [11]. Its portability, low cost, and minimal delay make it especially appealing in resource-constrained environments or when intraoperative MRI is unavailable [12].

21.4 Robotics in Microsurgery

Robotic technologies are gradually being integrated into cranial neurosurgery, offering submillimetric precision, enhanced tremor filtration, and ergonomic advantages during prolonged or deep-field procedures. Unlike conventional microsurgical manipulation, robotic platforms allow for instrumental stabilization, programmed trajectories, and repeatable micro-movements that are particularly beneficial in skull base, pineal, and ventricular regions where corridor constraints are narrow and critical structures are tightly clustered. Systems such as ROSA® and Modus V® the platforms are already employed for stereotatic procedures and endoscope assistance, while emerging tools aim to bring robotic control to microneurosurgical tasks such as tumor debulking or vascular clipping [13]. Although widespread adoption is still limited by cost, integration challenges, and the steep learning curve, robotic microsurgery is poised to augment human dexterity and redefine the technical boundaries of deep-seated cranial approaches [14].

21.5 Artificial Intelligence in Surgical Planning

Artificial intelligence (AI) is rapidly entering the neurosurgical arena, particularly in the domains of preoperative planning, imaging interpretation, and intraoperative decision support. Machine learning algorithms trained on large imaging datasets can now segment tumors, delineate eloquent cortex, and even stimulate optimal surgical corridors based on patient-specific anatomy and pathology [15]. Deep learning techniques have demonstrated comparable or superior performance to human experts in detecting radiological features such as midline shift, hemorrhage, and white matter invasion in gliomas, with applications expanding toward real-time surgical guidance systems [16]. AI-driven platforms may soon provide predictive analytics regarding surgical difficulty, potential complications, and long-term functional outcomes, allowing surgeons to tailor interventions based on risk-benefit modeling and objective data (Fig. 21.4).

Intraoperatively, AI is being explored for dynamic neuronavigation updates, gesture recognition, and automated workflow optimization. Integrating AI with intraoperative video and sensor data could enhance instrument tracking, flag potentially dangerous maneuvers, and even provide context-aware recommendations during dissection near critical structures. As these systems evolve, the role of the neurosurgeon may shift toward supervisory oversight—interpreting, validating, and guiding

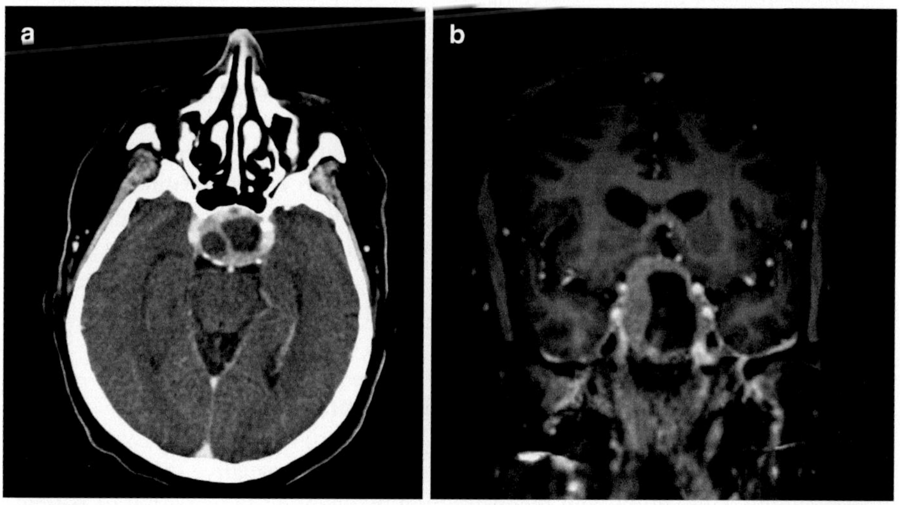

Fig. 21.4 Axial CT (**a**) and coronal contrast-enhanced MRI (**b**) of a sellar-suprasellar mass. While experienced neurosurgeons can quickly assess the anatomical boundaries and choose between a cranial or endoscopic transsphenoidal approach, artificial intelligence (AI) systems provide additional decision support by integrating imaging, lesion characteristics, prior outcomes, and anatomical constraints. For less experienced surgeons, AI tools can aid in surgical planning by suggesting the most appropriate corridor based on large datasets of similar cases, helping to optimize safety and efficacy while reducing variability in care

machine-generated insights within the framework of clinical judgment and experience. However, caution is warranted to avoid overreliance on opaque algorithms ("black box" models) without adequate validation. Ethical, legal, and safety frameworks must keep pace with technical advances to ensure that AI augments, rather than supplants, the nuanced decision-making central to neurosurgical craft [17].

21.6 Minimally Invasive and Tubular Technologies

Minimally invasive cranial techniques—especially those using tubular retractors and keyhole corridors—have significantly enhanced the neurosurgical armamentarium by providing safer, cosmetically favorable alternatives to traditional craniotomies. Systems are available for transsulcal or transcortical access to deep lesions, including thalamic hematomas, ventricular tumors, and subcortical metastases, while minimizing white matter disruption and retraction injury [18]. These techniques are especially beneficial in neuro-oncology and hemorrhagic stroke management, where precise trajectory planning and tissue preservation are crucial. Moreover, tubular and keyhole approaches are increasingly utilized in skull base surgery for meningiomas and epidermoids, as well as for hematoma evacuation in elderly or comorbid patients, where surgical morbidity must be tightly controlled [19].

Endoscopic-assisted surgeries have revolutionized visibility within narrow operative corridors, providing angled views of deep anatomical recesses that are otherwise hidden in traditional microscopic techniques. In cranial neurosurgery, endoscopic methods are particularly prominent in transsphenoidal pituitary surgery, intraventricular tumor resection, and skull base approaches to the clivus and craniovertebral junction [20]. Their application has also broadened in vascular surgery, where endoscopes aid in identifying aneurysm necks or perforators beyond the microscopic line of sight, and in tumor surgery to examine blind spots after resection. The areas most improved by minimally invasive, tubular, and endoscopic techniques include skull base surgery, intraventricular tumors, deep-seated gliomas, and hematoma evacuation, where constrained operative corridors necessitate maximal visualization with minimal disruption [21].

21.7 3D Printing and Anatomical Customization

Three-dimensional (3D) printing has emerged as a transformative tool in neurosurgical planning, simulation, and reconstruction by enabling the creation of patient-specific anatomical models from radiological data. These models allow surgeons to rehearse complex cranial approaches, evaluate the spatial relationships of lesions to critical neurovascular structures, and simulate osteotomies or drilling trajectories with unprecedented fidelity [22]. In skull base and pediatric craniofacial surgery, 3D-printed guides and implants facilitate precise bony reconstruction while enhancing cosmetic and functional outcomes. Beyond preoperative preparation, custom-designed prosthetics and cranial plates tailored to patient-specific defects have improved accuracy and reduced operative time in cranioplasty procedures. As printing technologies advance in resolution and material compatibility, their role is likely to expand into intraoperative navigation, bioprinting, and patient education [23].

Haptic Experiences Provided by 3D Models An important extension of 3D printing in neurosurgery lies in its ability to deliver tactile, or haptic, feedback that mimics the resistance, texture, and structural integrity of cranial and neurovascular tissues. Unlike purely visual simulations, haptic models allow surgeons—especially trainees—to rehearse drilling, cutting, and dissection maneuvers under conditions that approximate real surgical scenarios. Studies have demonstrated that haptic-enhanced 3D models improve spatial orientation, procedural confidence, and technical skull acquisition, particularly in skull base approaches, where complex bone anatomy and limited working angles demand nuanced hand-eye coordination [24]. These tactile simulations form a crucial pedagogical bridge between virtual reality training and the operating room, reinforcing muscle memory while minimizing patient risk. As materials science evolves, the fidelity of such models continues to improve, making them essential tools for competency-based microsurgical education and a natural prelude to broader simulation-based curricula [25] (Fig. 21.5).

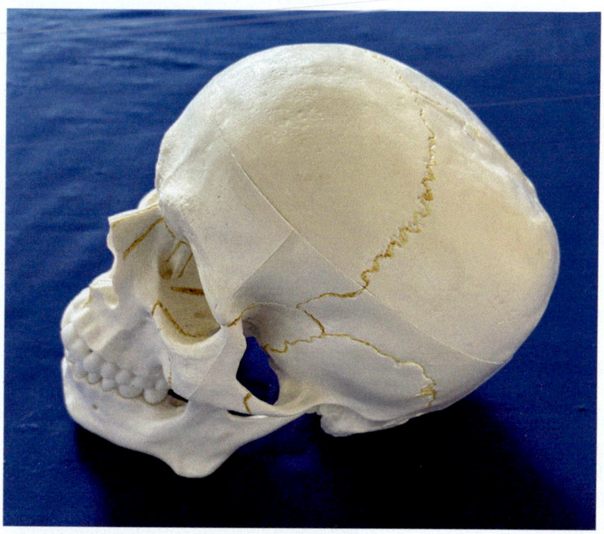

Fig. 21.5 This high-fidelity resin cranium served as a foundational model for planning and illustrating cranial approaches throughout this atlas. Its realistic anatomical detail and robust construction provided a valuable platform for haptic learning, replicating the tactile experience of bone drilling and exposure. Such physical models, like 3D-printed patient-specific replicas, play a crucial role in neurosurgical training by bridging visual knowledge with manual proficiency in a risk-free environment

21.8 Evolution of Training and Simulation

The landscape of neurosurgical education is experiencing a fundamental transformation with the integration of high-fidelity simulation platforms. Virtual reality (VR) simulators equipped with haptic feedback now enable immersive rehearsal of cranial approaches, aneurysm clipping, and tumor resection in a risk-free, repeatable environment. These systems are increasingly embedded in residency programs as objective tools for skull assessment and refinement, particularly in rare or high-risk procedures where hands-on experience may be limited [26]. Furthermore, simulation facilitates team-based training, fosters error recognition and correction, and accelerates the transition from conceptual knowledge to technical mastery. As neurosurgical procedures become more complex and technology-dependent, simulation-based learning is set to complement traditional cadaveric dissection and direct mentorship as a core pillar of operative training [27].

Photogrammetry for Neuroanatomical Studies and Neurosurgical Training Photogrammetry—the technique of constructing 3D models from a series of high-resolution photographs—has gained traction as a cost-effective, accessible method for building detailed neuroanatomical reconstructions (Fig. 21.6). When

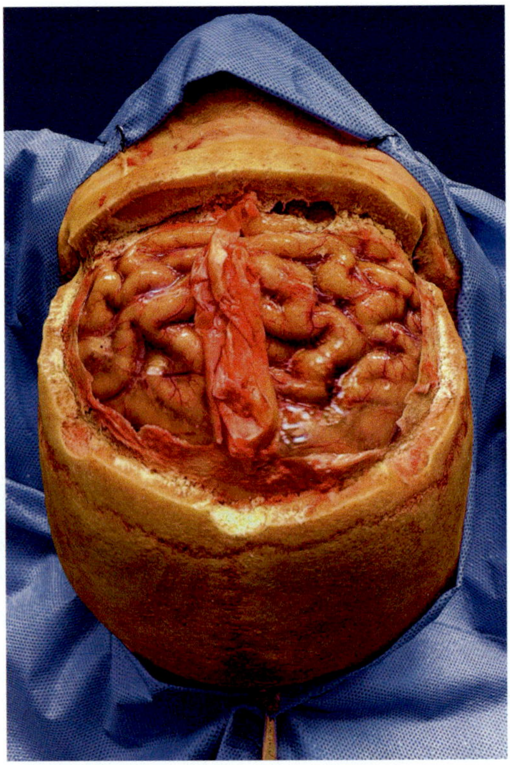

Fig. 21.6 Photogrammetric reconstruction of a cadaveric cranial dissection demonstrates the anatomical exposure achieved through a bifrontal craniotomy. This high-resolution 3D model exemplifies how photogrammetry can be used to digitally preserve complex surgical views for educational purposes. By capturing and reconstructing realistic dissections, this technique allows learners to explore microsurgical anatomy interactively, enhancing spatial understanding and surgical planning in a reproducible, low-cost, and globally accessible format

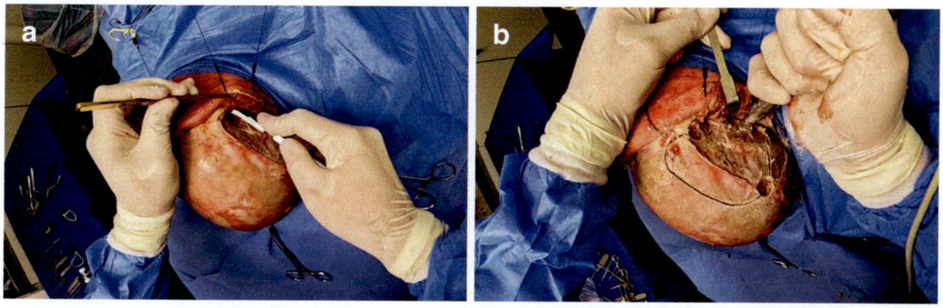

Fig. 21.7 Intraoperative perspective during a cadaveric demonstration of the pterional approach. (**a**) First-person view captured with a head-mounted GoPro camera, showing sharp dissection of the temporal muscle and exposure of the frontotemporal region. This angle simulates the surgeon's view, providing immersive visual feedback for training. (**b**) Completion of the pterional craniotomy, illustrating bone flap elevation and exposure of the sphenoid ridge. Together, these images highlight the procedural flow and technical details of the approach as experienced in real surgeries

applied to cadaveric dissections or surgical exposures, photogrammetry enables the creation of interactive, rotatable models that preserve spatial depth and structural context, thereby enhancing understanding of microsurgical anatomy [28]. These models can be integrated into digital atlases, used for virtual dissection planning, and even adapted into VR training environments. For institutions without access to advanced 3D printing or commercial VR platforms, photogrammetry provides a scalable alternative for generating high-quality educational content that supports anatomical learning and preoperative simulation in both cranial and spinal neurosurgery [29, 30].

Laboratory Training Cadaveric dissection remains the cornerstone of neurosurgical training, providing an unparalleled, risk-free environment for mastering complex cranial approaches. All procedures illustrated and recorded in this operative book and video atlas were developed and refined through decades of anatomical laboratory work. Unlike virtual platforms, cadaver labs offer tactile fidelity, true spatial orientation, and an appreciation of anatomical variability that no simulation can fully replicate. This controlled setting allows neurosurgeons to rehearse each movement, test new strategies, and develop the microsurgical discipline required for safe and effective operative performance (Fig. 21.7).

21.9 Ethical and Philosophical Considerations

As neurosurgery enters an era increasingly shaped by technology, it faces profound ethical and philosophical challenges that require critical reflection. The core values of the discipline—precision, safety, craftsmanship, and anatomical reverence—must be preserved as tools such as artificial intelligence, robotics, and immersive imaging become more integrated into daily practice. While innovation offers remarkable promise, it must be implemented with humility, rigorous validation, and ethical safeguards to ensure patient safety and maintain the central role of surgical judgment [31]. At its best, neurosurgery balances the mechanical with the humanistic, the technical with the intuitive, and the anatomical with the philosophical.

The Surgical Triangle: Window (Approach) Versus Light (Visualization) Versus Hand (Execution) Every neurosurgical act unfolds within a dynamic triad: the surgical *window* (approach), the *light* (microscopic or endoscopic visualization), and the *hand* (instrumentation). Ethical surgical planning arises from mastering the geometry and limitations of this triad. A poorly chosen approach may expose too little or too much; inadequate illumination may obscure vital structures; and imprecise hands may negate even the most elegant anatomical exposure. With increasing reliance on neuronavigation, exoscopes, and robotic arms, the surgeon must never surrender mastery over these three domains. Neurosurgical excellence lies not merely in adopting new tools, but in controlling them with full awareness of their benefits, limits, and potential consequences [32].

Evolution of Surgical Access Tools The progression of cranial access techniques reflects the broader evolution of neurosurgical precision. In the early phases of the field, neurosurgeons employed trephines and Gigli saws—manual and often imprecise instruments—to gain entry into the cranial vault. The development and standardization of powered craniotomes marked a significant leap forward, enabling faster, safer, and more controlled creation of bone flaps. Concurrently, technological advances provided neurosurgeons with increasingly sophisticated diagnostic tools: first cerebral angiography, followed by computed tomography (CT), and later magnetic resonance imaging (MRI). These modalities became essential in merging radiological insight with anatomical knowledge, transforming preoperative planning and facilitating safer, more effective treatment of intracranial disease. Collectively, these mechanical and imaging innovations laid the groundwork for the modern neurosurgical approach.

How Much Room Remains for Innovation in Neurosurgery? Despite the apparent maturity of cranial neurosurgical techniques, there remains significant opportunity for innovation—as long as it serves patient safety, anatomical fidelity, and therapeutic benefit. True innovation must address real clinical limitations: corridors that remain too traumatic, structures still too elusive, or tumors still too unsafe to access. It is not merely the addition of new tools but a transformation in how we consider exposure, preservation, and functional outcome. The ethical imperative is not to innovate for novelty but to refine what already exists, guided by long-term outcome data, anatomical validation, and peer scrutiny. Neurosurgery must evolve but not at the expense of its foundational principles [33].

References

1. Bliss M. Harvey Cushing: a life in surgery. Oxford University Press; 2005.
2. Yasargil MG. Microneurosurgery: an attempt to standardize microneurosurgical techniques, part I: microsurgical anatomy of the basal cisterns and vessels of the brain. Acta Neurochir. 1969;20(1–2):1–18.
3. Krayenbühl N, Yasargil MG. The use of the operating microscope in neurosurgery. Clin Neurosurg. 1970;17:267–85.
4. Fischer G, Brotchi J. History of microneurosurgery. In: Youmans JR, editor. Neurological surgery. 4th ed. Philadelphia: Saunders; 1996. p. 359–67.
5. Rhoton AL Jr. The supratentorial cranial space: microsurgical anatomy and surgical approaches. Neurosurgery. 2002;51(4 Suppl):S1–S272.
6. Kockro RA, Stadie A, Schwandt E, Reisch R, Charalampaki P, Perneczky A. A collaborative virtual reality environment for neurosurgical planning and training. Neurosurgery. 2007;61(5 Suppl 2):569–84.
7. Inoue D, Cho B, Mori H, et al. Preliminary study of the clinical application of augmented reality neuronavigation. J Neurosurg. 2013;119(3):639–46.
8. Wang MY, Green BA, Shah K, Vanni S, Levi AD. Augmented reality and artificial intelligence in neurosurgery: applications and future directions. World Neurosurg. 2018;114:466–73.
9. Essayed WI, Zhang F, Unadkat P, Cosgrove GR, Golby AJ, O'Donnell LJ. White matter tractography for neurosurgical planning: a topography-based review of the current state of the art. Neuroimage Clin. 2017;15:659–72.
10. Duffau H. The huge plastic potential of adult brain and the role of connectomics: new insights provided by serial mappings in glioma surgery. Cortex. 2014;58:325–37.
11. Prada F, Del Bene M, Mattei L, et al. Fusion imaging for intra-operative ultrasound-based navigation in neurosurgery. J Ultrasound. 2014;17(3):243–51.
12. Solheim O, Selbekk T, Jakola AS, Unsgård G. Ultrasound-guided operations in unselected high-grade gliomas–overall results, impact of image quality and patient selection. Acta Neurochir. 2010;152(11):1873–86.
13. Marcus HJ, Hughes-Hallett A, Cundy TP, et al. Technical advances in robotic neurosurgery. Ann R Coll Surg Engl. 2013;95(4):211–6.
14. Garnette D, Ebrahim Z, Arango MF, Parrent AG, Byrne JV. The role of robotics in neurosurgical practice: a review. Can J Neurol Sci. 2020;47(3):336–44.
15. Ravi D, Wong C, Deligianni F, et al. Deep learning for health informatics. IEEE J Biomed Health Inform. 2017;21(1):4–21.
16. Lao Z, Shen D, Liu D, Jawad AF, Melhem ER, Launer LJ, et al. Computer-assisted segmentation of white matter lesions in 3D MR images using support vector machine. Acad Radiol. 2008;15(3):300–13.
17. Senders JT, Zaki MM, Karhade AV, et al. An introduction and overview of machine learning in neurosurgical care. Acta Neurochir. 2018;160(1):29–38.
18. Labib MA, Shah M, Kassam AB, et al. The safety and feasibility of image-guided brainpath-mediated transsulcal hematoma evacuation: a multicenter study. Neurosurgery. 2017;80(4):515–24.
19. Reisch R, Perneczky A. Ten-year experience with the supraorbital subfrontal approach through an eyebrow skin incision. Neurosurgery. 2005;57(4 Suppl):242–55.
20. Jho HD, Carrau RL. Endoscopic endonasal transsphenoidal surgery: experience with 50 patients. J Neurosurg. 1997;87(1):44–51.
21. Cappabianca P, Cavallo LM, Colao A, et al. Endoscopic endonasal transsphenoidal surgery in recurrent and residual pituitary adenomas: technical note. Minim Invasive Neurosurg. 2002;45(4):193–200.

22. Mashiko T, Otani K, Kawano R, et al. Development of three-dimensional hollow cerebral aneurysm models for simulation of endovascular treatment. Neurosurgery. 2015;76(4):493–500.
23. Chae MP, Rozen WM, McMenamin PG, et al. Emerging applications of bedside 3D printing in plastic surgery. Front Surg. 2015;2:25.
24. Kockro RA, Amaxopoulou C, Killeen T, et al. Simulation of complex cranial neurosurgery with a patient-specific haptic temporal bone model. Neurosurgery. 2015;11(Suppl 2):285–98.
25. De Notaris M, Peris-Celda M, Cavallo LM, et al. Training and simulation in skull base surgery. Neurosurg Focus. 2012;33(3):E18.
26. Marcus HJ, Cundy TP, Hughes-Hallett A, et al. Systematic review of the role of simulation in neurosurgical education. Neurosurgery. 2013;72(5):829–39.
27. Winkler-Schwartz A, Yilmaz R, Mirchi N, et al. Machine learning identification of surgical and operative factors associated with surgical expertise in virtual reality simulation. JAMA Netw Open. 2019;2(8):e198363.
28. García-González U, Morais DF, Cavalcanti DD, et al. Use of photogrammetry to generate 3D models of neurosurgical anatomy: an affordable alternative to CT and MRI. World Neurosurg. 2020;134:e748–55.
29. Forster MT, Hattingen E, Senft C, et al. Virtual reality-based simulation as a training tool in neurosurgery. J Neurosurg Sci. 2018;62(3):229–36.
30. Palmiero OMH, Ribas EC, Carlotti CG Jr, Figueiredo EG. Anatomical assessment of cerebral sulci and gyri for neuroanatomy education using photogrammetry technique to generate 3D-tridimensional models. Neurosurg Rev. 2025;48(1):172.
31. Zuckerman SL, Neal MT, Englander ZK, et al. Ethical considerations in neurosurgical innovation. World Neurosurg. 2014;82(5):e541–8.
32. Spetzler RF. Surgical philosophy and the art of microneurosurgery. In: Winn HR, editor. Youmans and Winn neurological surgery. 7th ed. Philadelphia: Elsevier; 2017. p. 1465–70.
33. Rutka JT. The future of neurosurgery: are we looking far enough ahead? Neurosurgery. 2009;64(2):203–10.

Index

H. de Oliveira Manduca Palmiero, E. G. Figueiredo, *Neurosurgical Approaches Video Atlas*, https://doi.org/10.1007/978-3-032-04664-2

MIX
Papier aus verantwortungsvollen Quellen
Paper from responsible sources
FSC® C105338

If you have any concerns about our products,
you can contact us on
ProductSafety@springernature.com

In case Publisher is established outside the EU,
the EU authorized representative is:
Springer Nature Customer Service Center GmbH
Europaplatz 3, 69115 Heidelberg, Germany

Printed by Libri Plureos GmbH
in Hamburg, Germany